Memory and the
Human Lifespan

Steve Joordens, Ph.D.

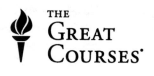

THE
GREAT
COURSES·

PUBLISHED BY:

THE GREAT COURSES
Corporate Headquarters
4840 Westfields Boulevard, Suite 500
Chantilly, Virginia 20151-2299
Phone: 1-800-832-2412
Fax: 703-378-3819
www.thegreatcourses.com

Steve Joordens, Ph.D.
Professor of Psychology
University of Toronto Scarborough

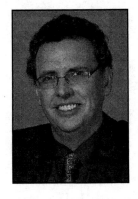

Professor Steve Joordens is Professor of Psychology, Associate Chair of Psychology, and Program Supervisor for the undergraduate program at the University of Toronto Scarborough. He received his undergraduate degree in Psychology from the University of New Brunswick and his master's and doctorate degrees in Cognitive Psychology from the University of Waterloo. After a brief postdoctoral fellowship at McMaster University, he joined the faculty of the University of Toronto Scarborough in 1995.

Professor Joordens's research includes developing and implementing technologies for learning. His innovation was honored when he and his Ph.D. student Dwayne Paré received a National Technology Innovation Award in 2009 for the creation of peerScholar (www.peerScholar.com), an Internet-based educational platform that supports the development of critical-thinking and communication skills in a classroom of any size. Through work conducted in his laboratory, he has published high-quality research related to teaching, learning, and the use of technology. Some of this work documents the functional and pedagogical validity of peerScholar, and some examines the use of technology to enhance traditional lectures.

More recently, Professor Joordens and his colleagues have been investigating the effective use of mobile applications as cognitive prosthetics to assist both the learning disabled and patients with Alzheimer's disease. This work has been presented at a range of international conferences and consistently wins "best in session" honors. In recognition of his work, he was invited to be a speaker for the Teaching of Psychology Section at the 2010 Canadian Psychological Association Convention, and he often gives keynote addresses at conferences related generally to effective teaching or specifically to the effective use of technology.

Professor Joordens continues to conduct research on human memory, consciousness, and attention and has many publications on these topics in top-rated empirical and theoretical psychology journals. This research has been consistently supported by grants from the Natural Sciences and Engineering Research Council of Canada. In recognition of his work on memory, Professor Joordens won a Premier's Research Excellence Award for the 2001–2006 period. The research relevant to this work provides the underpinnings of his more recent research on the effective use of technology to promote learning.

In addition to being recognized for his research and innovation, Professor Joordens received the Scarborough College Students' Union's Best Professor Award for 2002–2003 and 2010–2011. He has been nominated 4 times for Television Ontario's Best Lecturer Competition—once making the Top 30, once making the Top 20, and twice making the Top 10 list. He also won a provincially sponsored Leadership in Faculty Teaching Award in 2006–2007 in recognition of both his lecturing and his innovative approach to education. In 2010, Professor Joordens's teaching accomplishments were further recognized with a President's Teaching Award, the highest award for teaching at the University of Toronto. Along with a yearly research grant, this award makes Professor Joordens a member of the university's Teaching Academy, a group of 25 or fewer faculty who promote teaching initiatives and generally strive to enhance the learning experience for all students at the University of Toronto. ■

Table of Contents

Table of Contents

Table of Contents

Memory and the Human Lifespan

Scope:

Our memory allows us to remember and share past events, to function efficiently and intelligently in the present, and even to predict and prepare for the future. It is truly amazing that we can mentally relive events that occurred decades in the past. And yet this amazing memory system is also prone to failure, sometimes with embarrassing social consequences.

The goal of this course is to provide a rich and complete description of the cognitive and biological bases of human memory and to describe how they come together in everyday life. First, we shatter the illusory notion that memory is a single thing. In reality, influences of the past are carried forward by a number of different cognitive processes, each of which can be thought of as a distinct memory system. How we remember events of our lives differs from how we retrieve general knowledge about the world and how we remember a specific routine or skill. Each of our memory systems differs from the others in purpose and character, yet they also interact in complex and fascinating ways.

After a general introduction, the course begins with lectures on 2 techniques that have been used to enhance memory: ancient "art of memory" techniques, which date back to classical civilization, and rote memorization, which was central to the first scientific investigation of memory.

Subsequent lectures describe our various memory systems, including those that support our long-term memories of events (episodic memory), facts about the world (semantic memory), and skills we have learned (procedural memory). Short-term memory systems are also presented, including sensory memory systems and perhaps the most interesting and multifaceted memory systems, working memory. We also look at implicit memory, a system that allows us to learn and use the regularities of the world without even trying to learn them.

Sometimes these different memory systems work together, but sometimes they work at cross-purposes, and we'll take a look at situations in which habits, supported by procedural learning or implicit memory, can conflict with goals and produce unwanted behaviors. The importance of sleep to memory consolidation will also be highlighted, and we consider the extent to which our memory systems are, and are not, uniquely human. In addition, the development of memory systems in human infants is described.

Clearly, memory occurs in the brain, and we consider the links between brain systems and behavior both in intact memory systems and in various forms of brain damage, like the amnesias. Our understanding of memory and the brain has already been transformed by brain-imaging techniques such as functional magnetic resonance imaging; we'll look ahead to how attempts by some intrepid researchers to model brain systems using computer-based, artificial neural networks may offer further insights in the future.

With this scientific understanding of memory systems in place, we then consider the way these systems interact to produce important memory phenomena that influence us every day with or without our awareness. We consider the powerful influence of the simple repetition of experience, and in so doing we gain a better appreciation for why, for example, political candidates love seeing their names posted in every corner of your neighborhood. We visit the phenomenon of déjà vu as an illusion of memory to see what it might tell us about interactions of memory systems. We also consider the empirical evidence that it is possible to create false memories and the implications of this research for the controversy over recovered memories.

One critical point we will develop is that conscious memories are actually reconstructed, not simply retrieved, and that our conscious (i.e., episodic) memories are really created by weaving together accurately recalled information with the thread of semantic memory—things we simply know to be true of the world and thus assume to be true of new episodic memories. Within this framework, we must ask which details are accurately retrieved and what we might do to maximize the likelihood of accurate retrieval. In fact, we'll go over some clear tips for doing just that.

Other lectures focus on memory later in life in both Alzheimer's disease and normal aging. We consider the impact of Alzheimer's disease on caregivers as well as patients, taking care to distinguish early-stage Alzheimer's from normal changes during aging. We discuss factors that may help prevent Alzheimer's, look at research into cognitive prosthetics aimed at enhancing quality of life, and consider the overall implications of this devastating disease for our understanding of memory. We discuss how the changes of normal aging are often exaggerated, and we situate the real but small memory deterioration that does occur in the context of a broad cognitive transition, highlighting approaches for taking advantage of the transition while minimizing the deterioration.

Overall, the course describes the complex role that memory systems play at all stages in our life and highlights how critical these systems are for providing our sense of self. After all, who we are is ultimately defined by the experiences we have had, the things we know, and the skills we have acquired through life. Every aspect of who we are is embodied in memory systems, a better understanding of which can greatly enrich our lives. ■

Memory Is a Party
Lecture 1

Before we begin exploring human memory, we have to define what memory is. Rather than being a single entity, human memory is made up of multiple systems that interact in various ways. This complexity underlies both the power and fallibility of memory.

Human memory is truly amazing. Most of us can probably recall several strong decades-old memories. But memory can sometimes fail us, too. In fact, sometimes it can succeed and fail at the same time. How can the same system be simultaneously so amazing and so prone to error?

In a sense, we'll be answering that question throughout the course, but the short answer is, there is no single thing called memory. In fact, memory isn't really a "thing" at all but a group of cognitive processes that interrelate in complex ways.

The brain is divided into cortical regions and subcortical regions. The subcortex consists of small areas like the hippocampus and the amygdala that are critical for creating memories, especially emotional memories. It also comprises larger regions, like the whole cerebellum, which is involved in memory related to motor activity.

The cortex consists of 2 hemispheres of 4 lobes each, with a web of nerve fibers called the corpus collosum connecting the hemispheres. Three of each hemisphere's lobes analyze signals coming in from the world—seeing, hearing, and touching—and the fourth lobe, the frontal lobe, handles attention and self-control.

Memories involve a lot of coordination between the higher brain regions of the cortex and lower brain regions such as the hippocampus. Our memorial abilities actually reflect the orchestrated interaction of a number of different memory systems. Let's use some examples to look at the different memory systems.

If someone asks you, "What did you have for dinner last night?" that episode of your life likely replayed like a little movie in your mind; this is **episodic memory**. However, if someone asked you to calculate 5 times 4, it would probably feel like the answer just appeared, unaccompanied by an event. This is **semantic memory**, memory of facts you have learned about the world, detached from memory of an event or episode; your repeated exposure to this information has decontextualized it. Thus there seems to be a continuum between episodic and semantic memory systems.

The smooth and accurate performance of a physical routine—an athletic maneuver or dance number, for example—is the result of effective and repeated practice. The performer is using **procedural memory**, also called muscle memory, because the relevant muscles have learned how to orchestrate themselves. Procedural memory is also part of how we learn to speak a language fluidly. Learning words is an act of semantic memory,

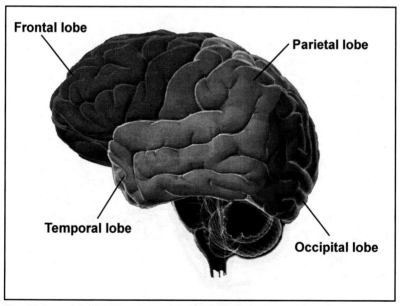

The 4 lobes of the brain are associated with different functions.

but the appropriate reproduction of sounds by the muscles of the throat is procedural memory.

From these examples, we can broadly define memory as any time when a past experience has an effect on current or future behavior. It doesn't matter whether or not you are trying to retrieve information from the past; whether the past affects the present is all that matters.

The memory systems we have discussed so far all belong to a general class called long-term memory. Other systems hold onto experiences for a short time, usually just long enough to accomplish some task.

Sensory memory is a fading copy of some stimulus that has impinged on our senses. For example, if someone asks you a question while you're thinking about something else, you might have said, "What?" But as the person repeats the question you say, "Sorry, never mind. I heard you." You stored the question in your sensory memory—specifically, your echoic memory—for a few seconds then replayed it.

Working memory, sometimes called short-term memory, allows you to hold a memory briefly until it can be used in some other way. A common example is repeating a phone number over and over while hunting for a paper and pen to write it down.

Working memory also plays a central role in the ability to combine information from other memory systems, often with the goal of solving some novel task or problem. When you gather information from various types of memory—episodic, semantic, and so forth—your working memory is where you process it, an act we tend to identify as conscious thought. ■

Terms to Know

episodic memory: Memories of specific, individual events, as opposed to general knowledge.

procedural memory: The body's mastery of a physical routine; often called muscle memory.

semantic memory: General knowledge about the world learned through repeated exposure to the information, as opposed to memories of specific events.

sensory memory: A temporarily retained impression of a sensory stimulus.

working memory: Sometimes called short-term memory, a memory system used for both temporary storage and as a mental workspace where information from other systems is processed.

Suggested Reading

Baddeley, *Essentials of Human Memory.*

Howard, *Learning and Memory.*

Loftus and Loftus, *Human Memory.*

Questions to Consider

1. How does the psychological definition of memory differ from the way you thought about memory before watching this lecture?

2. If you had to lose the use of just one memory system, which one would you choose to lose and why?

Exercise

Over the course of about 15 minutes, take note of how often you use memory to accomplish specific tasks and which memory systems you use.

Memory Is a Party
Lecture 1—Transcript

Human memory is absolutely amazing. It keeps us connected with our past while also preparing us for our future. It allows us to learn from our experiences and to share our experiences with others, and it literally defines who we are.

Think back to your childhood for a moment: What's your earliest memory of baking cookies? What do you remember about your childhood bedroom? Was there an object, maybe a toy, that you remember being fascinated by? Do you remember a childhood playmate? Or what about fear? Many childhood memories are related to fear. You may not recall such things right away, but think about them: It's just astonishing what we can recall. Even with just a little effort, we can recall events from literally decades ago.

But memory can also fail us. In fact, sometimes it can both succeed and fail at the very same time. Have you ever been in a situation where someone is recounting a memory to you, a memory that they have already told you about, perhaps many times? When they do that, they are remembering the experience they are relating, while also forgetting the experience of telling you about it previously. How can the same system be simultaneously so amazing and yet so prone to error?

Hi, my name is Steve Joordens. I'm a professor of psychology at the University of Toronto Scarborough, and I think memory is absolutely fascinating. I've been teaching about memory for over 10 years at the University, giving talks in the community. I also conduct research with my students to understand memory better. I am really thrilled to have this opportunity to share what I have learned with you, and I will try my very best to infect you with my fascination.

And while I am here as the expert on memory, I also want to confess right now that throughout my life I have been a generally forgetful guy. When I was a teenager, looking frantically for my car keys, or something else I had misplaced, my mother would tell me, "One day you will be a professor. I know this because you are so absent minded." The absent-minded professor. Sometimes stereotypes do come true.

But of course this is what we all do. We all forget our keys, our cell phones, our anniversaries, the names of people we've just met, and on and on. We are prone to the silliest-seeming memory errors, and I personally still feel really silly and embarrassed about it. But that's memory for you. It is a truly complex and fascinating beast. So my goal in this lecture is to convince you that the simplistic way that we often talk about memory is just that, very simplistic, in fact too simplistic. I personally feel that most humans have very little sense of just how interesting and amazing they themselves are. We take our abilities for granted, and we don't often think about them in much detail.

So, back to our question: How can our memory be simultaneously so impressive and yet also so prone to error? In a sense, we'll be answering that question throughout the course. We'll be building up a picture of how memory supports the conception of who we are, how memory declines (or changes) with age, and what sorts of things you might do to reduce this decline and even to improve your memory.

But the first step to a more accurate understanding of memory is to realize the following: There really is no single thing called memory. Yes, it's true that in colloquial speech we often use the term memory as though it were a "singular noun," that is, as if it represented one thing, so your memory is like your bed, a single thing that exists in a single place and performs essentially a single function. We say things like "my memory is getting bad," almost as though we're saying "my bed is becoming uncomfortable." However, memory isn't just one thing, and it isn't really a "thing" at all. Instead, remembering is a set of cognitive processes that occur within the biological matter of our brains. We'll cover brains in much more detail later in the course, but let's get an overview of how the brain handles remembering.

The brain has two hemispheres that are connected by a tangle of nerve fibers called the corpus collosum. These connecting fibers were the structure that was absent at birth from Kim Peek, the real person who was the basis for the movie character Rain Man. The absence of connecting fibers across the hemispheres may have fostered his extraordinary memory, and yet they also contributed to his difficulties on general IQ tests. These rare individuals with unusual brain features have historically been absolutely central to advances in what we know about how brains work in everyone. Each hemisphere of our brain has cortical regions (which are the higher, more outward regions), and subcortical regions (which are lower, more inward regions). The cortex is traditionally thought of as the seat of higher brain functions, while the subcortex handles lower brain functions.

The cortex consists of four lobes, three of which analyze signals coming in from the world—seeing, hearing, and touch—whereas the fourth, the frontal lobe handles how we direct our attention, what we choose to remember, and how we control our actions. If you wanted just one lobe to get you started, you might think first about the temporal lobes. You can get a sense of this region by putting your hands over your ears on both sides of your head while pointing your middle fingers toward the back of the head, until they almost touch. The temporal lobes are important for auditory memory, so they're critical for your ability to understand and remember what I'm saying to you right now.

And the inner region of those same temporal lobes (which is known as the medial region) are especially important for containing a small structure absolutely critical for creating any explicit memories at all. That structure is called the hippocampus. In fact, the hippocampus is one of the few brain locations that is constantly creating new neurons. That old myth you may have heard that adults never create new brain cells is refuted by the hippocampus.

The big picture is that stored memories involve lots of distributed representations spread across higher-brain regions of the cortex, working together with lower-brain regions such as the hippocampus. For example, the cerebellum (which is a large region in the back of the head) is responsible for helping us to remember to make our motor movements smooth and graceful. It was a defect in the cerebellum that contributed to the difficulties that Rain Man had in moving his body smoothly. The point is what we might recall our memorial abilities actually reflect the orchestrated interaction of a number of different brain systems. These complex brain processes allow for amazing feats, but they also allow for problems.

Thus by exploring these processes in detail, and by considering how they interact, you can gain a much stronger appreciation for your memory when it works. You can also have a deeper understanding of why and how memory sometimes fails, and how you can help your memory. Understanding how it all comes together also sheds new light on what goes into making possible who you are.

Let's make all this a little bit more concrete with a few fun examples that will introduce you, one by one, to some of your memory systems. In fact, why don't we make it more fun by imagining we are at a party, one in which the other guests are your memory systems. I will be your host, and I will introduce you to these systems and give you a very general sense of what they do, their professions if you like. Sometimes I will introduce them with a question, and that's to let you experience more personally what it is they are actually doing.

In fact, here's our first guest now. This is someone named Episodic Memory. Episodic Memory is a great guest to introduce via a question. So as I ask this question, pay attention to what is happening in your mind, because that will be important. OK. You ready? Here goes. Think about the last dinner that you remember. What was the meal? Notice what tends to happen. It's almost as though you have a little movie playing in your mind, one that includes the place of your dinner, the people you shared it with, perhaps the time of day, or maybe snippets of the conversation.

It is like that episode of your life was replayed. That's episodic memory. Oh, by the way, I need to warn you that some of these characters go by two names, which can make it a challenge to keep things straight. I'll try to be sensitive to that, and I'll generally stick with one name, but I might also mention the other occasionally as well. So, this episodic memory character also sometimes goes by the name Autobiographical Memory. Notice that both of these names relate to different aspects of the subjective experience that you just had. You replayed an episode in your mind, but it was an episode from your life, one in which you were the star. Thus it was an episode about you, making it both episodic and autobiographical.

So let's move on to the next guest then. Once again I'll introduce this guest with a question. Don't forget to introspect. Pay attention to what's in your mind. Question: What is 5 x 4?

What happened this time? You got the answer, but this time, it felt like the answer just appeared, unaccompanied by any other experience, right? What if I ask you what the baseball team from Boston is named? Again, just the answer, right? In 1972, a psychologist from the University of Toronto named Endel Tulving pointed out that this kind of memory feels different from our memory of episodes. He dubbed it "semantic memory," and characterized it as your memory of the facts that you have learned about the world. These facts were learned in the past and can subsequently be retrieved. Clearly this character belongs at the memory party. But this memory process does not involve the replaying of the event in which the information was learned. It doesn't feel like an episode from our life. It just feels like the facts, and when we want them they are retrieved and are available.

But if you are thinking ahead and organizing what we've been discussing and, by the way that's a really good thing to do. It helps to learn the new material well. You might say something like this: "Hey, wait a minute. The things that are in my semantic memory were learned via specific episodes. For example, if you'd asked me about the name of the Boston team just days after I had first learned it, I likely would have replayed that learning episode. It would have been an episodic memory."

If you thought this, you'd be right on. Episodic memories are when information is remembered within some specific context. Repeated exposure to information across a variety of contexts essentially de-contextualizes it. So yes, episodic and semantic memories do indeed dance together, sometimes in pretty complex ways. Memory isn't one of those parties where the characters just stand against the wall. No, they interact, and these interactions are critical to a full story of our more general memory abilities. So we'll talk about these interactions in some detail as we progress through the lectures.

OK. Let's now move along and meet the next guest. I can't really introduce this guest with a question per se, but I just ask you to consider the following. Think of some occasion when you've maybe watched an athlete, or a dancer, effortlessly performing some really complex motor movements. We all know, roughly speaking, how they come to be able to do that. The smooth and accurate performance that you see now has resulted from previous experience, specifically, from effective and repeated practice. At early stages this practice might have been informed by the learning of various "verbalized" routines, but the smoothness that you see now only comes with repetition.

Typically, the performer is no longer intentionally trying to use their memory in any way. They are just performing. But those previous experiences are indeed influencing their current behavior. The processes of memory are what bridge the gap between previous practice and the current fluidity of movement. This type of memory underlying the development and performance of these sorts of motor skills is called "procedural" memory or, sometimes, "muscle" memory. The "muscle memory" pseudonym reflects the fact that what one is learning in these situations is how to orchestrate muscles in appropriate sequences, that is a procedure, to perform some larger behavior.

Procedural memory is not just for athletes and dancers. Most of us speak our native languages as fluidly as an athlete performs their sport. Part of this involves learning words. And for that we need some assistance from semantic memory. But in addition, we also had to learn how to coordinate those muscles in our throat to produce the sounds of those words in an appropriate manner. In fact, when you hear babies babbling, that represents their very first attempts of babies to use their vocal muscles to produce speech-like sounds. This babbling slowly, over time, becomes much more defined and articulate as the muscles in the throat learn to coordinate themselves in an efficient and precise manner. Once again, this sort of development and orchestration of these interactions between muscles is procedural memory.

To again appreciate the extent to which these memory systems like to interact, let's consider how these memory systems might come into play when someone decides to learn a new language. Imagine you have decided you are going to learn how to speak French, so you take a class. After attending your first class you go home to work on the things you learned. At this point you are likely relying heavily on episodic memory. You're replaying the class itself and working on an exercise that the teacher introduced to you. Over time you will come to hear certain French words repeatedly, sometimes from the teacher, sometimes from books or the other study materials, and perhaps even from exposing yourself to French-speaking people. As you learn these words across a variety of contexts then they enter the domain of semantic memory.

This is similar to the transition from episodic to semantic memory described earlier, one of their favorite dances, if you will. But knowing the words, and knowing how to string them together to form sentences, is not enough to make you fluent in French. To be truly fluent, you need to say the words right. And what I mean by that is you need to learn the accent. For every language, the manner in which the vocal muscles coordinate to produce the accent of that language is a little different. If you keep using your English throat muscle procedures while speaking French, you will have a horrible English accent: Parlez-vous, le Française.

But if you keep exposing yourself to real French speakers, and keep mimicking the sounds as they make them, eventually your throat muscles will learn to coordinate in a French way. This is procedural memory, and marrying that with your new semantic knowledge, knowledge that was initially derived from episodic memories, is what will ultimately make you proficient in French. The dances that memory systems do are not limited to two participants at a time. I told you they were interesting characters.

While episodic and semantic memory likely seemed like things you thought of as memory, procedural memory might have seemed a little different to you. When you're performing some procedure you've practiced, it often doesn't feel like you are trying to remember anything. It feels to you like you are just performing. With this in mind, this is a good time to clarify what we mean when we say the word "memory." What are we including as phenomena that reflect the workings of memory? So if memory is a party, imagine we have a bouncer at the door of our party, and we have to give that bouncer some rule, something that clarifies who's allowed in and who's not.

What's that rule? Early psychologists struggled with this a little, but today we can use the following definition: Memory is active anytime some past experience has an effect on the way you think or behave now or in the future.

This is a very broad definition. It implies that anytime a past experience can be shown to affect you now in anyway then some sort of memory system must be preserving that experience over time. By this definition, it really doesn't matter whether one is trying to retrieve the information from the past or not. If the past affects the present, that is all that matters.

So, memory systems are the vehicles for transporting the effects of experience over time, and if we want to understand memory more fully we have to consider the full spectrum of the ways that this can happen. By now you can see that memory is indeed more like a party. So far you have met episodic, semantic, and procedural memory systems, and you have a sense of some of the ways they might interact. Is there even more to this party?

OK. The memory systems you have met so far all belong to a general class of memory systems called long-term memory. Long-term memory refers to any situation in which the initial experience occurred maybe days, weeks, months or years earlier. Thus, the experience causes some sort of long-term change in us that can affect us literally for the rest of our lives. When you learn French, you have that for life. The learning we performed left an enduring trace, and it supports our behavior even without us feeling that we are really remembering anything at all. We're just speaking.

But within this party of the brain, there are also memory systems that we use to hold onto experiences for much shorter time periods, usually just long enough to accomplish some task. These include very low level systems like this character over here named Sensory Memory. Sensory memories are fading copies of some stimulus, some stimulus that's impinged on our senses, for example, perhaps the slowly lingering trace of a touch, of a site, or a sound. There are at least two of these systems, and probably three.

But let me introduce you to the auditory version of sensory memory, Echoic Memory. Have you ever had someone ask you a question while you were thinking about something else? As you were clearing your mind you might have said "What?" But then as they begin repeating the question you say, "Yeah, sorry, never mind. I heard you." But you didn't really hear them. Instead you somehow stored the question while you were busy, then replayed it in your mind. It was the replay that you heard, not the initial question.

The initial question was held onto by our friend Echoic Memory, and echoic memory can hold onto auditory information for about three to five seconds. That's enough time to allow us to deal with distractions to switch our attention away from what we are currently involved in, and literally hear that event even though it happened in the past. Next time you ask someone a question and they say "What?" Just wait a few seconds. Let echoic memory do its thing before repeating your question. There may be no need.

Now we come to the most interesting character at the party. This next memory system sometimes goes by the name short-term memory, though I prefer its other name, working memory. So imagine the following situation. You're out for the evening, and you meet somebody who you think could really help you in some way. Maybe they could advance your career or, for whatever reason, they are somebody you'd like to keep in contact with. You have no paper or pen, or electronic device with you. They come up to you and chat for a while. It's your lucky day. But then after some point they say, "Hey, I have to go now. Call me sometime, and we'll continue our conversation. My number is 492-2085." And then they just walk away. What do you do? As soon as you can, without looking stupid about it, you likely start looking around for a pen and paper or some other way to record the number, and meanwhile, in your head, you repeat "492-2085, 492-2085," while you're looking around.

Notice what that voice in your head is doing. It is trying to hold onto that number over time as you search for paper. This is a form of memory, a very active form of memory. But it takes mental work to use this form of memory, which is why I often like the name working memory. Note also that while this working memory system can hold onto information for a while, it does not effectively hold onto information over longer periods. We know this from experience, and that's why we are so frantically looking for something to create a more permanent record.

While working memory can be used to hold onto information for a short period of time, it is actually a much more general purpose system that plays a very central role in our ability to combine information from the other memory systems. We often do this with the goal of solving some novel task or problem. For example, how high do you think you could reach if you were sitting on a camel?

In this case, you can't just rely on semantic memory to give you the answer, because you've likely never learned an answer to this question. Instead, you have to figure it out. Figuring it out is what working memory does best. Here are some of the thoughts that might go through your mind when trying to answer that question. You might think back to some time in your life when you saw a camel. Maybe you were in a zoo or on a vacation in the Middle East. You can relive that episodic memory, and pay attention then to how high the back of a camel was. So you replay that memory, maybe see yourself then and say, "Hmmmm. I think the camel was about 6 feet tall." OK. Cool. Now you start pulling in semantic memory. You probably know how tall you are. I'm six feet, three inches tall, for example, but of course that includes my legs.

From buying jeans or other pants, we know, that is, semantic memory tells me, what my inseam is: 36 inches. So I could calculate how high my head would be by subtracting my inseam from my total height, 6' 3" minus 3' 3". Aha. But now we have to take into account a little bit more. The camel is 6' tall, and my head is 3 above that. But I asked how high we could reach while sitting on a camel. So we have to take into account the reach. So if I say, "I don't know. Maybe that's about a foot and a half over my head. If I had to guess, I'd say I can reach about 11 feet tall. If I had to be more specific, I'd say 10' 9".

So information from both episodic and semantic memory was useful, but we also did new things with that information. We combined and transformed what we knew to come to a solution to a brand new problem. This is what working memory does. The thoughts you experienced were working memory doing its thing. I told you it was one hard-working memory system.

We do this kind of problem solving all the time, but have you ever been so tired, or perhaps so sick, that you felt you just couldn't think? It feels like t thoughts just won't work. Lack of sleep, or other forms of mental interference, tend to reduce how many things we can keep within our working memory, how many things we can literally hold onto, and if we can't hold onto many things, we simply cannot think about them deeply at all. We feel "zoned out."

I've been having a little fun depicting our memory systems as characters at a party. One thing you'll learn in this course is that imagery is one of the things that can help you to remember, and these characters, and their interactions, will be central in the dramatic interplay that underlies many of our truly amazing cognitive abilities. We will revisit and flesh out these characters as we move onwards in our story of your memory.

We will also visit the brain structures that underlie these memory systems, the homes where these character live if you will. And we'll get a sense of what life would be like when those systems are damaged. Of course none of us is getting younger, and the brain does deteriorate as we age. Given this, I will highlight the fact that while some forms of memory do become less effective as we age, others do not. Even those that do degrade, do so in the context of what can best be thought of as cognitive transformation, and this transformation includes both positive cognitive effects as well as the negative ones. As I'll also show, you can keep your memory strong while also enjoying the positive cognitive effects of aging.

We will also visit more extreme forms of memory impairment like amnesia and Alzheimer's disease, and I will highlight how technology may eventually be used to provide so-called cognitive prosthetics to step in when the brain fails. Having introduced you to your memory systems, I would like to make a general comment about the study of memory. As in many fields, researchers tend to create a lot of specialized vocabulary, with new terms being regarded almost like a toothbrush: everyone needs one, but no one wants to use anyone else's. Popular books on memory tend to be like the researchers: they, too, tend to fixate on just one or two aspects of the subject, and they ignore the rest.

In this course, by contrast, we are going to try to bring together the main insights of various research traditions literally from across the field. Our goal is to build an increasingly rich vocabulary for understanding memory in all its complexity, from mnemonics to the first experiments, to cognitive psychology, to cognitive neuroscience, neuropsychology, and beyond. Building that foundation will at times take us through some relatively academic terrain, where the connections to everyday life may not always be readily apparent. But I will try to highlight those where I can. My larger hope is that the journey as a whole will give you a far deeper understanding of memory than you would get from any of the parts considered in isolation from one another.

Understanding how our memory systems interact, sometimes together, sometime at cross-purposes, will be with us throughout this course. In the next lecture, we'll work on improving our ability to remember, using techniques that have been around since ancient times and that really do work. Do you wish your memory was better? Well, follow me as we retrace the steps of the ancients and encounter the ancient art of memory.

The Ancient "Art of Memory"
Lecture 2

Human beings have long pursued the "art of memory"—that is, developing and implementing techniques to enhance recall. The most successful of these so-called mnemonic strategies highlight the connection between strong encoding and successful retrieval through the techniques of organizing, associating, and dual coding.

It is possible to improve memory, but many books on memory improvement never address the issue of multiple memory systems. Usually, people are looking to improve their episodic memory—their ability to remember new bits of random information.

Let's start with a demonstration: Given a list of 14 unrelated words, my task is to remember those words in order over both a short and long time period. I can connect these words to a set of words that are meaningful and related to me. This is called the **method of loci**. ("Loci" is the plural of "locus," a Latin word meaning "place.")

The method of loci dates back to the great orators of the Roman Empire, who used it to demonstrate the accuracy and reliability of their memories (and thus of the news they brought from Rome to the far-

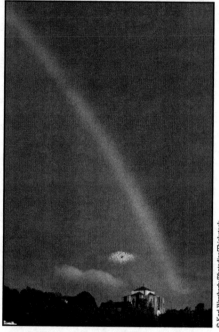

© Karl Weatherly/Photodisc/Thinkstock.

The ROY G. BIV acronym for remembering the colors of the rainbow is an example of multiple encoding—each color is associated with a letter, and the letters are encoded as a name.

flung provinces). They would associate the names of high-ranking listeners with familiar locations along their routes. This provided both associations between the familiar and unfamiliar and an organizational structure.

Often when people say they can't remember something, they are implying that the problem is with memory retrieval. Technically this is true, but our ability to remember something depends on the way we think about the information when we first encounter it—that is, on how well we encode it.

Research shows that we remember bizarre things better than we remember common things.

Organization at the time of encoding is the first critical variable that we can learn to use to enhance our memory. When you use the method of loci, you take the time to attach each new piece of information to a structure you already have in memory. This might be a list like the alphabet, the order of your morning routine, landmarks along your commute to work, and so on. You are using the familiar information to get to the right "area" of memory. Working memory is the system we use when bringing together information from the outer and inner worlds in this way.

Forming good associations is the second critical variable we can use to enhance our memory. Research shows that we remember bizarre things better than we remember common things. Turning each word into a picture also helps by making a sort of copy of the word: The word form is stored in the part of the brain that deals with linguistic stimuli; the picture form is stored in the part of the brain that deals with images. Psychologists call this **dual coding**.

Virtually all mnemonic strategies use organization, association, and dual coding in some manner. For example, in using the acronym ROY G. BIV to remember the colors of the rainbow, the name provides organization, the use of the first letter of the color word provides a strong associative link, and thinking of colors in terms of a name provides dual coding.

Unfortunately, many personal names do not lend themselves well to imagery, and that's partly why they are so hard to remember. Your best bet is to try multiple tricks. Some will be just playing around with words or well-known slogans, or you can search your memory for the most similar name you've ever heard. The more you know or notice about the person, the more possible connections you can make.

By using strong organization, forming good associations, and utilizing multiple codes when possible, your memory performance will improve. If you do all these things over and over, then it will become natural to put things into memory this way, so the effort involved will decrease. ∎

Important Terms

dual coding: The process of relating a new piece of information we wish to remember with both an image and a word to increase the ways we can retrieve the information later.

method of loci: A memory-encoding technique that relates an unfamiliar set of data to a familiar set of connected data, the most common example being places along a route; by recalling the familiar information, we can quickly bring to mind the new information.

Suggested Reading

Foer, *Moonwalking with Einstein*.

Haberlandt, *Human Memory*.

Higbee, *Your Memory*.

Lorayne and Lucas, *The Memory Book*.

1. In this lecture, organization, association, and the forming of images were highlighted as factors one can use to enhance episodic memory. Why might we remember images better than words?

2. If it's possible to improve our memories, why doesn't everyone do it?

Using the method of loci, create your own "memory palace" using places from your own life. As you do this, don't just create a list of place words; also take time to form a concrete image associated with each of your places. For example, if you were going to choose your house as a memory palace, actually walk through the rooms of your house in some specified order and take the time to really see each room. What things are in that room that you might later associate new concepts with? Maybe there is a piano in one room, a table in another, and so forth. The more you can enrich your image of each room, the easier it will be to subsequently associate things with that room.

Once you have your palace strong in your mind, mentally run through its locations at least once a day for a week, ensuring that this list is strong and easy to remember. Once your palace is firmly established, try using what you've created to remember a random list of words. Maybe write them out in the morning, commit them to your palace, then go about your day without further review. At the end of your day, try recounting the list of items. I bet you will be surprised at your success. It really works!

The next step is to use your new skill for something more practical. Maybe start with grocery lists and go from there.

The Ancient "Art of Memory"
Lecture 2—Transcript

Anytime I give a lecture on memory, one of the first questions I get goes something like this: "Sometimes I have a lot of trouble remembering things that I really want to remember, things like grocery lists, or the names of people I have recently met. Is there anything I can do to improve my memory?" It turns out this question is far from a new one. We know this because one of the very first strategies used to improve memory, the strategy I will highlight in this lecture, dates back to classical Rome and Greece. So to anticipate, yes it is possible to improve memory, and in this lecture I will show you some of the mental tricks you can use to improve your own memory.

But wait. If you've been paying attention so far you may be saying to yourself, "Wait a minute if there is no single memory but, rather, there are multiple memory systems, which one are we talking about improving?" I'm so glad you asked, because this is an important point, and one many books of memory improvement never address. Usually when people talk about improving their memory, they are talking about improving their memory for things like grocery lists, or to-do lists, or maybe for people's birthdays, or especially their memory for the names of people they have met but really don't know very well. It turns out we all have a lot of trouble remembering names, and it's a problem that seems to get even worse as we age. Well, by the end of this lecture you'll understand why that is, and maybe you won't feel quite so bad for yourself having so much trouble with names.

So let's go back to that question. Which memory system are we talking about? Because if we think about this a little bit it may help us to kind of congeal some of the information that I talked about in Lecture 1. For starters we're clearly talking about long-term memory. When we make a grocery list or a to-do list it's something we do now, but it's something we hope to retrieve later. So, given what we learned last lecture, that narrows it to episodic, semantic, or procedural memory. Well, this isn't about any sort of motor behavior like dancing or playing sports, so that rules out procedural. With respect to a person's name or birth date, well if we know that person well, say like a spouse or a child, then these things are semantic memories.

We just know their names or birthdays. Sure we sometimes forget, especially some of us who are men, and especially when the date in question is an anniversary.

But we all have the hardest time remembering newer information, new names, new dates, this week's grocery list. Those things are episodic memories, so mostly we will be focusing on improving episodic memory in this lecture. That said, we'll come back to the other memory systems in subsequent lectures, so dare I say I won't forget about them. But I just want to begin by focusing on our ability to remember new bits of essentially random information. That will be our context for now. Imagine that you've just been exposed to some new information, and you want to remember it later. What do you do?

Why don't we start with a demonstration, and then use that demonstration to highlight some of the relevant principles. Let's say you offer me the following challenge: You will give me a list of 14 unrelated words and my task is to not only remember those words but also to remember them in the order that you give them to me. And I have to this over both a short time period and also over a longer time period. So we'll test me just after I learn the list, and we'll also test me again at the end of this lecture. I can virtually guarantee you that I will be able to pull this off, and during the middle part of this lecture I will show you how it works so that you can do it too.

But you and I exist currently in a different time and place, and that will make it hard to interact directly. To do the demonstration, I have come up with another way. I'm going to start this demonstration with 14 words that reflect events or locations associated with my weekday routine. They really represent my morning ritual. It's a ritual that is pretty consistent. Basically, I wake up in "bed" (that's a good thing). I go downstairs for "breakfast," then I "walk" my two dogs, Lola and Layla. I "iron" my clothes, and take a "shower." I get "dressed," put on my "shoes," hop in my "car." I go past the "school," then a little later a "church," then a relatively famous landmark, Ted's "diner." Then I pull into the "university," grab a "coffee," and I go to "class." So I can think of these words—and just let me remind you what those words are again: bed, breakfast, walk, iron, shower, dress, shoes, car, school, church, diner, university, coffee, class. These words represent that ritual I just told you about. And these words are really going to be critical because they are what I will use to link new information to. What about that new information?

People here in the studio have come up with random words—these are the words for me to remember—and have placed them in this I guess what could best be described as an urn. I have not seen any of the words. I'm going to mix them up, and I will draw them out one at a time, and these will be the words that I will remember. What you'll see is that what I'm going to do is connect each of these words with one of those 14 words of my morning routine, and in so doing, I will be using a strategy called the method of loci. I'll explain that a little bit more in a moment. Once I have the words connected, once I've done the association, then I will be able to recall them accurately, and in order, without studying them any further. What's more, I will come back to them at the end of this class, about 25 minutes from now, and will still be able to recall them in order. So here goes.

Let me kind of tell a story here. We're going to take my morning ritual, and we're going to embellish it, thanks to the words in this urn. So, to start off, I wake up in bed. Let me pull out a word. The word is "sand." Oh, well, I obviously didn't sleep very well, because somebody kicked sand into my bed, made it very uncomfortable. But that's OK. I wake up and I go down to breakfast. "Ocean." Beautiful ocean. For some reason there's an ocean outside of my breakfast window. It wasn't there the night before. I don't know where the ocean came from, but for now going to eat my breakfast overlooking the ocean. What a fantastic image. Great. After breakfast I go for a walk with the wonder dogs, and I have the word "elbow." Hmmm. Walking with the wonder dogs-elbow. Well, let's just say the wonder dogs are a little feisty today, and they're pulling me this way and that, everywhere we go. By the time we get home, my elbows are really sore from all this. All right. Great. I'm home now, ironing my clothes, the next step. "Burglar." As I'm ironing the clothes, somebody has the nerve to start breaking into my window, while I'm right there ironing my clothes.

Luckily, Layla and Lola, the wonder dogs, kicked the burglar's butt. Cool. Now shower. I go into the shower. Problem. It's not water coming into the shower, it's glue. What a pain in the butt that is. Say no more. I get out of the shower and somehow I get the glue off me. Time to get dressed. And "shovel." OK. Well let's do a little bit of Groucho Marx or something as about to get dressed, and there's my clothes on the floor.

And I step, and there's a shovel jumps up and bangs me and hits me in the face. Why not? That works. But I get dressed anyway. Go to put my shoes on—"bacteria." Don't we all hate this? My shoes smell horrible. Clearly, it's bacteria. What can you do? This happens. I hop in the car, and "parade." Well, I opened the garage door. I'm about to back out but there's this parade on my street. And you know what parades are like. They don't allow you to kind of jump in, so I have to sit there and I have to wait for the whole parade to go by. Fine, do that. I hop back in my car. I pass the school, local school, "windmill." How about that? This school is really into energy conservation so there are a bunch of windmills on the roof. That's different. But pretty cool. Makes a lot of sense in this day and age.

Go past the church, the next destination, and it's "soccer." There's a bunch of priests and rabbi's playing soccer. It's a church. So it's a bunch of priests playing soccer against the nuns, priests versus the nuns. I'm curious to see who will win, but I drive on anyway, past the diner. At the diner, "lemon." OK. Well, the diner, for whatever reason, has decided to promote lemons, so all the specials today have lemons in them somehow. It doesn't sound very appetizing but why not? So I get to the university, "tarantula," ah. Don't you hate that? There's a tarantula infestation at the university. No big deal but when I drive my car over them, well, you get the idea. You get the image. Somehow I park, and manage to get around all the tarantulas, and go for my coffee. And here's the word "chess." So they won't give me my coffee until I beat them at chess first. Well that's easy enough, right? So I do that. And finally, I'm at my class in the morning, and "laser." OK. I get to class, and you know what happens. There are students with lasers and they're putting it on my forehead and such, while I'm trying to teach, and that's very annoying, but that's how it is.

So, 14 words. You saw how much I thought about them. I've formed all these associations. I will look at the words no more. They shall stay in this little urn over here. And to demonstrate that I have indeed learned the words, let me now recite them to you, quickly mentioning each step of my routine to show you how I use them to remember the words. All right, ready? Here goes.

I started in bed, sand, there was sand in my bed, made the bed really uncomfortable. Go down to breakfast. Ocean. Ocean view that was not there the night before. Fantastic. Took dogs out. Elbow. Pulling my elbows out every which way. Come back to iron. Burglar. Burglar was breaking in as I was ironing. Layla and Lola kicked his butt. After I iron, I have a shower, glue. Coming out of the shower to get dressed. Get hit with a shovel. Go down to put shoes on, bacteria. My shoes are smelly from the bacteria.

Hop in the car. Parade. I can't go anywhere because of the parade. Eventually the parade passes, and I start driving, and went by a school. The school had windmills on the roof, energy conversation. Excellent. Drive a little further. Nuns and priests playing soccer. So soccer was the church. A little further yet, passed Ted's Diner. Lemons. Lemons of the day. Drive to the university, tarantula infested. I hate when that happens, but I survive. Cool. Go for my coffee, have to play them a game of chess. So I beat them at chess. Get my coffee and go to my class. At class, those pesky students with their lasers, having a field day. OK. I think I got them all. I hope so. Are you impressed? Well don't be impressed yet. It's one thing to remember a list of items right after learning them; it's something else to remember them quite a while later when our mind is thinking about other issues. So let's see if what I did left a dribble enough of a trace for me to remember it at the end of this lecture.

But for now let me move on to an explanation of why this strategy works and what it tells us about memory. It turns out that this desire to improve our memory is far from new. The method I just demonstrated is called the method of loci, where *loci* is a just the Latin plural of "*locus*," meaning "place." So this procedure literally dates back to the glory days of Rome. At that time there were orators who traveled the land, stopping at various cities at banquets, their responsibility was to tell the leaders of the city about the news of the realm. What was going on in other places? Their credibility to do so was depended on others believing that the memory of those events was accurate. So to prove their memory strength, they would very quickly learn the names of the people at the banquet. They would learn this just before the banquet started, and then would literally introduce these people in the right order just before beginning to relay the news. So they would go table by table and introduce everyone that was there. This feat of memory would impress those there, so when the orators went on to tell the news, they would be much more trusted by the people who were hearing it. How did they do it?

These orators tended to follow familiar routes when they traveled through the land. They would go from city to city, locations to location. And when they were trying to learn these new names, they would take these new names and these people and would kind of imagine them in these different locations. So using imagery or anything else they could to strengthen that association, they could literally place these people along their normally traveled routes. So then when they had to retrieve those names, they would mentally travel that route again. And along the way they would essentially collect the people, and say their names as they did. If the associations they formed were strong enough, then retrieving the locations would provide a cue that would allow them to retrieve the name. So the locations played a critical role in organizing this new information.

By the way, this is pretty much what Simonides the poet did in Greece in the 5th century B.C. Simonides was the sole survivor of a roof collapse that killed all of the other guests at a large banquet he was attending. He was able to actually reproduce the guest list by imagining each table and remembering who he had observed sitting there. So he didn't really do the kind of encoding I did, but because the people were pretty organized at the tables and because he knew them, he was would associate people to tables and then literally go table by table, the same general process. In his case it was the environment that provided the organization, and his knowledge allowed him to form those associations. But when the environment doesn't provide the organization, we can still do it ourselves. And that's exactly what I did with you in the demonstration I just performed.

This is all really important, because often when people say they can't remember something, they are implying that the problem they're having is with respect to retrieving the information out of memory, literally the retrieval stage. They know they originally heard the information, for example, maybe some person's name that they met. Or maybe they know that they thought about the chores they wanted to do, but when they needed to remember them, they couldn't, and they assume the problem is with respect to retrieval. Technically it's true; retrieval can fail. But the real lesson we learn from mnemonic strategies is that it is often not enough to just listen to something or to think about something. We really need to think about it deeply. Our ability to remember depends heavily on the way that we think about the information when we first encounter it, that is, when we encode it. If we encode the information well, we will have a much better chance of retrieving it later.

Remember when we spoke of working memory, and I told you that it's a memory system that we often use to combine information from different sources to solve some new goal we have, some new task. I also told you it's very strongly linked to consciousness and our mental thoughts. Anytime that we encounter some new information that we want to remember subsequently, we have a new goal. That is a goal, and therefore it is working memory that we can best use to reach that goal. It was working memory that we were using in the demonstration that I just gave to you. It is literally taking information, combining it, and helping us to remember it better for later.

If you think about that information properly at the time of encoding, that is, if you engage in the right techniques using your working memory, then you can in fact, indeed, remember the information better. Interestingly, these techniques mostly have to do with encoding. It has to do with how you put the information into memory, and if you put it in the right way, then it is easier to get it back out again later.

To make this kind of make sense, imagine the following. Imagine we have two boxes, one is pretty large, the other is much smaller. And imagine we have some recipes that we might want to use later, and we've written them down on small recipe cards, and we've made two copies of each recipe. One copy we just throw into the large box. The other copy we "file" into the smaller box, perhaps sorting it as we do, maybe according to the alphabet so apple pie might be first, and zucchini casserole might be last. Tonight we decide that we would like to make the Portabella Pasta recipe, and we know that we've written it down. We also know that we put it in both boxes. We tossed a copy into the big box, and we filed it in the appropriate spot in the small box. Now what happens if we want to find this? Well, it will be much easier to find this recipe in the smaller box, that is, both the time to find it, and the likelihood of actually finding it before we give up will be higher if we look in the smaller sorted box. In fact, if we had a whole bunch of recipes in that big box, we might find it almost impossible to ever find the recipe we want. We would know it's there, but we just couldn't "bring it back." And this is a lot like when we know we listened to a name or some chore we want to do, but we just can't remember it later.

Putting things in the right way helps you get them out. Now it takes more time and effort of course to put things into the recipe box and into memory in an organized way, but there is good dividends to be paid for this. So the point is it's not about the size of your memory. It's not about making your memory bigger, it's about storing information in your memory in a more efficient way that helps you get it out.

So the first kind of variable that will help us do that is organization. If we organize information at the time of encoding, we can learn to use that organization to enhance our memory. So what sort of things can we do during encoding that will help us to do that? Well, let's return to the sorted recipe box. In that case what we used to provide the organization was the alphabet. And think about how we actually found the Portabella Pasta. We used the alphabet. It gave structure to the information, and we could use that structure to later retrieve the information that we want. So we know that portabella begins with a p, so we can search that small recipe box, find the p area. Even if we only sorted by the first letter, we would already be in the right area of memory. If we alphabetized a lot more detail right through the letter, we could hone right in to exactly where that recipe is. It would be very efficient to be able to find it when it was put in in a highly organized way.

So now let's think about the method of the loci. We had new information to put into memory, for example, the words given to me to remember. But I didn't just throw them into memory. Instead, I took the time to attach each new piece of information to a structure, a structure that I already had in my memory. Not the alphabet, but my morning routine. By associating each piece of new information with something I can already retrieve easily from memory, I am essentially using my routine to get me to that right area of memory, just like the alphabet lets us get to the right part of the recipe card file.

Right now is a great time for you to pause this lecture and come up with your own list like the one I used. Come up with your own morning routine or whatever it is. Make it long enough so you can store lots of items if you need to. You can always just use only part of that list. I prefer the lists tied to my daily routine because I live a pretty consistent sort of life on weekdays. So that listing is quite ingrained in my mind. But maybe there is something else for you. You can choose anything, anything in which certain steps occur in a very specific order, as long as you know these steps, and you know the order in which they occur, that's fantastic. So pause me for a minute and go write a list like that.

So let's talk about what your list of cues can do for you. By having these well structured memory cues we can organize the information better in memory, and we can use this organization at retrieval to get us in the right general area of memory. Now how do we get the information we want? This is where associations come in, as forming good associations is the second critical variable we can use to enhance our memory.

You likely noticed that when I was associating the new information with my cues I often made use of bizarre images. That is, I turned the words into images, and joined the two bits of information in ways that were either slightly humorous or downright odd, like glue coming out of shower. I did this because research show that we remember bizarre things better than we remember common things. Thus by forming strong associations between a set of organized cues, my morning ritual, and some new information, I not only can get to roughly the right place in memory, but I also can use the association to get the specific information I want. Now that you have your list of cues, let's practice using them. Either by writing your cues down, or by working through them in your head, use them to memorize the following list of words: newsletter, harpoon, window, chap stick, calamari, Elvis, pachyderm, tuba, donut, Popeye.

Basically, do what I did. Generate bizarre images that is very important, and that is to link the words to your cues. You can pause me again right now while you try that if you like. So how did you do? You can learn even from trying this just once, but you can start to get really good at it with a few tries.

By the way, there's another aspect of bizarre images that is important, and that is the very fact that I turned each word into a picture in the first place. In so doing, I was creating a copy of the item, and I was storing the copy and the original in different parts of my brain. A word is in the linguistics department. It goes into the linguistic part of the brain. The picture is stored in the picture area. So I literally have two copies, almost like two recipes in one box, which will make it even easier to find. Psychologists call this the dual-coding hypothesis and, based on it, they generally encourage people whenever possible to form multiple copies of a stimulus. This dual-coding is yet another variable that can help us to enhance our memory. Organization, association, and dual coding.

As another example of a different strategy that also utilizes these three factors, you likely learned from your teacher this acronym, ROY G. BIV, and it's what you can use to remember the colors of the rainbow. Now notice this ROY G. BIV as being this imaginary character. Each letter in the name is associated with a color in the rainbow, r-red, o-orange, y-yellow, g-green, b-blue, i-indigo, and v-violet. So the name provided the structure; the letters of the name provided cues to the association. And the fact that we've now taken color information and stored it as a name provides dual coding.

So now let's just return to those pesky names. Well, think of those critical variables. And now think of yourself as trying to remember names. Well, if you are introduced to someone named Bill, maybe you can form a bizarre image of "Bill" running out of a restaurant to avoid paying the "bill." So now we've used association and dual coding to remember that name. That should help. Ah, but here's the real problem. That's fine with Bill, but what about George? Alicia? Frederick? Or Ajmal? Many names simply do not lend themselves well to imagery, and that's a big reason why they are so hard to remember. But Ajmal? That's a challenge. Your best bet is to try multiple tricks. Some might be just playing around with words and well-known slogans. So we can think of something like "The great Aj Mal, almost as great as the Taj Mahal, and, ah, he went to the "mall" to play "dodge ball." You can also search your memory for maybe a similar name you've ever heard before, like, "Ajmal and Jemal had a great "fall," anything you can use to help you to remember that name and, of course, the more that you know the person and more about the person, the more that that can give you other possible associations. You can think, "Ajmal, so tall" or "Ajmal, in the hall."

This is precisely why we have the trouble remembering names. The names are so random that they are hard to organize, often hard to form associations with, and harder to code in more than one way. Of course, you can and should still try, but don't be surprised if names always remain a more difficult thing to remember. They just are. By the way, this technique may seem like a lot of work, but you do these things over and over, it will become very natural to put things in memory this way. The effort involved will decrease. For example, that demo I did with you, I've done many times and in many different talks so the words I use, that routine, it's actually second nature to me. And I can jump right into the process of forming associations. Yes it still takes time and effort, but the amount of effort reduces, and heck forming these associations and especially these bizarre images is kind of fun. So, all in all, not a negative experience. Of course the most critical point is that these things work. It's actually called the art of memory and has been used a couple of thousand years in a lot of different names. So give it a try. Remember, the main steps are organize, associate, and duel coding. You'll be taking part in a long tradition. You'll be improving your memory at the same time, your episodic memory, remember. So now the moment of truth. Let's see if I can still remember those items from earlier in the lecture. Bed-sand. Breakfast-ocean. Walk dogs-elbow. Iron-burglar. Shower-glue. Dressed-shovel. Shoes-bacteria. Car-parade. School-windmills. Church-soccer. Diner-lemons. University-tarantula. Coffee-chess. Class-lasers. Think I got them all. How about you? I think if you try it yourself, you'll find it's pretty easy. And it's kind of cool. I'm thinking you can do it. Give it a go. And try it in many different circumstances if you like. It's something you can really use to enhance your memory. Enjoy.

Rote Memorization and a Science of Forgetting
Lecture 3

All art of memory methods require expending most of your effort up front, when you first encounter a piece of information. But traditionally, people have memorized general knowledge through repetition—rote memorization. Rote learning requires more ongoing effort but less extreme effort at any given time.

Rote memorization is interesting for 2 reasons. First, it has an interesting past and present and, to some extent, provides a great basis for comparison with art of memory strategies. Second, it played a key role in the birth of a true science of memory, in that it was the subject of the very first scientific memory experiments.

Rote learning and mnemonics almost seem like opposites. Mnemonic strategies require plenty of up-front effort, but thereafter the memories are retained rather effortlessly. By contrast, rote learning requires more sustained but less intense effort. Mnemonics are associated with episodic memory, whereas rote memorization is more strongly associated with semantic memory.

Repetition of facts might occur within some specific context, such as when a teacher drills us on multiplication tables, or we might have heard the same fact repeated across different contexts, like multiple people calling Florida the Sunshine State. If we do hear something enough, it becomes committed to our semantic memory, and over time we may forget the specific context in which we heard it. This is why politicians and political parties use talking points, so the same message is heard again and again across a variety of news formats.

Rote learning is probably quite ancient; we know that today's most important religious texts were originally transmitted orally, because there were few copies of the texts in existence. In Victorian Europe, rote memorization skills were regarded as evidence of a strong work ethic and strength of character. Rote memorization remains part of our education system.

Virtually all of the earliest psychologists studied perception, but German psychologist Hermann von Ebbinghaus published the world's first scientific study of memory, *Memory: A Contribution to Experimental Psychology*, in 1885. Using himself as a test subject, Ebbinghaus measured the time it took to learn, forget, and relearn a list of 2000 nonsense syllables using rote memorization. He ultimately produced a mathematical function called the **forgetting curve**.

Ebbinghaus's main discoveries were that memory decays exponentially, with most of the losses occurring right away, and that meaningless syllables were more quickly forgotten than meaningful words. Memory for real-world

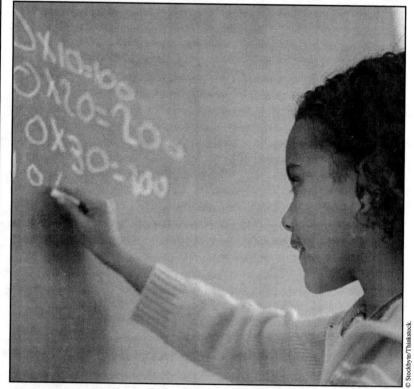

Facts learned through rote memorization, such as the multiplication tables, are stored in semantic memory.

experiences is likely not this dramatically affected, as we tend to process stimuli in a deeper, more meaningful way.

Subsequent research has suggested a number of reasons why we forget, or at least fail to recall, information. Sometimes we don't encode it well enough in the first place. Interference theory suggests that similar experiences, either before (**proactive interference**) or after (**retroactive interference**) you try to encode a memory, can interfere with encoding and recall.

Retrieval failure holds the most promise as a general explanation for memory failure; this occurs when memories are encoded without good retrieval cues and more recent memories seem to bury it in one big pile of information. The theory of retrieval failure fits Ebbinghaus's discovery that it was faster to relearn information than to learn it. His findings also support a distinction between conscious and unconscious or subconscious knowledge.

Both mnemonic techniques and rote memorization can be useful at the same time. Consider actors learning their parts for a play: They must learn very specific lines and movements. They could use their positions as location cues associated with a trigger word carrying the gist of the appropriate line, but rote learning might be best to memorize the lines themselves. We can use this combination in everyday life as well. In general, a key to creating a very lasting memory is to use more than one memory system. ■

Important Terms

forgetting curve: A mathematical function that predicts the time required to memorize, forget, and re-encode a set of data through rote memorization.

proactive interference: A previous experience that prevents successful encoding or recall of a similar piece of information.

retrieval failure: Forgetting; that is, when we cannot recall a piece of information, usually because it was encoded without good retrieval cues.

retroactive interference: An experience that weakens the encoding or recall of a previously memorized piece of information.

rote memorization: Memorization through repetition.

Suggested Reading

Ebbinghaus, *Memory*.

Herrmann and Chaffin, *Memory in Historical Perspective*.

Questions to Consider

1. List some contexts where you think rote memorization might be the best way to learn and remember. What, if anything, do those contexts have in common, and how widely do they differ from one another?

2. Why do you think Ebbinghaus's research failed to spawn a rigorous investigation of memory?

3. On another shopping trip, try learning your grocery list by rote. Don't think about it deeply, just repeat the items to yourself over and over.

Rote Memorization and a Science of Forgetting
Lecture 3—Transcript

If you want to remember a lecture, you could listen to it over and over. Suppose you listened to a lecture 10 times. How much more likely do you think it would be that you would remember it? And how much longer would you remember it?

In the previous lecture, we looked at what is sometimes called the art of memory, essentially, pre-scientific ways to be smart about ways to use your memory. Mnemonic strategies, such as the method of loci have been relied on since the classical period, especially for enhancing episodic memory. What all of these sorts of art of memory techniques have in common is that you expend extra effort up front: You need to use organization, association, and dual coding. And the extra effort pays off by producing a deep and strong memory trace, even for random stimuli.

But when you are listening to a lecture, you want to acquire and remember general knowledge, and for that, the traditional and most basic memory technique is quite different. Whether with a book or a lecture, the most basic way to remember general knowledge has traditionally been to repeat it over and over and over, what is called rote learning, or rote memorization.

Rote memorization is interesting for two reasons. First, it has an interesting past and present and, to some extent, it provides a fantastic basis for comparison to the art of memory. Second, it also turns out that rote memorization played a key role in the birth of a science of memory, in the sense that the very first memory experiments were performed, were actually performed in the context of rote memorization. Thus, the subject of rote memorization is a great complement to what we've already learned, and it makes a natural transition from pre-scientific approaches to memory, into the scientific studies of memory that we will be focusing on for the remainder of this course.

Rote memorization is very different from mnemonic strategies and from the art of memory. Rote and mnemonics almost seem like opposites. Mnemonic strategies require plenty of up-front effort, but thereafter the memories are retained almost effortlessly. By contrast, rote learning seems to require lots more ongoing effort, although the effort at any given time is required less. All that ongoing effort is why some parents and teachers like rote learning, even apart from how well it works as a memory technique.

Anyway, rote is different, and that difference results in rote memorization being more strongly associated with semantic memory, our general knowledge of the world, things like the number we get when we multiply 4 by 6, or the knowledge that the panhandle state is Florida. How did we come to know these things? Well, mostly we learned them just from hearing these facts repeated over and over and over. This repetition often occurs in different contexts, but it may even occur in a very specific context, such as when a teacher "drills" us on the multiplication tables, or usually it occurs because we simply have heard those facts repeated in many different contexts. So perhaps we have heard a number of different people refer to Florida as the panhandle state.

Of course, if you hear some claim enough, you will eventually believe it's true. If you hear some claim enough, you will eventually believe it's true. Sorry. That felt like it bore repeating. But of course it is true. When you hear something enough, it becomes committed to memory, semantic memory. It becomes part of our general storehouse of knowledge of the world. Over time, we often forget the specific context in which we heard it. It just becomes a "fact." This is why politicians, of course, like to repeat their so-called talking points, and why a given political party will often send out a number of its members to utter the same talking points across a variety of news formats. This repetition across a variety of formats, when it's combined with variation in the details of where we heard the message, makes it all seem more like the truth.

This relationship between repetition and memory has deep roots, probably going back to human beings even before the invention of writing. We do know that rote learning was very important once writing had been invented. As you know, most religions have some book they consider sacred, be it the Bible for Christians, the Torah for Jews, or the Qur'an for Muslims. Prior to print, there were only limited copies of these texts in existence, not enough for every religious scholar to have their own a copy. In addition, the specific wording of these texts is considered extremely important, as they are often viewed as representing the word of God or Allah. It would not be sufficient for a religious reader to just convey the gist of what they read to their faithful. They are expected to deliver the word as represented in the texts.

Even just reading the texts aloud posed a challenge, given that writing didn't yet include such conveniences as spaces to separate words, commas to separate phrases, periods to separate sentences, or anything like paragraphs or sections. The letters just went on and on. Reading today is far easier than it was in ancient times. So even for the purpose of just reading aloud, having some type of familiarity with the text was a really big help, and verbatim memorization, well that was even better. Traditional scholars would literally read passages over and over in an effort to become more familiar with the text, as well as to commit more and more of the precise wording to memory. In some cases those who were able to memorize the entire religious texts were afforded some sort of special status. For example, one who has memorized the entire Qur'an is known as Hafiz, which literally means a "guardian," a "guardian" of the word of Allah.

However, as printed books spread, the premium placed on memorizing an entire book gradually declined. On the other hand, a premium for learning specific facts began to rise. By the 19th century, there was an extraordinary passion for rote memorization of specific facts. We can see that strong emphasis on rote memorization in many parts of the world even today.

And rote memorization still remains part of our education system, too. For example, our multiplication tables in mathematics and periodic tables in chemistry are still often taught via rote memorization. However, in North America our education system has moved away from a heavy use rote memorization as a general learning strategy, instead focusing more heavily on deeper learning approaches. We'll see reasons for that, both in this lecture, and elsewhere in the course.

But in the 19th century, rote memorization had a special place in the Victorian era on the European continent. At that time, a keen ability at rote memorization was viewed essentially as a virtue. One who was able to recite poetry from memory was highly regarded, the notion being was that they had to put a lot of work to do that and they must have true strength of character to do that. Thus, it is fair to say, that if you lived in Europe during the Victorian era, and if you were interested in memory, you likely viewed rote learning as a viable method for getting information into memory. This is an important point because it is within this context that the very first scientific researcher of memory began. This work by a German psychologist named Hermann von Ebbinghaus. Before we talk about the details of Ebbinghaus' work on memory, let me situate it within the context of psychology as a science. While a philosophical interest in the mind dates back to ancient civilizations, the birth of psychology as an independent science did not really occur until the mid to late 1870s. At that time Wilhelm Wundt established the first dedicated psychology lab in 1879, less than 150 years ago.

This late birth is primarily due to a resistance by humans to view human behavior as determined by material processes, processes open to understanding via scientific inquiry. Given this resistance, nearly all of the early psychologists, Wundt included, focused their research on the study of perception, our ability to internally represent external events as they occur. In many ways, perception can be viewed as one of the very first steps of a mind's interaction with its environment, and one that's not too far removed from the scientific study of external objects, that is, physics. In fact, many psychologists refer to themselves as people studying psycho-physics. So perception was a cautious first step into a scientific study of mind.

In fact, virtually all of the earliest psychologists also studied perception. However the hero of our current lecture, Hermann von Ebbinghaus, was a bolder scientist. Ebbinghaus was interested in memory. Memory is a somewhat abstract concept, and it was definitely far removed from the sorts of topics studied by scientists prior to Ebbinghaus's time. There were serious questions about whether one could scientifically study memory at all. And Ebbinghaus was determined to show that, yes one could, and if one can study memory with empirical rigor, then perhaps one could study any aspect of the mind.

Ebbinghaus was specifically interested in a few questions about memory. How long does it take us to learn something? How long does it take then to forget those things? And when we seem to have forgotten something, have we really forgotten? In 1885, at the age of just 35, he published the first scientific book on memory. It was translated as "Memory: A Contribution to Experimental Psychology." Now recall that Ebbinghaus lived in the Victorian era, a time when the conception of memory was heavily influenced by the process of rote memorization. Thus, it should not be surprising that the experiments he performed reflect this influence.

Ebbinghaus began his research the same year that Wundt had opened the world's first psychology lab over in Leipzig, Germany. And Ebbinghaus was just as determined to approach memory in the same scientific way. To get a sense of this, one only needs to consider the procedures that he used. Now Ebbinghaus didn't have a lab. At the start of his research, he didn't even have a full-time university position. So he kind of knew from the outset that if he wanted to study memory, he would have to study his own memory. So his plan was to see how long it took him to learn various materials, then how long it took to forget what he had learned, and then how long it took him to relearn what he had apparently forgotten. But what sort of material would he memorize?

For Ebbinghaus, words would not do. He saw them as possessing way too much baggage, too many pre-existing associations with other words, with images, and with our lives. Of course, in the mnemonic strategies that I discussed earlier I emphasized how images and associations could be used to enhance one's memory, but this is exactly the sort of thing that Ebbinghaus did not want to happen. He viewed such things as complicating factors, and he wanted to eliminate them in order to study a more pure form of the processes related to memory. So instead of using words he created nonsense syllables composed of a consonant, a vowel, and a consonant. So items like nim, kop, or lef. He saw these items as much more neutral, and therefore more appropriate to use in the context of a scientific investigation of memory.

So he first created a very large set of these consonant, vowel, consonant strings, and essentially put them in a hat. During the learning phase he would then pull out syllables and write them down in a notebook, perhaps creating a list of, let's say, 20 items or so. This would be his learning set. He then read them aloud, one at a time, in a neutral voice, to the beat of a metronome trying to remember them as he did so. To give you a sense of this, let's imagine Ebbinghaus learning a list as follows. Here's our metronome. And you would hear Ebbinghaus doing something like this: dek, pim, nis, vot, rup, tog, bek, kem, lun, hib. You get the idea.

Clearly he was using rote memorization to encode the items. He would then go through his list fully, and then he would attempt to recall the list. He did this repeatedly over and over until he could correctly recall the list twice in a row, and he recorded how many repetitions it took to get to that point. That was his measure of learning time.

For his experiments on forgetting, he would learn a list well enough to recall it twice, then put he would just put it away. He would literally try very hard not to think about the list in any way. After some amount of time had passed, he would then attempt to retrieve the list from his memory. And he would score himself in terms of how many items he could recall. He did this over and over, with different lists, and allowing different amounts of time to pass, really, anything from 20 minutes to 31 days. By looking at his accuracy then, he was able to examine how much information he forgot as a function of time. By doing so, he ultimately produced the forgetting curve, a depiction of forgetting over time, and one that he is now quite famous for. What's more, he was able to calculate the formula suggested by the forgetting curve, a mathematical function that captures forgetting. Now this was really important because by adding math to this, he was providing compelling evidence that memory processes can be quantified experimentally, and that they seem to follow natural laws that conform to mathematical description. So that was very important. Many of the early psychologists were trying to show they could study psychology scientifically. Here was Ebbinghaus doing exactly that in the context of memory. So that was fantastic.

One startling aspect of Ebbinghaus's forgetting curve was that he, himself, at least, tended to forget half of the information he had learned, really in just a matter of days or weeks. He forget the rest more slowly. That is, memory was obviously decaying exponentially, with most of the losses occurring almost right away. That said, Ebbinghaus also showed that part of the steepness, I should say the onset of the curve, was due to the fact that he had used nonsense syllables, these CVC strings. When he instead tried it with words, he found that he could retain the original level a little longer. When memories began to drop, they still dropped precipitously. So there was still roughly an exponential drop, it was just shifted to a little later in time.

Keep in mind that even when Ebbinghaus used meaningful stimuli, he still encoded the information in a rote memorization fashion. That is, while the meaningfulness of the stimuli might have spontaneously brought to mind images or associations, Ebbinghaus certainly did not try to strategically use this information in any way, definitely not in any way as described in the lecture on mnemonics. So yes, the forgetting curves look pretty ominous, but they depict relatively extreme cases of pure rote memorization. Memory for real-world experiences is likely not as dramatically affected, as we tend to process stimuli in a deeper more meaningful way.

That said, even in the context of much richer real world stimuli, we still can often feel like we forget things very quickly after we learn them. For example, given that you're watching or listening to this course, it's quite possible that you have experienced other examples of the Great Courses. Have you ever had the feeling that while you were learning a lot at the time, you seem to have forgotten virtually everything you learned within days after watching or listening?

Perhaps you also have that feeling with books. As you read them you might think, "Ah, that was an interesting part. I want to remember that." But then after you've read the book you don't feel like you can remember any of those interesting parts. Why can we no longer remember information shortly after learning it? Is that information really gone? Is memory really so fleeting?

Ebbinghaus did not go into detail about why we forget, or at least fail to recall. But subsequent research has suggested a number of relevant possibilities. One reason people fail to remember some experience is because they just didn't encode it well enough in the first place. For example, you may find you need to listen to a lecture more than once just to encode it properly. But in the case of Ebbinghaus' experiments, we know that he made sure he could first recall the list twice, at least right after learning it. So even though his approach to encoding might not have been very rich, it was at least rich enough to support memory just after learning. Still, had he tested himself more than twice, or have distributed his learning over time, he presumably would have come closer to the longer-lasting results we get from practicing something many times, the kind of results we get from rote memorization with multiplication tables.

Another concept, though, that is sometimes presented when thinking about forgetting, is the concept of decay over time. So as we think about forgetting, this is sometimes the natural thing we want to say, that memory just decays over time. But it's important to note, however, that time, itself, doesn't cause decay. It really just provides a temporal space in which other processes might occur. So, for example, it's not really correct to say something like, "The pyramids are deteriorating over time." Pyramids may be deteriorating by friction of the sand slowly eroding them. That sort of process unfolds over time. That's the true cause of the degradation, not time itself. So, when we get to memory then, we want the same kind of thing. What is it that's actually causing a decay in memory?

Well, there's really two types of processes that we've talked about that hold promise for getting a better understanding of forgetting. The first process is called interference theory, and the second is retrieval theory. Interference theory suggests that sometimes experiences that occur before or after some experience can interfere with our ability to remember. Let me give you an example to make that clear. Suppose you take a French course for the first time, but then you switch to a Spanish course. Although having started on a similar language may help you in some ways, but you may also feel that learning Spanish was a little more difficult because some of the details you learned in the French course keep coming to mind. This is called proactive interference, and it's when a memory from the past is messes with your ability to remember subsequent events.

Or suppose you learn French well, set it aside, and then you learn Spanish. You might find that when you try to go back to French, you have some Spanish words coming to mind instead. This is called retroactive interference, when a memory for a later event interferes with your ability to remember some earlier event. So sometimes interference effects of this sort can make it difficult to either remember, or to separate, similar sorts of experiences.

While interference can explain how two similar experiences can reduce the ability to kind of separate, and possibly even recall either one, it doesn't explain why we sometimes have trouble remembering something when we haven't subsequently encoded something similar. And that's where retrieval failure holds the most promise as a general explanation. Here is how I explain retrieval failure to my students. Imagine you are the sort of person who changes clothes several times a day, and every time you change clothes you just toss the dirty clothes on the floor. You do this day after day, and eventually what you have is a layer of clothes on your floor. One day you want a shirt, a shirt that you wore many days ago. But when you look at your floor, all you can see is a mass of clothes, with the clothes that you wore most recently on the top.

Is that shirt you want gone? No, it's not gone. But it may seem to be gone. It's there somewhere. But if you don't know where to look, it might take you a long time to find it. It is not gone. It's just buried under the new clothes, and the only way to get it is to search all the way through. Depending on how large your floor is and how many clothes you have tossed on over the shirt you want, the search could be very difficult. Unless you know something about where the shirt is, something that helps you to look for it, it could seem like you just can't find it. It must be gone.

Well, memory encoding never stops. It keeps encoding, and it keeps putting things into memory. So it's kind of like the clothes being tossed on the floor. If you encode some new experience and then don't think about it for a bit, it also can become buried under the new experiences that you encode thereafter. As time progresses, these new experiences build up, and the older experience becomes more and more buried. Before long, that experience may seem to be completely gone. Unless you know where to look, that is, unless you have a good retrieval cue to guide you in your memory search. If you don't, you might not be able to retrieve it at all. It may seem like the information is forgotten when really it is just impossible to get to without the right cue.

While Ebbinghaus did not propose this retrieval failure, but he did perform additional experiments that seem to fit with the notion very well. Recall that when he had learned a list, he noted how long it took him. Then he had put it away for some period of time, then tested himself to see how much he remembered. All that formed the basis of his forgetting function that I told you about earlier.

But here's the new twist. He then went back to work re-learning the list. That is, just as he had done initially, he went through that list one at a time with the metronome, and counted how many repetitions he needed to re-learn the entire list, once again, to the point where he could correctly recall the list twice in a row. And what he showed was that he could re-learn that list much faster than it had originally taken to learn, and he referred to that difference as "savings."

This finding was important for two reasons. First, they were perhaps the first experimental results that suggested a distinction between knowledge that is conscious and knowledge that is not. After all, it was "as if" some learning episode was futile because you could not bring it to mind. It felt like it was gone. But clearly it wasn't gone. It was there. It just could not be consciously retrieved. So that was an important implication of his results.

Second, on a more practical level, it means that even if you cannot remember some experience, even if it seems to go away after a few days or weeks, that does not mean the experience was in vain. The knowledge is potentially there. And, in fact, is probably there. And should you ever need to you could bring it back, perhaps quite quickly, with just a little bit of relearning. In a sense, if you find that shirt you were looking for and then toss it back on the top of the pile, it will be easy to find, at least until you bury it again. That should come as some consolation. Maybe you don't remember all the details of the courses you have watched or listened to, but really that information is just sitting there in your brain just waiting to be refreshed.

OK. Let's take a moment now to integrate what we learned about mnemonics and the art of memory in the second lecture, and what we have learned here about rote memorization and the early science of memory. If we are willing to do some serious mental work, when we experience some new information, we can encode it in a way that organizes that new information well, associate it with things we already know, and maybe even store multiple copies of it. If we do all that work, it will make it possible to remember that encoding experience, and it does so in a way that gives us really strong access to the new information even though we have only encoded it once. That's the art of memory.

In contrast, rote memorization relies on heavy repetition of information to literally stamp that information into our memories. Because the repetitions occur over several distinct episodes, we don't tend to recall the specific learning episode associated with the information. Instead we just remember what we learned, often in a very precise or verbatim way. That information becomes part of what we simply assume to be true, and this sort of memory is called semantic memory.

There are times when both forms of memory enhancement can be useful. And we want to combine these perhaps. Let me give you an example. Let's consider actors learning their parts for a play. The actors must learn very specific lines, of course, but they also have to learn specific movements. They have to be at certain points of the stage at certain times. So maybe just like the ancient Romans, they could use these places as loci. Each location then could be used as a sort of "trigger word." If they've associated a word with each location, and then when they're at that location, that trigger word could be used to cue them about the gist of what they have to say. However, just like the religious scholars of old, they of course can't just give the gist of their lines. They have to speak the precise lines. So given this need for specificity, rote learning might be the best way to memorize the necessary lines. So they can use the method of loci as a cue that could begin a set of lines learned by rote. A beautiful orchestration of different memory enhancement techniques.

Of course, this is true not just for actors, but for remembering more generally. You can try this yourself. Start looking for ways to combine the memory enhancement techniques we've discussed so far. First, look for episodic cues you create for yourself, the more vivid the better. For instance, if you are going to use flashcards to do some rote learning, start by trying to create vivid mnemonics for each flashcard.

Or suppose you want to remember a lecture better: In that case, you could take the time to do some deeper encoding. That is, to organize the new information well, associate that information with things you already know, and maybe even store copies of that information in more than one way.

Then you could try to use vivid cues you've already created even when you go back to the material. That combination of vivid episodic cues together with the additional episodes provided by rote learning will transform an already durable episodic memory into semantic memory, backed by multiple episodes. But "multiple episodes" doesn't mean listening to the same lecture 10 times; most of the episodes helping you remember can come from thinking and talking about the material yourself.

In general, the key to creating a very lasting memory is to use more than one memory system. So, in the next lecture we'll begin a discussion of our memory systems in much more detail. Yes, Ebbinghaus got the memory research ball rolling in the late 19th century, but no researchers really followed his lead until much later. Specifically, many continued to see memory as too vague a concept to think about scientifically, despite the data Ebbinghaus provided. Even Ebbinghaus himself switched his research to perception later in his career. He turned instead to a study of color vision.

So the scientific approach to human memory that Ebbinghaus pioneered, really lay dormant for eight decades, until the late 1950s. That's when research on human memory suddenly began to flourish. So let's hop in our time machine and set the dials for the late 1950s, the heyday when memory research really began to take off, and let's see what they were doing back then.

Sensory Memory—Brief Traces of the Past
Lecture 4

Sensory memory is a short-lived memory buffer that retains sensory stimuli for a brief period, giving a person time to switch attention to the new stimulus even though it is no longer present. Whatever our conscious mind may be engaged with, we seem to be constantly storing incoming visual and auditory information and, at some level, processing it for potential importance.

Perhaps you or someone you know has the ability to focus on a task to the point where the rest of the world drops away. This is an extreme example of human single-mindedness; that is, people find it hard to consciously think about more than a single thing at a time. We're all familiar with the idea of multitasking, but the truth is that most evidence indicates we're not actually doing 2 things at once; we're switching our attention rapidly between the 2 or more tasks.

Rapid attention switching is made possible by our sensory memory, which acts like a very short-lived memory buffer, retaining a sensory stimulus (a sight, sound, smell, taste, or feeling) for a brief period after it occurs. This buffer gives us the time to switch our attention; more importantly, it maximizes the likelihood of us catching important stimuli when focused on something else.

The basic principle of this sensory memory buffer is straightforward, at least with respect to visual and auditory stimuli. (Little research has been done on the other senses.) A copy of the stimulus is briefly retained, giving us enough time to switch our attention and then process the copy. Switches of attention happen quickly, so the copy doesn't have to be saved for very long.

The visual form of sensory memory is called **iconic memory**. It is related to the persistence of vision—the phenomenon that makes a series of still pictures running through a movie projector imitate continuous motion and causes a light attached to a bicycle wheel to leave a trail as the wheel is spun. The buffer of our iconic memory allows the light to live on in a certain spatial position even after the light source has moved on.

Iconic memory was first studied in detail by psychologist George Sperling in the 1960s. He used a device like a film projector, called a tachistoscope, to briefly show grids of letters to his subjects and measure how much they could recall and for how long. His results indicated that the subjects saw every letter in the grid initially, but the memory only lasted about 1 second—only long enough for subjects to specifically recall half of them. So the raw iconic memory fades quickly, but some part of the information can be transferred to another system, likely working memory. In fact, it seems that that purpose of iconic memory is to keep the raw image around in case some components of it are important.

Sensory memory—iconic memory in particular—also plays a role in keeping our sensory representations of the world intact and rich. Our eyes take in a scene not all at once but in 200-millisecond bursts called **saccades**. Each one gives us a snapshot of one part of the world; our iconic memory buffers allow us to piece these together like a mosaic. Our sense of hearing also has this sort of short-term memory storage, called **echoic memory**. Formal experiments indicate that echoic memory lasts for about 4 or 5 seconds, much longer than iconic memory, which is likely why we notice it much more.

Scientists think echoic memory lasts longer than iconic memory because of the importance of speech to human functioning. Speech is serial, with one word following another. We need to remember a whole sentence to process its meaning accurately; therefore, we need to hold words in our memory for several seconds at a time. Visual information does not have the same structured unfolding over time.

Do our other senses have short sensory memories as well? For taste and smell, the answer seems to be both yes and no. Smells and tastes do not suddenly appear and suddenly disappear; the natural fading of olfactory chemicals and the span of time food spends in our mouths gives us plenty of time to switch our attention to them. **Tactile memory**, or **haptic memory**, allows us to feel a touch gradually fade away as well. ■

Important Terms

echoic memory: The ability to hold or recall a sound in one's mind; the auditory form of sensory memory.

iconic memory: The ability to hold or recall an image in one's mind; the visual form of sensory memory.

saccades: Swift glances moving from object to object in a scene that our iconic memories use to piece together a whole.

tactile memory (a.k.a. **haptic memory**): The lingering impression of something we have touched or been touched by; a form of sensory memory.

Suggested Reading

Braisby and Gellatly, *Cognitive Psychology*.

Foster, *Memory*.

Luck and Hollingworth, *Visual Memory*.

Questions to Consider

1. When a dog goes outside, it smells lampposts and such because doing so tells the dog which other dogs have been there and when. How is a dog's sense of smell like human sensory memory? How is it different?

2. What if iconic memory lasted for 10 seconds and echoic memory for 30 seconds? Do you think that would be better? Can you imagine ways it could be problematic?

Pay attention to what happens when you speak to someone who is deeply focused on something else. When they ask what you said, wait for a bit, and see if they realize what you asked without you repeating it.

Sensory Memory—Brief Traces of the Past
Lecture 4—Transcript

Welcome back. In the first lecture I introduced you to the different forms of memory, and I promised that I would reintroduced you to each, and give you many more details. We then took a trip into mnemonics, rote memorization, and the very beginnings of the science of memory by Hermann Ebbinghaus. So now I want to get back to my promise. I want to begin to describe each of our memory systems in more detail. I'd want to give you a better sense of the data that supports the existence of each, and tell you more about the contexts in which each system plays a role. We will also discuss the manner in which these systems interact.

We're going to start by talking in this lecture about a kind of memory called sensory memory. To introduce you to the relevance of sensory memory I'd like to tell you a little story about my Dad. When we grew up, we had one television. My father was a very hard working man. He had his full time job, and he always had hobbies to ensure he did not have "idle hands." But when he relaxed, the TV was his way of doing so. He would watch TV shows intently, and the rest of the world simply vanished. If any of us spoke while he was watching, it was like we didn't exist. Whatever we said just disappeared into the ether. If we wanted to communicate with Dad, we waited for a commercial. Perhaps you know people like this. Perhaps you are such are a person.

My Dad's behavior while watching TV is an extreme example of the limitations we have with respect to processing information. The world we live in is extremely rich and complex and at any given moment, there are all sorts of things we could either look at, or listen to, or feel, taste, or smell. However, humans are largely single-minded animals. By that, I mean that we tend to find it very hard to consciously think about more than a single thing at a time.

Yes we can multi-task, that is, we can apparently do multiple things at once. But do we really? Or, instead, do we simply switch our attention between tasks? Most of the existing evidence favors the attentional switching hypothesis. That is, those who are good at multi-tasking are usually good at moving their attention back and forth between a variety of tasks or sources of stimulation. At any given moment though, it seems they, like the rest of us, can really only deeply think about one thing at a time. Some people, like my Dad, don't even try to multi-task, and instead deeply engage in one mental activity while ignoring all others.

This limitation to focus on only one source of stimulation at a time could pose some major problems for us. If we're thinking deeply about something, say that we are looking at, what if someone says something that is critical? We could miss it completely, and sometimes, in fact, we do miss things in that way. If anyone said anything to Dad while he was watching TV, he would miss it. But this usually only happens when we insist on "locking on" to one thing as my Dad did.

More commonly we switch our attention from whatever it is we were concentrating on, and then we're able to kind of hear what was said to us. But wait. How can this be? How does this work? If after some of the words were already said, then how can we switch our attention to hear what was already said?

We are able to do this thanks to sensory memory, a very short-term memory buffer that really holds onto sensory stimuli for a brief period after they occur. This buffer gives us the time to switch attention to some other stimulus, and to still see or hear it, even though that precise stimulus is no longer present in the environment. Sensory memory is what compensates for our inability to think about two things at once; better still, sensory memory maximizes the likelihood of us catching stimuli that might be important to us, even if we were distracted when they appeared.

In a way it's almost as if the information coming into our sensory systems was set up to allow a time delay when we switch our attention. For example, if one were to think of the information coming into our sensory systems as streams of information, then we are only able to attend to one stream at a time. But we can switch between streams like a time delay. Let me be clear about that. We can only attend to one thing at a time. If somebody was talking to us, of course we could see, hear, and maybe even smell them all at once, all at the same time. All of this information is being processed, but our attention is primarily focused on one sense. In most cases this would be to the words that are being said. In fact, if we did begin to notice, say, that this person didn't smell so good we might also have the sense that we are not listening well anymore because we are being distracted, that is, attention is being captured by the less than pleasant smell.

But if something catches our attention in a stream we are not attending to, we are able to switch to that stream in an almost time-delayed manner. That is, we don't start where the stream is now, but rather we start a little before where the stream was when it caught our attention. Somehow that information that grabbed our attention in the first place is retained just long enough for us to switch, rewind, and catch what it was that caused us to switch in the first place. Seriously, that's pretty cool.

The basic principle of sensory memory is straightforward. If each of our sensory systems had a buffer system that allowed stimulation to be preserved for a while after it occurs, then if we were concentrating on some visual stimulus when an important auditory stimulus appeared, a copy of that auditory stimulus is briefly retained, giving us enough time to switch our attention and then "listen" to the copy. Switches of attention happen quickly, so the copy doesn't have to be saved for very long.

This seems to be exactly what the brain does, especially when it come to visual and auditory stimulation. It's probably also true of the other sensory systems, but there has been little research done on them. So let's focus on the visual and auditory streams right now, and I'm going to tell you about some of the relevant research. We're going to begin with the visual form of sensory memory, remember? It's the kind of memory called iconic memory.

In 1740, a physicist and mathematician named Johann Segner fixed a burning coal to a wagon wheel and spun the wheel. As the wheel spun Johann perceived a streak of light behind the coal's position. When the wheel spun at about 10 revolutions per second he perceived a complete circle of light, as if the light that had left the coal 100 ms previously was still there when the coal made it back to the same position. Well, we don't have a wagon wheel, but what we do have is a bicycle with a light attached to the back wheel. So I'm going to get that wheel spinning. Let's see the trail we make, and let's see if I can actually get a complete circle of light. OK. So here we go. You can try this at home with a string and a light.

Anyway, I think you'll agree that the light can only be in a single location at a single point in time so the trail of light that we see cannot really be occurring in the real world. Instead, that trail reflects our perception of the event as coded by our brain. Somehow, within that perception, some component of memory is allowing the light to live on in a specific spatial position even after it has moved on. That component is iconic memory. This might remind you of what is called "persistence of vision" when you watch a movie in a theater. The actual movie is a series of distinct frames, projected at say 60 frames per second. But your iconic memory holds each frame long enough after it's gone that you don't notice the gaps between the frames. What you see instead is a continuous picture.

When iconic memory was first studied in detail by George Sperling 1960, he used a device somewhat like a film projector, something called a tachistoscope. Sperling's experiments involved a contrast between two experimental conditions; one which was called the full report condition, and the other of which was called the partial report condition. While these conditions themselves are pretty simple, the logic that links them to conclusions about iconic memory is a little complex. So I want to kind of walk through these rather slowly.

In the full report condition, letters would be presented as 3 rows of 3 letters, so a 3 x 3 grid of letters. Participants in the experiment would see the letters flash briefly, and would then be asked to report what they did see. Typically they report about 4 or 5 letters on average, and this is a number consistent with experiments performed by James Cattell back in the 1800s.

But many of the participants claimed that they actually saw more, at least initially. That is, they said it felt like they had seen all 9 letters, but as they began reporting letters this visual image faded, kind of the way a dream fades when you wake up in the morning. By the time they had reported let's say four or five letters, the visual image was completely gone, so they could report no more.

Sperling was intrigued by what these participants said, and he wanted to see if he could actually confirm that they had originally seen many more letters than what they could eventually report. To test this he devised a partial report condition that worked as follows. Once again, a 3 x 3 matrix of letters was flashed briefly, but after it was removed, a tone was sounded, and that tone was used to determine which row the participant was asked to retrieve. A high tone told them to retrieve the top row, a middle tone the middle row, and low tone the lowest row. When he did this he found that most participants could report at least two and often all three letters of the cued row. So here's the logical part that can be a little tricky. If they could report two or three items from any row without knowing which row would be cued, and the fact that the letters were gone when it was cued, but they could still report two or three, that kind of when the letters were presented, that suggests that they could actually see between six and nine letters. That's two to three x three. Theoretically they could do that from any of the rows that were cued. Thus, it does indeed seem as though the participants' reports were correct. Initially they could see most of the letters, even after the letters were removed. But this visual image faded quickly, and was gone by the time they had specified what some of those letters were.

With Sperling's technique, he was also able to ascertain how long this visual trace of this stimulus lasted, and he did this by varying the time between when the letters disappeared and when the cue was presented. After just one second, performance in the partial report condition was no better than in the full report condition, that is, people could report only about 1.5 items of the cued row in the partial report condition which implies that they could report about 4.5 items overall, and that's obviously right smack in the middle of the four to five letters participants could report in the full report condition. So it seems the image is completely gone after just 1 second.

Of course, even in the full report condition, the participants can report four or five items, and once those items are selected, participants can remember them for quite a while thereafter. So there is an implication here that there are really two memory systems at play. One is that raw sensory image of all the presented items. But as participants start to sample that and report those items, the items they were reporting seemed to be transferred to another system, and that system is most likely working memory.

In fact, it seems that the purpose of iconic memory is to literally keep the raw image around long enough just in case some components of it are important enough to deserve such a recoding, such a more enduring memory. It is almost like a sort of sensory "holding cell" in which a wide net is cast across all items presented so that some might be detained as others are allowed to leave.

In everyday life then, the purpose of iconic memory is to help us to not miss important things when our attention is engaged on some other sense, or even on some internal thought. In fact, as I was preparing this part of the lecture I paused my writing at one point, and I went for a hike with my wife and my two dogs. As we were walking, I was sort of deeply thinking about the lecture and where I wanted to go with it. Of course, I was also watching where I was going, but my mind was really on my thoughts, not on the visual scene in front of me. However at some point, I noticed a quick movement, which grabbed my attention, then I kind of re-watched with my iconic memory and saw the blue jay fly across our path. My wife then said, "Hey, did you see that blue jay?" and, thanks to my iconic memory, I was able to say that yes, I had. I hadn't missed it.

Sensory memory, and iconic memory in specific, also plays a role in keeping our sensory representations of the world intact and rich. For example, when it comes to vision we feel like we are seeing a complete representation of what is in front of us. However, the truth is that our eyes dart all over the visual scene. Our eyes make little jumps that are called "saccades," and each jump is about 200 ms or a fifth of a second. Each one of these jumps gives us essentially a basically a small snapshot of what's in the world in front of us, but somehow, all of these snapshots were able to form an internal representation, in which all of these snapshots are essentially pieced together in a mosaic, and it's that mosaic that underlies the illusion we have of a complete representation. This is almost like David Hockney photo collages that you may have seen.

Iconic memory allows this integration of parts to happen more smoothly, even though each snapshot remains for a second or more, and then gradually fades as we continue to sample new areas, we don't just have one snapshot active at a given time. We actually have one sort of currently active and up to five or so that are in various stages of degradation. So iconic memory ends up giving us much more visual information and, without it, it's not clear that we really would have the illusion of seeing the entire scene in front of us at any given time. Thus, iconic memory really serves two functions for visual stimuli. When we are attending to vision, it supports our perception of a rich and detailed representation of our world. When we are not attending to vision, but some important visual event occurs, it allows us enough time to switch our attention to that event and still see a copy of it. In both cases, it really is making our perceptual processing of our world much more fluid and seamless.

At least one of our other senses also has this sort of short-term memory storage, that sense is audition, or hearing, and that form of sensory memory is called echoic memory. Think of it as echo, what was said. We've all experienced echoic memory frequently, and it is likely more familiar to you than iconic memory is. Here is a typical situation, one it's one that I mentioned in the initial lecture. So, again, imagine you are reading a novel or watching TV. A family member comes into the room and says something to you. You stop attending to the novel or maybe you're deep into a television show, or perhaps even deep into your own thoughts. A family member enters the room and says something to you. You stop attending to the novel or the TV or your thoughts, and automatically say "What?" But then as start to repeat what they said, and you say "Oh, sorry. Never mind I heard you. You don't have to repeat yourself." But the fact is you didn't actually hear them, at least not when they originally spoke to you. Once you switched your attention though, you were able to replay the question which was still stored in your echoic memory. Thus you heard the echo, not the original communication.

It's actually rather easy to experience echoic memory, and to get a sense for how much information it can hold. Why don't we try it now? I'll read to you a list of numbers. At some point I will say "stop." Just listen to the numbers. Don't try to memorize them. Just listen to them. When I say stop, tell me what the last few numbers were. Ready? Here goes: 6, 7, 6, 5, 9, 4, 2, 3, 7, 0, 2, stop. I tried to read the numbers at a rate of about 1 per second, and most of you could likely replay something like 3-7-0-2 about the last five seconds of the list. There have been more formal experiments for measuring the duration of echoic memory, and they also typically suggest that it lasts for about 4 or 5 seconds. This is much longer than iconic memory, which is only about a second. That's why we likely notice echoic memory more. So this brings up the question, Why? Why is echoic memory longer lasting than iconic memory? We're not exactly sure of the answer to that, but it's a good issue to consider. It's one of the ways scientists think about questions like this.

Since the time of Charles Darwin, scientists have begun to think more in terms of a function of certain attributes or processes. I'm sure you've heard about the finches that were so important to Darwin's original thoughts on evolution. He noticed that two distinct species of finches lived on the same island, but on different parts of that island. But the two kinds of finches looked different. One had a short strong beak, whereas the other had a long narrow beak. The finches with the short strong beaks lived in an area that had lots of berries and nuts, the sort of food that a strong beak would be really useful for eating. The finches with the long narrow beaks lived in areas where there were many insects furrowed in dead trees. The long beaks would allow them to get at and eat these insects. Thus the shape of the beak was not purely aesthetic, but rather it had real functional significance.

With functions in mind then, we can ask questions of the following sort: Given the environment we live in, the human environment, why would our echoic memory last longer than our iconic memory? One possible answer would go something like this. For humans, speech is highly important. Our ability to communicate via speech allows us to share information in rich and powerful ways. We're doing it right now. Given this importance, it is not at all surprising that we have large parts of our brains devoted just to the processing of speech. In fact, we have an entire area we call Broca's area for producing speech and another whole separate area we call Wernicke's that is used for understanding.

Speech is serial, one word following another slowly over time. What's more, the ends of sentences often don't make much sense unless you know the beginning. So if someone is talking to us, and we must switch our attention to begin listening to them, it would be very beneficial to have as much of their previous speech in memory as is possible. Hence an echoic memory that can hold a lot of information would be highly beneficial.

In contrast, visual images are just that, visual images. They do not tend to have the same structure unfolding over time, and usually we just want to see something, not an entire related process. Yes, we might all like to have our own personal instant replay of an entire process once in a while. But that's kind of something television has taught us to want, and having that running all the time might actually be overwhelming, or at least really inefficient. Thus, a short-lived visual memory may be perfectly sufficient.

What about our other senses? Do they have short sensory memories as well? For taste and smell, the answer is sort of a qualified yes. In a sense there is a sensory memory, but it's one supported by the environment and not supported by the brain. What I mean by that is the following. Smell and tastes are chemical senses and they tend to automatically kind of fade in and fade out as a function of those chemicals. For example, skunk had been hit.

For example, imagine if you were driving down a road where a skunk had been hit. As you approach that smell, the concentration of that chemical gradually increases, so it builds up. And then as you drive away from it, it gradually decreases, kind of like a fading iconic memory. So we don't really need the brain to do this. The concentration level of the chemicals kind of does it naturally. So it's not at all clear that we would have the same sort of iconic memory for smelling, or that we would even need it. But for something like vision, it seems to perform important functions, things like letting us see a blue jay.

What about touch then? That would be called tactile or haptic memory. If we have short-term memories for other senses, we might have them for touch as well. Remember when I told you that psychology was a very young science? Well, very few studies have examined whether there is a short-term memory for touch. Personally, I think there is. If I simply touch my cheeks and then let go, it feels to me as though the touch gradually fades as though the sensation of the touch lives on for a while. One thing to know about touch is that it's a relatively slow system. Another thing is that it's sequential, like hearing. A third thing is that touch often involves not only the skin but also our kinesthetic system. So there's a lot going on with touch.

So far there has been some really very preliminary research. And interestingly this research was done with both blind subjects and sighted subjects. For example, it's possible to either create familiar objects or unfamiliar patterns using what are called raised lines. And these are things which blind people can feel as well as sighted subjects. You could ask the subjects to feel these lines and then remember what they experienced.

An entirely preliminary view from this research is that a sensory system for touch may indeed exist. However, if so, it appears to be very brief, possibly even briefer than for iconic memory, and possibly limited to just two or three items. So what do I hope you have learned about yourself from today's lecture? Well, one important point is the following; The world literally bombards us with information and, at any given time, we can only really attend to, and think deeply about, one source of information. This could be information about the external world as it comes in from one of our senses, or it could be information about the internal world, our thoughts. Perhaps we are lost in a memory, or working out a plan for the future, or engaging in a pleasurable daydream or fantasy.

Whatever our conscious mind may be engaged with, we seem to be constantly storing at least the visual and auditory information that is coming into our senses. Not only are we storing it, but at some level that information is being processed for its potential importance. If it is deemed important, then our attention may be pulled from wherever it is, to the iconic or the echoic trace, and that allows us to see or hear that information despite the fact that it is actually no longer there. Unless of course you're my Dad watching his favorite TV program. In that case, other information can try pulling you all it wants, but your mind is not paying attention, and the sensory memories are lost. But if you do turn some attention to new information from sensory memory, then that information can be saved, and it can be passed on to a far more powerful system. And that's the subject of our next lecture, the system of working memory.

The Conveyor Belt of Working Memory
Lecture 5

Working memory is a collection of mental processes that allow us to work with information, often to solve some problem. These processes can also be used to keep information "in mind" for a brief period; doing so, however, takes effort and is vulnerable to interference. Working memory is also limited in capacity, and that limit seems to determine how richly we can think about things.

Working memory plays a critical role in nearly everything we do. Pioneering psychologist William James called it primary memory, while he referred to everything we now call long-term memory as secondary memory. But working memory is much more than a memory system; in fact, it may literally be the part of our minds where "I" exists and interacts with our mental worlds.

Brain studies have shown that many areas across the cortex can be activated in support of working memory depending on the task at hand. The prefrontal cortex, for example, seems to maintain attention and manage distractions to make working memory more effective.

Working memory has 2 basic functions: First, it keeps information from fading away for short periods of time. Second, it is the gateway for putting information into long-term memory. In this lecture, we'll look at the first function.

Making and exploring mental re-creations is what psychologists call using the **visual-spatial sketchpad**. This part of working memory can deal with numbers, words, and images. Mentally reciting words or numbers to hold them in memory is also a function of working memory; that internal voice is called the **phonological loop**.

How long can working memory keep information alive? That depends. If you kept repeating a list of items to yourself forever, you could keep them alive forever, but you wouldn't be able to do much else. The main reason things leave working memory is because we need to stop the repetition to think about something else. Thus, working memory is very fragile and easily disrupted.

Do things disappear from working memory by fading over time, or do they get pushed out by the new information? This is not an easy question to answer, but most evidence points to the latter—that older information gets pushed out of memory like items on a conveyor belt. Time is not the important factor; rather, the number of intervening items is most important.

A person's working memory capacity has been shown to correlate with his or her intelligence.

All this implies that working memory can only hold so much information at any given time. This raises some obvious questions: What is the working memory's capacity, can it be increased, and is increasing its capacity important or useful for daily functioning? Psychologist George Miller has found that humans, on average, can hold 7 items, plus or minus 2, in working memory at any one time. Across a number of studies, a person's working memory capacity has been shown to correlate with his or her intelligence and successfulness. This makes some sense, as a greater working memory capacity enables you to hold more relevant data in mind from which to make any decision, and thus the more accurate you would expect those decisions to be.

Can you increase the capacity of your working memory? In a sense, you can, if you can learn to chunk several bits of information into a single item. For example, you can think of the individual string of numbers 7, 4, 7, 1, 4, 9, 4 as seven bits of information, or you can use mnemonic strategies to remember them as "airplane" (747) and "Columbus" (1492). Now there are only 2 pieces of information to remember—and room for a lot more. So it's not the amount of information per se; it's the number of chunks that sets the limit for working memory. ■

phonological loop: The ability of the working memory system to recall and repeat a sound; one's inner voice.

visual-spatial sketchpad: The ability of the working memory system to re-create and explore a place or object in iconic memory.

Suggested Reading

Baddeley, *Working Memory, Thought, and Action.*

Gilhooly and Logie, *Working Memory and Thinking.*

Vandierendonck and Szmalec, *Spatial Working Memory.*

Questions to Consider

1. Imagine you could only hold 2 pieces of knowledge in your mind at any given time. How far do you think you could get on the "How high you could reach sitting on a camel?" problem?

2. Imagine you had an intact working memory for the first 16 years of life and then it stopped working. What would life be like? Would it be like you are a zombie who could only react to things in an automatic or habitual manner? Or would it be that you just didn't seem very smart?

Exercise

One of the challenges at the World Memory Competition requires contestants to learn the order of the cards in one or more shuffled decks. To do this, contestants use chunking in combination with some of the mnemonic techniques described earlier. The chunking typically works like this: Before trying to remember the order of cards in a particular deck, contestants first practice associating 3 cues with each card: a person, an action, and a place.

Coming up with vivid and distinct items for each card is key. Maybe the jack of hearts would be Prince William, his activity might be polo playing, and his location might be the Mall in London. The queen of hearts might be Angelina Jolie, adopting a child, and the Hollywood sign; the king of clubs might be Tiger Woods, riding a golf cart, and a golf course in Scotland. Competitors do this for all 52 cards; then, during the competition, they use this information to chunk 3 cards into one image. So, for example, if the first 3 cards in the deck happened to be the queen of hearts, the king of clubs, and the jack of hearts, one could imagine Angelina Jolie riding a golf cart along the Mall.

Try it! If you cut a deck down to just 20 or 21 cards (e.g., start with the 10, jack, queen, king, and ace of all 4 suits) and create and remember 3 aspects of each card (name, activity, place), you can impress your friends at your ability to remember the precise order of all 21, which of course will be just 7 chunks.

The Conveyor Belt of Working Memory
Lecture 5—Transcript

In the previous lecture you learned most of what there is to know about our sensory memories. Those forms of memory do keep information alive, but only for very brief amounts of time. They are really all about allowing us to function well "in the present," and they do that by ensuring that we don't miss some bit of critical information while we're attending to something else. In effect, they allow us to move our attention from one sense, or thought, to another in a smooth way, almost "as if" we move our attention on the new source even before it left the previous one. When you started watching this course you likely didn't even know about sensory memory and didn't think of it as a memory system at all.

The next memory system we are going to talk about is called working memory and, again, it is a memory system you might never have thought about when you thought about human memory. But, as you'll see, it plays a really critical role in nearly everything we do. In fact, it's so important that William James actually called it "primary" memory, while he referred to everything we now call long-term memory as "secondary memory."

We've discussed working memory a little already in both the first and the second lectures. Remember how high could you reach if you were sitting on a camel? When I discussed that example before, I was using it to show how working memory can be used to bring together all sorts of information with the goal of solving some new problem. Sometimes it seems kind of strange to call working memory a memory system, in the same sense that it would seem strange to call a car a form of furniture. Sure you can sit and relax in a car it certainly can serve as furniture if one should wish, but a car is so much more than just furniture.

Similarly, working memory, is so much more than just a memory system. In fact, working memory may literally be that part of our mind that we are most familiar with, the part where "we" seem to exist and interact with our mental worlds. Memory is who we are in lots of senses, but working memory is who we are right now. That includes everything from whatever specific information we are holding in our mind to how we are managing our attention. Brain studies have shown that many areas across the cortex can be activated in support of working memory, depending on the specific task, and especially the prefrontal cortex may be involved in maintaining attention and managing distractions, so that working memory can be more effective.

Let me give you another example of working memory to make its general power more apparent. Let's suppose you grew up in a detached house that you think of as home; if no house comes to mind, think of some other relatively small building that you know well, perhaps a close friend's home. So now pay attention to what happens in your mind as you answer the following question: How many windows does that house have? Try to come up with an exact answer.

OK. What happened? You likely experienced a mental re-creation of that house. That house was somehow retrieved from your memory and rebuilt in visual form. You were able then to inspect it. Not only inspect it, but even do things like walk around it, looking at the various walls, counting the number of windows. This example shows the rich process that is possible using our working memory. The specific process you were using as you walked around the house was something psychologists call the visual-spatial sketchpad, the part of working memory that deals with visual elements. It can work with numbers; it can work with words, and images. If you are good at mental math, you are probably good at using your visual-spatial sketchpad to do that.

While working memory is indeed powerful, and it's really a general purpose system, our focus here and in this lecture is how it contributes to memory. In this respect it actually has two functions. First, working memory is a memory system that can keep information from fading away for short periods of time. It can hold onto information. And it's in this respect that it has sometimes been labeled "short-term memory." But for this course I will stick to the broader label of working memory. Second, as we already discussed when talking about mnemonic strategies, working memory is also used to store information in long-term memory, making that information available to us long after the original experience. Thus, working memory is both a memory system—and more in and of itself, and it is also the gateway for putting things into long-term memory.

In this lecture we will focus on working memory as a memory system in and of itself. Let's begin with a really simple example to let you feel your working memory well working. Unless you are driving, you may actually want to pause this recording right now to grab some paper and a writing implement, because we are going to do a few experiments in today's lecture and occasionally you might want to write things down if you want to play along.

For this first experiment I am going to read out a list of words, then I will pause for a little while, then I will say "go." Using just your mental powers, try to remember the words, keeping them in your mind until I say go. Then tell me what you remember. So you can write down if you like or speak out loud what you remember. I'll give you some time to think about it. All the while, of course, pay attention to what is happening in your mind. Ready? Here comes the list: Pay some attention to your mind, and remember all of the items you can: "boat, justice, speaker, keyboard, cloud, pink, mankind, carpet, hollow, thrill." OK. Go.

So, how many did you remember? There were ten words altogether, chances are that most of you remembered between five and nine words. I'll get back to that in a minute. But for now, what was happening in your mind as you tried to remember the words? For most of you, it probably felt something like this. The first word I read was "boat," and when you heard it you likely began repeating it to yourself "boat, boat, boat..." Then I read "justice," and you likely repeated "boat, justice, boat, justice, boat, justice." Then I said "speakers. You probably thought "boat, justice, speaker, boat, justice, speaker." At some point I had read too many words for you to continue stringing them along for you to repeat them all, so you probably just did what you could at that point.

Eventually, when I said "go," you likely still had the last few items echoing in your mind. Those items would have been "carpet, hollow, and thrill" And they would have been in your echoic memory. Then you had to wait in silence during the pause, in which you likely continued to repeat words to yourself, but perhaps now the words were more the latter ones given that were freshly heard. So maybe you were saying, "carpet, hollow, thrill." Of course a few other items might also have been in there all of them being repeated in your mind as though you were kind of reading to yourself.

When I finally did say go, whatever words you were repeating to yourself are the first to be remembered. Then you think about others. Probably those items from the beginning of the list come to mind. They were repeated quite a lot, at least initially. So you likely remember the last few items in the list, some of the first items, and maybe one or two from the middle of the list. OK. Given all that. Let me remind you what the complete list was and you can see which items you recalled and where they were on the list. So the complete list was "boat, justice, speaker, keyboard, cloud, pink, mankind, carpet, hollow, thrill."

Maybe my description I just gave didn't perfectly match your subjective experience, at least in terms of the specific items that you ended up repeating. What I've presented to you is the typical description people give, but people always differ a little from this typical description. We are individuals after all. But I can say with pretty much virtual certainty that you did repeat words to yourself and that you did hear some internal voice doing that. Previously I mentioned that one of the processes that working memory uses is that visual-spatial sketchpad. Well, it has other processes that it uses too. Another is called the phonological loop. Phonology is a word that refers to the sounds we make when reading words. So the phonological loop refers to the process we use to speak to ourselves within our mind. That's what you heard as you tried to remember those words. By speaking the words over and over, as you did, you were able to keep them alive in memory, at least for a little while. It's kind of like every time we speak a word, we breathe a little life into it, keeping it active in working memory and keeping it available to be recalled.

One really fascinating aspect of all this is that a skill that we usually use for external communication, spoken language, also has an apparent internal analogue. We use it to speak to ourselves. We see this in small children all the time, but it's true of adults, too. In fact, in one really interesting study, a psychologist performed the same sort of experiment we just did, but he did it with congenitally deaf participants, participants who communicate with one another using American sign language. (I'd like to demonstrate this for you, but unfortunately, I don't know sign language.) When those participants were trying to keep the words in their minds during the pause, they produced muted sign movements for the words. Your quiet inner voice was their muted hand signs. So what it suggests is that humans rely on their language abilities when trying to remember items in working memory, but the exact way they do that depends on the way they usually use language.

So now you have felt your working memory in action. Now let's talk about some of its characteristics as a memory system. First, we talk about working memory as keeping information alive for a short period. I've told you it's sometimes called short-term memory, but how short? Well, this is one of those questions where the answer is, it depends. I said above that each time you read a word to yourself it is essentially as though you are breathing life into that word, keeping it alive for another few minutes. If I gave you a really short list of words to remember say, "eggs, bread, tomatoes, and cereal." If you kept repeating those items to yourself, you could probably keep them alive forever. So much for short term. Of course, the problem is, you wouldn't be able to do much else except walk around repeating those words. The system you use for thought would be totally occupied making it impossible to think about anything else. In fact, the main reason things leave our working memory is because we often can't help but think about something else and, when we do, the repetition stops and as we think of other things the items that we had in working memory are replaced by these thoughts. Thus, working memory is really a very fragile form of memory. It's easily disrupted by other events that try to capture your thoughts, and this fragility is what makes it successful as a memory system only over short intervals.

How about another quick demonstration that will hopefully let me illustrate this fragility to you? I'll read another list, but this time when I pause, we won't all just be silent. Instead, at the end of the list, I going to give you a two-digit number, and as you try to remember the list of words I want you to count backwards, by threes, from the number I give you. So, for example, if the number was 48 you would say 45, 42, 39, 36, etc. Keep counting backwards until I say "go." And of course, all the while, I want you to be introspecting, noticing what is going on in your mind. Here comes the list: "kick, corn, police, heavy, fresh, grill, jump, sick, break, whisker, 77, 74, 71, 68, 65, 62, 59, 56, 53, 50." Go.

Once again feel free to pause the tape if you need more time. I will go on. How did you do this time? I expect you recalled far fewer items. Which items did you remember? Well I suspect you remember the first few items in the list. Once again, let me remind you of the list. The list was "kick, corn, police, heavy, fresh, grill, jump, sick, break, whisker." Why was this so much harder? Well, in order to count backwards by threes you need to use the phonological loop, which means it can't be used to keep repeating the items in your mind. Without repetition, the items fade from memory. By the way, you can also do this experiment with deaf people. If you literally hold their hands after presenting the list then they can't use them to sign the words to themselves, and they also can't remember as many. Without signing, their memory also fades.

The experiment we just performed was originally performed by Peterson and Peterson in 1959. They found that if you make people count backwards by threes during the retention interval, that is, the time between when you end the list and when you give the cue to recall, then the correct recall of a short list of items drops from 90 percent when recall is immediate to under 50 percent after just three seconds of counting. After 12 seconds of counting recall is below 10 percent. Thus, when rehearsal is prevented, and when one must use phonological loop, thus their working memory for the backwards counting task, things disappear from working memory quite quickly.

Of course, this raises the next obvious question. How do things disappear from working memory? Do they simply kind of fade like we talked about sensory memory? Or do they get pushed out of working memory by the new information that comes in? This latter notion, the notion of getting pushed out, is sometimes described as analogous to a conveyor belt. Imagine a conveyor belt moving from right to left. As the words come in they are put on the belt, but then as each new word comes in we shift the words over. So if we're given a word, it keeps moving across the belt. Of course, this belt can only hold so many items. So if we load too much up, then things will start falling off the end of the belt. In the case of that backwards counting experiment, the notion is that you load the words up when they are read, but then when you start counting you need to hold on to some information to do that task. For example, you need to know the number you are on so you can count backwards from it. Then you need to know the number you get once count backwards, etc. So you're loading now these numbers onto the conveyor belt, which pushes some of the words off the other end. If we load up enough numbers, then there are few or maybe even no words left. They have all fallen out of working memory.

OK. It's a nice analogy. But how can we really tell if it's right or maybe words do just decay. It turns out this is not an easy question to answer. But most of the evidence favors that conveyor belt notion I just explained to you. For example, consider the following experiment. Participants are read a list of words. Some of these words begin with the letter "b." When a word beginning with the letter "b" is presented, participants are asked to recall the previous word that began with a "b," and one of the variables that we manipulate is how many items occur between the "b" words. So how many intervening items are there?

As you might expect, performance decreases when there are more intervening items, which makes sense according to the conveyor belt notion because each time a new item comes up, you have to pay enough attention to it, at least to know if it starts with a "b." You have to put it on the conveyor belt. The more items you put on the conveyor belt, the more likely that that previously "b" item will have fallen off by the time you have a new one. Of course, it also fits with the decay theory because the more intervening items, the more that time passes. It could just be that over time that the previous "b" item has just decayed. So how do we know which one is correct?

This is where the interesting twist comes into our experiment. Sometimes the words are read at a rate of one word per second, but sometimes they were read at a rate of four words per second. I don't know if I could even do four words per second but it would sound like this. Click. Click. Click. Click. So they come really fast. So after eight intervening items, for example, only two seconds have passed, whereas eight seconds have passed in the one word per second condition. So if time is what matters, there should be less decay in the four words per second condition, and that should show through as a higher recall performance. However, the decline in recall that we see as a function of intervening items is, in fact, very similar across those two conditions, and this really suggests that time is not the important factor, rather, it's all about the number of intervening items. That kind of result really supports the conveyor belt notion. And in a more general sense, it supports that idea I already suggested to you, that working memory can hold onto something until something new pushes it out.

Alright, so we know that we can use the phonological loop to keep items alive. And if we don't, then they will leave working memory. We're pretty sure that's because something is pushing them out, this sort of conveyor belt notion. What's implied by all this is that working memory can only hold so much, that there is some sort of limit in terms of the number of things that it can work with at a given time. This raises some obvious questions. What is this capacity? Can it be increased? And is the capacity of my working memory really important to my abilities to function in daily life?

In the first that experiment we did, the one at the very beginning of this lecture, you may recall that I gave you a list of 10 words and then there was just a silent retention interval. I then told you to recall the words, and I predicted that most of you could recall between five and nine items. Where did that prediction come from? Well, a researcher named George Miller did a famous experiment, actually a number of experiments, over and over with many different people, and what he found was that on average, people can remember seven plus or minus two items, so there's my five to nine item prediction. In fact, following his famous title, this capacity of working memory is now often described as the magic number seven, plus or minus two. So I suspect that for most of you, your memory fell within that range, five to nine items. For those of you who remembered ten items, fantastic. Consider yourself doing very well.

So why's the capacity of working memory important? Well, I can tell you this, across a number of studies a person's working memory capacity has been shown to correlate very well with their intelligence and their success in life. And if you think about it this really makes a lot of sense. If working memory is the system we use to combine information from all sorts of sources with the goal of solving some problems, it makes sense that someone who can work with more information might end up with richer solutions. That is, anytime you have to make a decision, the more information you can bring into your decision the more accurate we would expect your ultimate decision to be. So yes indeed, it does seem that the capacity of working memory is important.

Can we increase the capacity of our working memory then? Well, here's another one of those yes and no answers. In a sense you can. You see, when Miller said we could remember seven plus or minus two items of information, he also pointed out that not all items are created equal. That is, if one is clever it is possible to chunk (and I'll get to that word "chunk") several bits of information into a single item, so those seven items may actually reflect more than seven bits of information. Let me give you an example. Imagine I gave you the following list of number to remember: 7, 4, 7, 1, 4, 9, 4. Seven numbers. Most of you could likely hold all seven numbers in your working memory, but it would likely be a challenge. But think of those numbers in the following way, and it becomes easy: big plane (747), two years after Columbus (1494). So, what was originally seven numbers has become two chunks of information: big plane and two years after Columbus sailed the ocean blue. When Miller said we could remember seven plus or minus two, he meant seven plus or minus two chunks, so by chunking information effectively one can hold onto more information.

Let's consider this notion of chunking in the context of the first list that I asked you to remember. Just to remind you that list was "boat, justice, speaker, keyboard, cloud, pink, mankind, carpet, hollow, thrill." If we think about them that way that's ten items. But we could combine the items in some way in pairs. Let me just show. We'll just go through the words. "Boat" and "justice." So we might think of a judge on a boat, and we try to remember that image, and we try repeatedly seeing that image in our visual-spatial sketchpad just as we repeated the word before. Cool. Judge on a boat. Got it. How about a keyboard with an embedded speaker? Think about that. Got it. Then, well, a pink cloud. Those two are easy. Excellent. Judge on a boat, keyboard with a speaker, pink cloud, so far so good. Now, hmmm, some vague notion which we kind of see as "mankind," and he's laying on a "carpet," like a scene out of CSI. Ah, and a "hollow thrill." Sounds like an excellent B. B. King song—the thrill is gone. A judge on a boat, a keyboard with an embedded speaker, a pink cloud, a mankind on a carpet, and B. B. King singing hollow thrill. Poof. The 10 items are now five, and it's relatively easy to keep five items in mind. That's the idea of chunking.

So yes, the capacity of your working memory is indeed important, but with work, it is possible to increase the capacity of working memory, increase beyond what's normal for you. Does this sound familiar at all? It might remind you of the lecture on mnemonics. In that lecture I pointed out that with some work you could increase the accuracy of your long-term memory. And clearly there is a relation here.

To give you a taste of this, let me tell you about the following. There are actually memory competitions, national memory competitions and international memory competitions. Competitors in these competitions are given a range of memory tasks, all of which seem really, honestly, very ridiculous. But they can do them, and they can do them well. One of these tasks, for example, requires the competitors to memorize the order of cards in 10 shuffled decks. So they have 10 decks that are shuffled, and they have to memorize the order of the cards. And they have to do this in an hour or less. How is this possible? Well, first of all, it is possible. They do it. Well the way the competitors do that is they first take each card in a deck, and they associate it with three different names, a person, a verb, and an object, kind of like the way I used the routine in the mnemonic lecture. But it will be a little different. So they remember these aspects that are memorized prior to the competition and stay constant, kind of like person, object, and verb associated with them. Then when they are in the competition, they chunk them together. For example, when 23 year old Grand Master of Memory Edward Cooke saw a 3 of hearts, a 9 of clubs, and a 9 of spades, to him that would conjure up an image of Brazilian lingerie model Adriana Lima in a Biggles biplane shooting at his old public-school headmaster in a suit of armor. How's that for a nice bizarre image, bizarre and interesting. So he's condensed the three cards into one chunk—an enormous chunk, but still one chunk—and that frees up space in his working memory. He also obviously is making use of heavy, bizarre imagery to ensure transfer to long-term memory. This relation between working memory and long-term memory will form the basis of our next lecture.

Before going there though, here are the things I hope you got from this lecture. What we call working memory is actually a collection of mental processes that allow us to work with information, often with the goal of solving some problem. However these same processes can also be used to keep information "in mind" for a brief period of time. Doing so, though, is effortful, and it's prone to interference. That is, anything that pulls the mind away from rehearsing the information will bump things out of working memory. Working memory is also limited in capacity, and that limit seems to determine how richly we can think about things. The limit can be increased by chunking information, so that it's not really the amount of information per se, it's the number of chunks, really, that sets the limit for working memory. If you got all that, a fantastic lecture. Thank you.

Encoding—Our Gateway into Long-Term Memory
Lecture 6

Encoding is the gateway where your present communicates with your future. One of the major functions of working memory is to perform this encoding in a way that makes memory retrieval easier. If you take time to use it correctly, working memory can even encode information in ways that cue you to remember that information at a specific time.

The **hippocampus** is the brain structure that allows working memory to perform the second of its 2 major functions—the transfer of information into long-term memory. In a general sense, the process that gets information from the external world into our long-term memory is called encoding.

We've seen how information that is deliberately organized and carefully encoded by working memory is easier to recall. Most of our memories do not go through such deliberate encoding, yet they are successfully moved to long-term memory anyway. In this lecture, we'll examine how this is possible and why certain experiences are more memorable—that is, easier to recall—than others.

Generally, people remember the beginnings and ends of things better. Better memory for the beginning is called the **primacy effect**, and better memory for the end is called the **recency effect**. Beginnings are well encoded because they spend the most time in working memory; endings are easier to retrieve because they may still be in working memory at the time of recall.

The evidence for this process comes mostly from dissociations—experimental manipulations that affect one component of the memory but not the other. These experiments may involve reversing the order of items in working memory or changing the speed of item presentation rate, for example. The results indicate that the recency effect occurs in working memory and the primacy effect in long-term memory.

These effects also clarify how rote memorization works: Using working memory to repeat items over and over doesn't promote a strong transfer to long-term memory unless a lot of repetitions are performed. If one thinks deeply about the information instead and elaborates on it in some way, even in a simple way, then the transfer to long-term memory—the encoding—is much stronger. This sort of deep processing can be accomplished without a lot of elaborative rehearsal. Good-versus-bad categorization is one of the easiest ways to encourage deep processing, perhaps the fastest way to enhance memory on the fly.

What other factors affect the likelihood of remembering something we have encoded? Re-creating the context of the original experience—such as revisiting the original location—has been shown to improve recall. Fascinatingly, re-creating the internal context—that is, your mood—can be just as important as re-creating the external context; this phenomenon is called **state-dependent memory**.

Encoding information in a way that leads to strong memory recall takes a lot of cognitive effort. The more you practice deep encoding, the easier it will get, but it will never be perfectly easy or automatic. Sometimes expending even a little cognitive effort can be difficult. Exhaustion, stress, and distractions are among the everyday challenges to successful encoding.

Prospective memory—reminding ourselves to do something in the future—is difficult for most people. It can fail even over extremely short time intervals. The classic "tie a string around your finger" and similar external retrieval cues can be inconvenient, and over long periods they may not even work. The ideal prospective memory cue is one that suddenly appears at the moment we

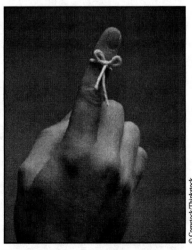

There are far better ways to aid prospective memory than the traditional string on the finger.

need to remember the instructions. For example, if you need to remember to bring a certain book to work, try associating that book with the image of your front door and the sound of your jangling house keys. ∎

Important Terms

hippocampus: A region of the midbrain that allows the transfer of working memory into permanent storage and may coordinate the simultaneous activation of various memory systems.

primacy effect: Better encoding and recall of the beginning of a list or series of events.

prospective memory: Giving oneself instructions to remember or do something in the future.

recency effect: Better recall of the most recently encoded information.

state-dependent memory: A memory whose recall is improved by re-creating the emotional context in which it was learned.

Suggested Reading

Benjamin, *Secrets of Mental Math*.

Mason and Smith, *The Memory Doctor*.

Parker, Bussey, and Wilding, *The Cognitive Neuroscience of Memory*.

Payne and Conrad, *Intersections in Basic and Applied Memory Research*.

Questions to Consider

1. If you think about the brain in evolutionary terms, does it make sense that it might remember images, and even bizarre images, especially well?

2. Research shows that depressed people tend to think a lot about the negative events that happen in a day, but they don't think much about the good things. Can you see how the resulting memories of the past could actually feed into the depression and make it worse?

3. Recite the alphabet in your mind. You can't help but sing it, can you? This is a good example of how dual coding can aid memory retrieval—the letters become linked sequentially by a melody and by the appropriate use of rhyme. Can you think of other examples? Can you create one yourself?

Exercise

Categorizing in terms of good versus bad may have seemed like a simple point, but it actually represents perhaps the best trade-off between using labor-intensive mnemonic techniques and minimal time and effort. Next time you come into contact with some things, or perhaps even names, you want to remember, think of each one and quickly decide whether you would categorize it as a good thing or a bad thing. Which way you categorize each item isn't critical, but notice how images and associations come to mind naturally, effortlessly, and notice that this does make those items easier to remember.

Encoding—Our Gateway into Long-Term Memory
Lecture 6—Transcript

Clive Wearing was a very successful musician, conductor, and singer. He married the love of his life and was apparently a very happy, friendly soul. Unfortunately Clive had Herpes Simplex. Now usually, that just causes sporadic sores or rashes. But occasionally, it can give rise to infections, infections of the brain, and that's what happened to Clive. Clive's infection, in fact, was so severe that it resulted in damage to both his frontal lobes and part of his midbrain called the hippocampus, and both damaged quite dramatically. Clive survived the infection, but he was a very different man thereafter.

When Clive describes what it is like to be Clive, he says things like the following. "Do you know that moment when you first wake up, and you see everything around you, and you slowly realize who and where you are? Well, that's what it's like for me all the time." In fact, he keeps a journal, and in that journal he will write the time, and then he writes something like "I am now awake for the first time today." Two minutes later he crosses that out, and writes it down again, with a new time. Clive literally lives in an eternal present.

Clive is extremely lucky. He has a devoted wife, who loves him very much. In fact, if there is one image that really captures the reality of what it is like to be Clive it is perhaps the following. Each time his wife leaves the room he forgets she exists. But somehow, when she returns, he does recognize her, but he simultaneously feels like he cannot remember the last time he saw her, almost as if this is the first time he has seen her. So he embraces her as we might embrace a loved one that we haven't seen for years. And when you see it, it's very loving and it's very warm. The problem is he does this over and over again each day, every time his wife leaves his sight.

So what did that infection do to Clive's brain? What caused such a dramatic change? As we will discuss at a number of points in this course, the hippocampus plays a critical role with respect to the transfer of information from working memory to long-term memory. The damage to Clive's hippocampus has created a serious problem.

In the previous lecture I told you that working memory plays in fact two roles related to memory. First it can hold information itself using the phonological loop or the visual-spatial sketchpad, and our last lecture discussed working memory from that perspective. But in addition it also provides at least one gateway for information to enter long-term memory. That is, often when we process things in working memory they can find their way into long-term memory. For Clive, thanks to the damage to his hippocampus, that gateway was closed for good. Other than the transfer to long-term memory aspect, his working memory seems largely intact. But as soon as his working memory gets pulled to some new information, some new stimulus, whatever was in it prior is gone. Clive shows us what life would be like if information from our working memory was in fact never transferred to long-term memory. As this example shows, clearly this transfer is critical to how we live and who we are.

In this lecture we will be focusing on this crucial gateway function of working memory. In a general sense, the process that gets information from the external world into our long-term memory is called encoding. That is, we somehow encode the experiences we have into our memory, allowing us to consciously relive those experiences later. Of course, that's in the case of episodic memory. It also helps to transfer information to semantic memory. And in that case, we just have the information.

We've already discussed the role of working memory with respect to encoding when we discussed mnemonic strategies. In that case, the main point was that if the information was deliberately organized, and if effective associations and dual-coding is used, then it will be much easier to recall the information from long-term memory later.

However, most of our memories did not go through such deliberate encoding, and yet they do still get successfully stored in long-term memory. How does that happen? In this lecture we'll flesh out this gateway function of working memory in a much broader way, leaving you with a much more well-rounded notion of why certain experiences end up more memorable than others.

In the last lecture, I read you ten words and asked you to recall them after a brief retention interval. When you did, I suggested that you likely recalled the first few words on the list, the last few words on the list, but perhaps only one or two from all the words in the middle of the list. I was basing that prediction on something called the primacy and recency effects in recall. That is, it's generally true that people remember the beginning of things and the ends of things better. The memory for the beginning is called the primacy effect, and the memory for the end is called the recency effect.

For example, in one study participants were given a list of 15 items to remember. After a brief retention interval, memory for the first three items was in the 25–30 percent range; memory for the middle nine items was down in the 15–20 percent range; and memory for the last 3 items was up again in the 25–40 percent range. So the first three items and the last three items were recalled much better than the middle nine.

This is one of those findings that has actually found its way into the popular culture. If it is true that people remember better at the beginning and ending of things, then if we are creating say a movie or play, and if we hope to gain some promotion via word of mouth then we'd better make the beginning and the end especially good. A really pointed example of this were the early James Bond movies. At that time, many movies began by rolling credits, showing credits as to who was going to be in the movie and such. But not James Bond movies. They tended to start right away with an action sequence. No story, no character development, just fast skiing downhill or jumping out of airplane. Nice exciting beginning, dramatic beginning. This is the way to maximize the primacy effect, and it is a method that is now quite common in all sorts of situations: start strong and end strong, because the beginnings and endings are remembered best. And even though most people don't watch the closing credits, you'll have noticed that some movie makers are even trying to spice up their closing credits too, trying to take advantage of that recency effect.

In the scientific context the primacy and recency effect has been used to provide convincing evidence for the distinction between working memory and long-term memory. The general idea goes like this: As the list is read people begin to repeat the items to themselves using working memory. The first few items will be the ones that they repeat the most so they spend the most time in working memory, and if working memory is the gateway to long-term memory, then those initial items have the best chance for getting through the gate. The last few items are still in echoic memory when the list ends, and so they can be quickly transferred into working memory and rehearsed until the recall prompt is given. So they are well recalled because they are still in working memory at the time of recall. In fact, when most people recall items, they first recall the last few items, the recency effect. And then they start to think. This usually results in the first few items of the list coming to mind. And that's theoretical again because the first few items had the best chance to make it into long-term memory.

Well, it's a bit of a complicated story. How do we know it's true? The evidence that favors this account comes mostly from what are called dissociations, experimental manipulations that affect one component of the memory effect but not the other. For example, remember when we did that counting backwards by threes experiment during the retention interval? Well, if you do that then the recency effect often disappears, but the primacy effect remains, so you still remember those first few items. And that of course is because those are the items that are supposed to be in long-term memory. But the recency effect was supported by the items still being in working memory, and when you're using your working memory to count backwards by threes, it is no longer possible to hold those items.

Dissociation also occurs the other way as well. If you read items more slowly, this does not affect the recency effect. But it increases the primacy effect. It makes it stronger. Why? A slower presentation rate does magnify the differential practice for early items on the list. You can get more practice in during those longer times. So the more you practice, the longer the item is in working memory, and the better the chance that these multiply-repeated items will make their way into long-term memory. And so if the primacy effect reflects that long-term memory, that's why you see the stronger primacy effect.

So taken together then, these findings support this distinction between working memory, which is what's responsible for the recency effect, and long-term memory, which is responsible for the primacy effect. And that was very important in early science in establishing the difference between these two memory systems.

In addition to these findings also clarify how rote memorization works. Remember Ebbinghaus? Rote rehearsal does get things into long-term memory, but it's also prone to quick forgetting. That is, all forms of rehearsal really are not created equal. When you just repeat items over and over in working memory, that form of rehearsal is called maintenance rehearsal. It's a way of maintaining the item in working memory, but it doesn't promote a strong transfer to long-term memory unless a lot of repetitions are performed. That's exactly why rote memorization is often referred to as "drilling," like a military drill; for repetition to be effective, one must drill the information into one's head by hearing it over and over and over.

If, however, one thinks deeply about the information instead, and if we elaborate on it in some way, even if we elaborate in a simple way, the transfer to long-term memory can be much stronger. For example, let's return to the list I gave you at the beginning of the last lecture. Let me remind you that list was "boat, justice, speaker, keyboard, cloud, pink, mankind, carpet, hollow, thrill."

Instead of associating those words with a second set of mnemonic cues, as I did last time, I could instead just as quickly associate them with each other and try to make a story out of them. So there was this "boat" that sank, which represented a sort of "justice" because the captain had mounted a huge "speaker" that would amplify every click of his keyboard. The boat sank when a "cloud" that happened to be "pink" rained down hail of the like never seen by "mankind," so thick that it left a "carpet" of hail on the water leaving me feeling a somewhat "hollow thrill." OK. There's the 10 words in a story. Weird, I know, but you get the sense I am elaborating on the information, connecting it together in some way. This sort of elaborative rehearsal leads to a better transfer to long-term memory, better encoding.

Another way to make this distinction between maintenance rehearsal and elaborative rehearsal is in terms of depth of processing. Items that are processed more deeply are subsequently remembered better. And, deep processing can sometimes be even simpler, without a lot of elaborative rehearsal. For example, imagine we present a list of words for people to remember. And we're going to do so in two different conditions. In one condition, I simply ask them to look at each word and notice, and not to themselves, how many vowels in that word. That's what is called shallow encoding, that's looking at the structure of the word. Now in another condition, we just ask them to categorize the word as "good" or "bad." Well, the good versus bad sounds innocent enough. It sounds like it would be an easy decision. But actually you can produce really deep coding in a very simple way. So for example, imagine that one of the words on the list is the word "rust." In the vowel condition, someone would just say, "rust," one vowel. That's the depth of their processing.

However, in the good versus bad condition, most people would probably think something like this: "rust." And they would imagine some car with rust all over it. It looks ugly." Andy they would say, "Rust is bad." Well what do we have? We have an image there. And we know imagery is good right? I, myself, might think a little differently. I might say, "*Rust?*" Neil Young's live *Rust* album. I like that album. Rust is good." Of course, it doesn't really matter whether a person ends up thinking of rust as good or bad. What matters is that they tend to form stronger associations, maybe with images or even with songs heard in their head. So that good versus bad categorization is an easy way to encourage deep processing, and it will almost always lead to better memory than will a more shallow task like thinking about how many vowels a word has. What's more, it's fast and easy, perhaps the fastest way to enhance memory "on the fly."

OK. We've talked about deep encoding a lot. And now I want to talk about some other factors that affect our likelihood of remembering something we have encoded. Have you ever had the chance of returning to someplace that you hadn't been to for a long time. Maybe your old school or something like that. And when you get there you experience the flooding of memories. Those old-familiar cues and context that you're in suddenly make it much easier to retrieve memories that were coded in that context. It turns out this is a general effect on memory. If you think of memory retrieval as re-creating some past experience, it makes sense that this re-creation is performed more readily if the re-creation context is similar to the context of the initial experience. The greater the match between your study context and your retrieval context, the better retrieval will be.

There's an experiment demonstrating this, a demonstration using scuba diving. Scuba divers have this tablet, and they can write on them. They can write on a beach or under the water. So it makes it easy enough to do memory tests with scuba divers. In this experiment, some of the scuba divers learned a list of words on the beach and were re-tested on the beach. Others learned under water, and were tested under water. Under those two conditions, learning context and retrieval context matched. But in two other conditions they mixed and matched. So one group learned a list of items on the beach and their memory was tested under water. The fourth group learned them under water, and they were tested on the beach. What you find in that study is that memory performance is better when the retrieval context, the place where their memory is tested, matches the learning context. So the beach/beach or under water/under water. It is almost like the context itself becomes an effective retrieval, so that you can effectively pull that item out of your memory.

Perhaps even more fascinating, is the fact that what matches in our internal context can be just as important as matches in our external context. For example, let's talk about emotion for a second. You can use music to actually induce certain mood states in participants. And psychologists do this. So for example, it's very hard to listen to the *William Tell Overture* without feeling happy and energized. You know the *William Tell Overture*. That rally kind of can't help but to energize you. Slower music, on the other hand, especially if played a in minor key, can make people feel sad. So psychologists use this to create conditions, where people are, for example, happy when they encode and happy when they retrieve, sad and then sad, happy and then sad, or sad and then happy.

And just like the scuba study, if you're happy when you encode, you will remember better if you're also happy when you retrieve. So to the extent your emotional state matches, you will remember better. Just like external context, internal emotional context can assist you when it matters. This is also true in other situations. In general, it's called state dependent memory. So for example, it's not just the emotions.

Generally speaking, a drunk person will not remember as well as a sober person. But a drunk person will remember things they learned drunk better than the sober person will remember what they learned when they were drunk. That matching internal/external context goes for alcohol and virtually any other drug you can think of, whatever. If you match the test context with the study context, you get better memory. So this is a general truism for memory. Matching helps you retrieve.

One thing to take from all this is the following. If you are ever in a situation where you have to study some material for a later test, then here are some things you should think about. What will be your physiological state at the time of the test? Do you expect to be very nervous and maybe pumped up on caffeine? If so, then you might want match that state. Drink lots of coffee when you study.

Do you know the context in which the exam will occur? Perhaps you want to try to re-create that context when you study, at least as much as you can. Do you have any sense of the way questions will be asked? As you study, you might want to create your own questions of that type or try to find practice questions that are similar. And of course, once you have matched your study context to your test context, both internally and externally, then you want to encode the information as deeply as you possibly can, perhaps even employing the sorts of strategies discussed in the mnemonics lecture. Wow, that's a lot of work for good memory.

You know, that's really an important point, and it's worth repeating. Encoding information in a way that leads to very strong memory takes a lot of cognitive effort. Yes, it is true, the more you practice deep encoding, the easier it will get, but you should never expect to ever reach a point where you can remember all of the events in your life, even just the noteworthy events, without some serious cognitive effort at the encoding stage.

But expending even a little cognitive effort can sometimes be difficult. For example, at the end of a long day, we feel exhausted. As a result, our ability to encode events will be impaired. You will therefore have trouble remembering the details of events that occurred simply because you were exhausted. Remember also that working memory is very prone to interference. In order to think deeply about some experience that we wish to remember we need to be able to focus our mind on it. Sometimes this can be hard to do, even when you have enough mental resources. Maybe very stressful things are going on, and every time you try to think about something deeply, those stressful things pull your mind away. In fact if you ever speak to someone who's stressed out in this way, you can almost sense that they are really not encoding the things you are saying to them. Even when we are not stressed, the world is full of all sorts of distractions, and so sometimes maybe we're trying to focus, and e-mails come in or text messages or whatever. The world is always trying to pull us away. And those types of distractions make it very difficult to deeply process information even when our intentions are pure.

These are the challenges that come with successfully encoding information in our daily lives. It sounds easy to say that all you need to do is think very deeply about the material you want to remember well. However, thinking deeply requires that you have enough mental resources, that you can focus your working memory on that material, and that you guard your working memory against distracting forces. If any of these things fail, then encoding fails, and if encoding fails, the gateway is closed. Conversely, when all those things fall into place, then memory is on the way to working the way we all want. All this really emphasizes is the importance of working memory, so at least now you have some excuses to fall back on when your memory fails. That's something. "Hey, I know we met before. I can't remember your name. I think that's because my working memory was distracted by your beautiful smile." Keep that one in your back pocket.

So far we've really been talking about encoding in way that might generally support retrieval anytime in the future. If we return to our recipe card example, the one I presented earlier, the idea is that if we simply put information into memory well, then whenever we want it, it should be easier to find. But now I want to talk about a sort of special case. Sometimes, we want to do something more specific at the time of encoding. For example, maybe we are at work, and we are talking to a colleague about some book we read. And we're kind of gushing about how great the book is. The friend sounds interested, and so we offer to lend the book. We say hey, this seems like a nice thing for me to do. Confidently we say things like "I will bring that book in for you tomorrow." Tomorrow comes, and we forgot. And maybe we even forget the next day, and the next. To both our friend's annoyance and to our own annoyance, we keep forgetting to bring in this book. Why is it so hard to remember to do something in the future?

This specific problem is sometimes characterized as the prospective memory problem trying to encode some instruction to ourselves to remember to do something in the future. It's almost like setting some device to tape a program we want to watch. Just set the timer, and all is fine. Well, it seems to work well for mechanical devices, but it doesn't work well for humans. We seem to have a lot of trouble with this kind of encoding for future retrieval.

One really salient example of our difficulties with prospective memory is how often we initiate some e-mail, and the whole reason for initiating that e-mail was the intent of sending someone an attachment. But then we also decide to write them a little note so we do so. And then we send the e-mail, without the attachment. to accompany the attachment. Diligently we write the note, perhaps even referring heavily to the attachment as we do so, and then we send the e-mail without attaching the attachment. We all do this commonly. And of course, one of the things to learn from that is to attach first, and write the note second. But it's a good example of our prospective memory. Even though working memory was on task, and even though the time between initiating the e-mail and ultimately sending it might be quite short, still we sometimes forget that primary purpose, the reason we sent the e-mail.

If prospective memory can fail at such a short time interval, it shouldn't be surprising that any of us is even worse when the event we want to remember is hours or days away, like remembering to bring that book in for your friend. The classic remedy for this problem, of course, is to simply tie a string around your finger. This is one of those remedies you hear about, but almost never see anybody using. Why? Well for one thing the retrieval cue is with you all day, and maybe all night, in the case of lending the book. And so you do this the whole time and that's annoying as all heck. Plus we might even become so used to having that string on our finger, that it doesn't even cue us when we need it. So is there any way that we can do something else? Is there any way we can use working memory to encode this sort of intent for future retrieval?

Well, what we would really like to do is think of some cue that will suddenly appear in our world at the time when we want to remember, and we want to associate that cue with what it is that we're trying to remember. So let's do the novel one. Let's say I want to remember to bring that novel in tomorrow. I need to think about this as I'm leaving the house. So maybe I do the following. Maybe I Perhaps I can use my working memory, and my visual-spatial scratchpad in specific, to imagine the door to my house from the inside, but to imagine it as the cover of the novel. So I may actually literally imagine myself reaching for the doorknob of this giant novel. Maybe I want to go a little further, imagining opening the novel. Walking through. Closing it. And as I'm locking it behind me, I imagine putting the key right into the novel itself. If I do all that well, if I deeply encode that image, then maybe, just maybe, that image will come to mind as I leave my house tomorrow morning. If it does, then I will succeed.

So let's take stock of where we are so far. Encoding is the gateway where the you of the present is communicating with the you of the future, and by so doing, building all the potential connections between your past and your future. One of the major functions of working memory is to perform this encoding in a way that will make life easier for the future you but storing the information in a way that will make it relatively easy to find later whenever we might want to access it. However, because working memory is such a flexible and powerful memory system, if one takes the time to use it right, it can even be used to encode information in ways that not only make that information available later, but that literally can cue us to remember that information at a specific time, solving the prospective memory problem. Most of the time we don't expend the effort to use it in this way. We leave some of the abilities of working memory untapped and instead put up with the annoyance of forgetting. But to the determined user, working memory has the potential to reduce these annoyances.

If working memory is the gateway to long-term memory, I now suggest that we walk through that gateway and enter into a discussion of long-term memory itself. I'll meet you on the other side, at the next lecture, that is.

Episodic and Semantic Long-Term Memory
Lecture 7

Episodic memory and semantic memory are both types of long-term memory, but episodic memory is more context dependent, whereas semantic memory is more independent. Both interact with the conscious self via working memory. Interestingly, good encoding of long-term memory seems to alter the neurological paths in our brains and even change the size of the hippocampus.

Long-term memory systems allow experiences to affect behavior over longer temporal windows. We have already encountered 3 kinds of long-term memory—episodic, semantic, and procedural. Here, we'll take a deeper look into how these systems function.

The true virtuoso of multiple long-term memory system interaction is the licensed London taxi driver, who must know hundreds of detailed routes, landmarks, and points of interest. The cabbies' semantic memory supplies their general knowledge of the city's convoluted streets learned across hundreds or thousands of drives around the city; their episodic memories keep them apprised of countless current events, like road closures or traffic accidents, that affect their performance; and their procedural memory controls the muscle movements used in driving.

The relationship between working memory and long-term memory can be described like a library: The stacks are like long-term memory; books (information) are placed there and left alone until needed. The patron desks are like working memory; books are taken from the stacks and brought there, accessed, analyzed, and combined to create some new product. That new product might even be stored in the "stacks" if it's important enough to become a new "book."

Although these 2 forms of memory interact all the time, they are distinct. Long-term memory is mostly about static storage. Working memory is about results. One could argue that consciousness is the experience of what is occurring in working memory.

The defining trait of an episodic memory is that the information is recalled with contextual details. In a way, episodic memory is autobiographical, although we can also have episodic memories where we are not the "star" of the show, like the taxi driver hearing about some 1-day event. If the taxi driver combines several episodes to form a new piece of general knowledge, that will become part of his semantic memory. Episodes where we are not the star may be the most natural contributors to semantic memory.

Working memory allows us to create virtual worlds within our minds. For example, when we read a novel, we visualize its characters. We use this reality simulator for things other than memory: We can speculate about events taking place elsewhere or events in the future; we use it to daydream and to make plans.

Semantic memory is generally much less personal; it is information about the world at large. When we attempt to retrieve it, it arrives in our working memory without context. Semantic memory recall is likely to improve

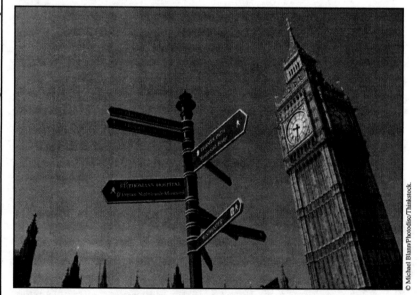

© Michael Blann/Photodisc/Thinkstock.

Memorizing the complicated geography of London's streets has been shown to change the brain structure of London's taxi drivers.

through use of mnemonic tricks. But everything in our semantic memory also got there through episodes of contact with that knowledge. Thus, in some cases, a given memory experience includes aspects of both semantic and episodic memory.

Working memory allows us to create virtual worlds within our minds.

In 1948, psychologist Donald Hebb suggested that the human brain has **neural plasticity**—it undergoes changes, namely enhanced connectivity, as a result of new experiences. In 1973, physiologists Tim Bliss and Terje Lømo induced this enhanced connectivity in the rabbit hippocampus and called the phenomenon **long-term potentiation**. Research has shown that London cab drivers have enlarged hippocampi, adding to the evidence for neural plasticity. Long-term potentiation is now viewed as the primary neural basis of learning. ∎

Important Terms

long-term potentiation: Enhanced connectivity between brain regions as a result of new experiences.

neural plasticity: The idea that the brain undergoes physical changes, specifically enhanced connections between brain regions, as a result of learning.

Suggested Reading

Baddeley, Eysenck, and Anderson, *Memory*.

Dere et al., *Handbook of Episodic Memory*.

Tulving, *Elements of Episodic Memory*.

1. If someone had damage to working memory, might that person still show an intact semantic memory or episodic memory? Which would most likely be impaired?

2. If you have recently exposed yourself to some sort of learning activity, consider some facts you have learned about that activity, including facts you have learned recently and others that you learned some time ago. Are the recent facts more likely to produce episodic memories of the actual learning experience?

Exercise

Imagine someplace that is relatively close to your house, say within a few miles. Using just your spatial memory, draw a map from that place to your house, including as many details about side roads and interesting locations as you can. Then go online for a map to see the actual layout of the area you mapped. How accurate was your map? Did you draw some streets straighter than they actually are? This is called a regularization error and, as we discuss later in the course, this is one of the sorts of errors our memory systems often commit.

Episodic and Semantic Long-Term Memory
Lecture 7—Transcript

I was one of those kids who just kept changing what I wanted to be when I grew up. Just after getting my driver's license I was thinking, "Wow. Being a taxi driver wouldn't be so bad. You get to drive your car around all day. As long as you don't have fares, you can crank up your music as loud as you want. A dream for a 16 year old, right?

Once I read more about the challenges of being a taxi driver, the image kind of changed a little bit. Of course the goal of any good taxi driver is to get as many fares as possible, and then to officially ferry them around the city without getting lost. So, in order to do this, first you have to be in the right places at the right time, the places where people who want a cab tend to be. It also requires great knowledge of the city and how things work in the city. You know, what's the best route to go down, and which way should you be driving down that route to most efficiently get from point A to point B? They also learn the rhythm of the city pretty well, so they know, for example, to be around office places at the end of the day, or maybe to visit restaurant districts around the time when people are done eating, and to be around clubs and bars at the time they let out.

Taxi drivers also pay a lot of attention to specific events that might be going on in the city. Perhaps there is a concert, or a home show, or some other one-day event that is expected to attract many people. If they remember that this event is going on, they may decide to also visit its location, especially if the event ends at some specific time.

Remember when I first introduced the psychological definition of memory? I said that anytime past experiences affect your current behavior, then memory is at work. Already you have learned that there are many ways in which the past can linger in our minds, including very short-duration sensory memories, and the more effortful working memory system that we use for all sorts of purposes. In this lecture, we are going to turn our attention to long-term memory systems, the systems that allow experiences to affect behavior over longer temporal windows.

In my little story about the life of taxi drivers I included three different examples of long-term memory. I had introduced these previously, and we will discuss more of this in this and subsequent lectures. I mentioned that taxi drivers have to know the roads of their city. To take perhaps an extreme example, aspiring taxi drivers in London, are advised to study for 2–4 years, learning hundreds of detailed routes, including virtually all of the landmarks and points of interest, and they have to this and then write a qualifying exam, an exam simply known as "the knowledge."

Taxi drivers also just come to know certain parts of the city, and they tend to be in good places to pick up fares at certain times. So all of this kind of knowledge, knowledge of the city and knowledge of where to be is represented in their semantic memory, their general knowledge of the world learned across a range of experiences. I also mentioned that taxi drivers will take into account specific one-time events. Presumably they would have heard of these events via a radio advertisement or they read it in a newspaper, and if they remember learning about that event at the right time, that is, as it's about to let out, then they will go to the appropriate location. This form of memory would be an episodic memory. It's related to some specific episode in their lives, the episode of hearing about that event, for example, the date and when it might let out.

Of course, all the while they also have to drive, and that requires remembering the muscle movements related to driving, and that's procedural memory. All three of those types of memory reflect the influence of events that occurred sometime ago, perhaps hours, days, months, or years. And all three are considered different types of long-term memory.

But before we get to that, let's begin with two analogies that will allow us to think about the relation between working memory and long-term memory in general. The analogies won't be perfect, they seldom are. But some of these imperfections will actually allow me to highlight some important aspects of long-term memory, so the imperfections are useful.

The first analogy is a library analogy. Let's say you have some sort of project you are working on and you need to do some research. You go to the library and find a table where you can work. You then begin searching the library stacks for relevant books. When you find some then you bring them back to your table, and you combine those parts of various books that are relevant to your project. In this example, the stacks are like long-term memory. Information is placed there and essentially left alone until it's needed by working memory.

Before we get to that let's begin with two analogies that will really help us to think about the relation between long-term memory and working memory. The analogies won't be perfect. They seldom are. But some of these imperfections will actually allow me to highlight some important aspects of long-term memory. So even the imperfections will be useful. The first analogy is a library analogy. Let's say you have some sort of project, and you need to do some research to accomplish this project. So you go to the library, and you find a table, where you're going to work. You then begin to go to the stacks and search through the stacks to find books related to your project and bring them back to your table. Once you bring them back, you search through the books, find the stuff that's relevant and probably combine information from various books, to ultimately produce your project.

In this example, the desk that you're working at is essentially your working memory; it represents your working memory. The stacks represent your long-term memory. So the working memory is a sort of a dynamic place, where a lot of things are coming together. Information from long-term memory is brought there. It's accessed. It's analyzed. And it's combined with other information to create some sort of new product. If that new product is something that we may want later, then perhaps we work on it enough such that it itself becomes a new book, and we essentially take it and place it in our long-term memory, almost as if we added a new book to the library. So as that analogy suggests, working memory sometimes uses information from long-term memory, but it can also put new information back into long-term memory, very interactive.

For those of you who prefer computers to libraries, computers also provide an interesting analogy. Let's say you want to write a letter using some program like Microsoft Word, for example. That program has previous installed on your computer and, thus, a copy of it is on the hard drive. The hard drive of a computer is something like our long-term memory system.

Once something is copied to it, it just stays there and essentially does nothing until that program is activated, which we typically do by double-clicking on some icon.

Once we do that, the program is loaded into what is called RAM, random access memory. Now, RAM is like working memory. It is the place where items from long-term memory, like programs or previous versions of files that were on the hard drive, are loaded into RAM so that the user can work with them. Perhaps the use creates new content, or updates old content, or maybe they're combining previous content and new ideas to produce something completely new. Like our working memory, only so much information can be active in RAM at a given time. And once again, if we create something that we might want later, we can then save it to the hard drive, which is akin to placing the newly created information into long-term memory.

Both these analogies are good in the sense that they highlight the following points. Working memory and long-term memory are very interactive in the sense that information from long-term memory may be copied into working memory, usually with the goal of solving some problem we have or task, and the solution to that problem may also be copied back into long-term memory as a new bit of information that might affect future performance.

At the same time, these two forms of memory are distinct. Long-term memory is more about static storage, although as I say that you'll see that statement kind of too strong of a claim, really. But for now, let's think of it that way. Long-term memory: static storage. It stays there until we need it. Working memory, in contrast, is much more about accomplishing something, something we need to get done. I mentioned earlier that working memory is related to the notion of consciousness. More strongly, one could argue that our conscious experience is really the experience of what is happening in working memory. This will be especially important as we discuss the first kind of long-term memory I want to focus on, episodic memory.

Of course I introduced you to episodic memory in the first lecture, but let me re-introduce you through another question similar to the one I asked you then. They are a little different. Here's the question. When was the last time that you went shopping? If you were able to remember, I expect again you remembered much more than just the answer to that question.

What likely happened is that as you searched your memory to remember one or more shopping trips, and as you remembered each they were replayed in your mind like short movies, movies in which you are typically the star, but the movies probably also included all sorts of other details, like maybe the people who were with you, some details of the place in which you were shopping and the people you interacted with there, and perhaps even images of what you purchased or other random events that occurred.

So the answer to the question also came with all sorts of other contextual information. Part of that information probably included when you went shopping, and if multiple shopping episodes came to mind you might have to sort through which was the most recent. In order to do this you also had to explicitly remember something about the event and when it occurred specifically.

The critical point here is that the subjective or conscious experience of episodic memory is really critical. In fact, it's called "episodic memory" precisely because it involves the replaying of some episode from your life. It is sometimes called autobiographical memory because it is about your life, much as an autobiography is the story of your life, autobiographical memories are episodes from your life, chapters in that story.

There is a slight caveat to all this, and that caveat is as follows. One can also mentally replay episodes from your life in which you are really not the star. Perhaps you saw a fascinating play or a great concert once, and you can mentally replay the events of that play or concert. You are still in that memory, but you're playing more the role of spectator. So in that sense, it is still an autobiographical memory, a memory of your life, but it is one in which you are not really the star. In fact, that taxi driver example I gave you, the one about the taxi driver hearing about some event, maybe from a newspaper or radio ad.

In that case the taxi cab driver's really isn't the star; he's more of a spectator. But it's still considered episodic because it's still an episode from that person's life. And if the taxi driver starts to combine these sources of information and form a new piece of general knowledge, like when and where to look for fares, that will become part of his semantic knowledge. Episodes where we are not the star maybe the most natural contributors to semantic memory.

So the conscious experience is what makes an episodic memory an episodic memory, and working memory is the place where conscious experiences happen. The best way to understand this relationship is by way of a concept that I like to call the reality simulator, and it's a concept very similar to notions of virtual reality, and especially similar to the holodeck notion that was often described in the Star Trek series in which Patrick Stewart starred as the captain.

The idea behind the holodeck was as follows. The characters on the show were all on a spaceship in deep space for long periods of time. And as you can imagine, this could give rise to inevitable cabin fever of the worst sort. The holodeck was a room that could be used to create settings in a virtual reality sort of way, complete with contexts and characters acting in appropriate ways.

So for example, if someone felt the need to escape to a 1950s-era jazz bar, the holodeck could be used to create a virtual jazz bar within which that person could interact with other patrons, maybe watch live music if they wanted, and perhaps even play live music, along with these artificially generated characters. So it was a virtual reality that could be used to provide a "get away."

To some extent, working memory is our own personal mental holodeck. It allows us to create virtual worlds within our minds. So, for example, when we read a novel we literally see the people and the places as we read about them. We envision the interactions as they are described. In fact, many of us are disappointed when we see the movie, if there's a version movie of this novel. When we go and see that, somehow it just doesn't seem as personal or as relevant. The people and places we created in our minds were somehow superior to those presented in the movie.

We use this reality simulator for all sorts of things other than memory. For example, imagine the following. You are a mother. It's midnight. Your daughter's not home, and your daughter has an 11 pm curfew. What do you think is happening in your mind? Chances are you are creating all sorts of terrible movies in your mind, movies that portray all these horrible things that could be happening to your daughter right now, the various things that she might be experiencing. This kind of mental experience is what we call worry.

Note than in this situation, you yourself are not represented in the simulation at all. This is a simulation about your daughter, not about something you did or that you experienced. Interestingly, it also has nothing to do with memory per se, although clearly your knowledge about your daughter and her friends could help form that simulation that you create. The simulation itself is a simulation about your daughter, and it's about things that might be happening now. It's not a simulation related to memory, certainly not a memory of your life.

I could tell you similar stories relating to daydreaming, fantasies, or maybe even planning some event like a future trip. All of these internal events involve you simulating some sort of event within your mind and watching that event unfold, and working memory is the system within which such events are experienced. So really, working memory is about a whole lot more than memory, which is why I described it as such a central cognitive process.

From this perspective then, episodic memory is simply another of the sorts of simulations that working memory can provide. We set our reality simulators, our internal holodecks if you will, to simulate some context we experienced in the past. Yes these contexts tend to be autobiographical, with you playing the role of either the star, or occasionally the observer. We then replay the events we recall occurring within that context and, in so doing, we experience the event as a conscious memory. Thus, working memory is the system that gives episodic memory a conscious quality. That's why we're still talking about working memory in this lecture about long-term memory.

Let's contrast all this with semantic memory. Just to re-introduce you to semantic memory, let me ask you some questions that are the sort you would use semantic memory to answer. So here goes. This is like the quick round in a trivia game show on TV. What comes after March? What is 8 x 3? What is the capital city of Germany? Is Ontario east or west of British Columbia? Do more or less of 10 percent of Canadians still live in igloos? What is the name of the American national anthem? OK. How did you do? Notice that these questions were general, much less personal. I didn't ask you about any event in your life, but rather I asked you about some information that you either did or did not know.

Again, these are the sort of questions that might be asked on trivia game shows. And generally, when we see people do well on such shows, we might describe them as "book smart" or intelligent. They have acquired a whole lot of information about the world. When we attempt to retrieve information about the world, information we clearly learned on some earlier occasion, the subjective experience tends to be very different. Usually we feel like the information just arrives in our working memory without much help. What month comes after March? Well, April. We remember it. That's it. It just comes to mind. Perhaps it mnemonically comes to mind. For example, which months have 30 days? Well, 30 days has September, April, June, and November. That perhaps might come to mind, but there's no movie in our mind. It's just the answer retrieved from memory.

So really, the primary distinction between semantic memory and episodic memory is the lack of an episode, an autobiographical episode to be exact, in the case of semantic memory. A secondary distinction is that items in semantic memory are most likely to benefit from fun and simple mnemonic tricks. Maybe you learned the number of humps on Bactrian camel versus a dromedary camel by thinking of a capital B versus a capital D, with both letters lying face up.

Clearly episodic and semantic memory are related. Virtually everything that is in our semantic memory got there through episodes of our lives in which we had contact with the world knowledge. In fact, together, episodic and semantic memory are often call "declarative memory" because whether we retrieve an episode or a semantic memory, in both cases the retrieval feels intentional and the result is a product that can then be declared. Thus the two kinds of memory have much in common. They differ in terms of the subjective experience. Episodic memories come tied to a bunch of contextual details that make us feel like we are reliving the experience whereas semantic memories do not.

So perhaps the question becomes the following, when I ask you a question like 8 × 3, for example, why don't you have an episodic replaying of the event when you first learned that? I mean, such an event occurred. At some point in time there was a teacher who initially taught you that problem. We know that occurred, so I ask you to think back a little bit. Try to remember that experience. Can you do it? No. Right? It's really hard. Why are you having so much trouble retrieving that particular episode? Of course, there were also other episodes. Other teachers probably taught you that problem too, perhaps in different context. There are all sorts of problems that you have likely encountered in your learning that required you to multiply 8 by 3. You may have also encountered that problem in the context of homework you were doing with your parents' help, or maybe it even came in the context of a problem outside the educational sense in general. Maybe you wanted to buy three T-shirts at one point, and they cost $8 each. And you had to know if you had enough money. And that required the same multiplication problem. Why is it that you can't remember any of these episodes when I ask you that question? Why do none of them come to mind?

In a sense, I have answered that question by asking it the way I did. The claim is this. In order for some experience to become an episodic memory it needs to be somewhat unique, and it needs to be tied to some relatively rich and singular experience. If we experience some piece of information over and over again, and we do so across a range of different contexts, then it becomes generalized knowledge, knowledge that is linked by so many varying contexts, that it loses any association to any one of them. That is what semantic memory is, and that is why it typically does not bring to mind any specific contextual information when you try to retrieve it. It is linked to so many different contexts, that no one of them is especially linked to it.

So, when I ask you what you had for dinner last night, I am asking you about a unique event linked to the food you remember, and many of the details of the event are likely to come to mind. But if I ask you if you like potatoes, that is a very different question. No unique event is implied. You have eaten potatoes in many episodes of your life, and chances are none of them will particularly come to mind.

Now, lest I sound too black and white about this, there are some cases where given memories include both semantic and episodic memory. You may still remember the moment when a teacher or someone else first helped you remember some semantic information. For example a guy I know told me the following story. Whenever he wants to remember some of the geological periods that he learned in school—and of course, we all want to remember our geological periods now and then, right? Anyway, whenever he has such a desire, he remembers a female classmate from a long-ago class saying something that started with, "Please Cover Our Salad Dish with Carrots…," which obviously corresponds to the Precambrian, the Cambrian, the Ordovician, the Silurian, the Devonian, and the Carboniferous periods respectively.

So he is able to access this bit of knowledge of the world. And in a sense, that is a semantic memory. It is his knowledge of the world. But he accesses via episodic memory. Most of our semantic memories do not come to us in this manner, but some might, especially if the context in which we learned it was unique. I certainly have never heard that little acronym before, sounds very vegetarian to me.

This all ties into our previous discussion of rote memorization. Yes. Cases of rote memorization do often occur in some specific context, typically a classroom. But again, they involve a simple repetition of fact. The fact is not tied into any sort of rich context. It is just presented as a fact, and re-presented in that same dry manner over and over. When we learn information in this manner it can go directly into our semantic memory we learn the fact but the context in which we learned it might not come to mind when we retrieve it.

When most of us complain that our memories are poor, we are most often referring to our declarative memories, semantic and episodic memory. In previous lectures I suggested that by practicing strong encoding strategies, especially those that use organization, association, and dual coding, you can improve your declarative memory. Of course, that all makes sense at an intuitive level, but let's take a moment to look at how that might actually happen.

One notion that is a truly fascinating idea is an idea related to something called neural plasticity. The basic idea here is that our brains, even fully developed adult brains, still alter their structure as a function of their experience. One mechanism for doing this was originally hypothesized in 1948 by Donald Hebb. Hebb suggested that learning experiences could lead to enhanced connectivity between different brain areas. For example, let's return to our cabbies from London.

They have to first learn all the streets of London. They then have to learn all the points of interest that lie on those streets. One can imagine the streets as representative of certain regions, and these points of interest represented another brain region. When one has to learn to put these two things together one has to co-activate the two regions and, perhaps, when these brain areas are co-active, connections are formed. That was the notion the Hebb initially suggested, but he couldn't provide any evidence that this was the case.

However in 1973, not long ago Tim Bliss and Terje Lomo described a phenomenon that they observed in a rabbit hippocampus, a phenomenon that they termed long-term potentiation. Specifically, here's what they did. They would first stimulate two different locations in the hippocampus at the same time across a number of trials. As they did this, occasionally they would stimulate just one [location] and they would record the amount stimulus passed the other electrode. So this was the bigger picture. They would stimulate both/both, and then every now and then stimulate just one and measured. And then both/both/both. Then just one and measure. So this would allow them to look at how the transfer of activation may have changed as an action of co-activation over time.

What they observed was that the transfer actually became stronger, so the more often two brain regions were co-active, the stronger the link between them came, either because of an increased number of connections between these regions or because an actual strengthening of the connections. So the process that they observed fit exactly with Hebb's proposal, and long-term potentiation is now viewed as the primary neural basis of learning.

So when you are forming associations, you are literally strengthening the connections between brain regions. Of course, I just assumed that what is true of the rabbit brain is also true of the human brain. Is this assumption justified? Well, thanks to some imaging techniques, that I will describe shortly, researchers were able to examine the hippocampi of a number of our London cab drivers.

Remember, those who want to be taxi drivers typically spend two or more years learning all the routes, and the locations on those routes that a customer may wish to go to. They do this learning through books and also from getting out on the streets on these little scooters, and that's to attach their kind of book knowledge to direct experience.

Well guess what? Those who passed the London taxi driver test and have been driving for a while tend to have larger than average hippocampi. What's more, the longer a driver has been driving, the bigger their hippocampus is.

This implies something truly fascinating by working hard to encode information you are actually strengthening and (in more unusual cases) perhaps even enlarging that part of your brain that performs this function, making it generally more effective. In some ways then, your brain is not that different from the rest of your body. If you want to be able to run faster, practice running and the biological tissue that supports that will be strengthened. If you want to remember more, practice remembering, and the biological tissue underlying the formation of declarative memory will be similarly strengthened.

So working memory is the gateway that allows the formation of declarative memories, both episodic and semantic, and now I suspect you have a pretty good sense of the sorts of things you can be doing to essentially oil that gate so it allows information to flow more readily. But guess what? While working memory is the primary gateway to long-term memory, there is also a secret passage. That secret passage is called implicit learning, and that's what we'll talk about next.

The Secret Passage—Implicit Memory
Lecture 8

Implicit memory is a system that allows humans to learn the structures and patterns underlying many aspects of daily life, from grammar to music to etiquette. Through encoding these structures, it also allows us to make predictions about events in the near future and to draw attention to events that do not fit these patterns so we can act on them if necessary.

The **implicit memory** system contains memories encoded by repeated experience within some context but without any explicit attempt to learn. It is sometimes called the secret passage to long-term memory. The implicit memory system plays a major role in shaping appropriate human behavior.

The kinds of information we can encode in an unintentional manner are different from the kinds we can learn using intentional strategies. Intentional learning strategies are best for remembering specific content and information. The things we can learn unintentionally relate to the structure that underlies that information.

Grammar is one common example of an implicitly learned structure. We learn how to properly form a sentence in our native language years before we ever set foot in a grammar class. Perhaps we couldn't explain these rules, but we could use them. We learn how to speak by hearing speech but also by talking and getting feedback—sometimes explicit, sometimes subtle. Processing that feedback requires tiny bursts of conscious effort.

Psychologists study implicit memory by creating artificial grammars and testing how people learn them. In a typical experiment, subjects are shown "legal" strings of symbols over and over without being told what makes the strings legal. Afterward, subjects are able to distinguish legal strings from illegal ones about 70–80 percent of the time. In follow-up experiments, participants are explicitly taught the grammar before they see the strings. Afterward, they are reliably worse at distinguishing between legal and illegal strings, as if conscious knowledge of the structure made it harder to use implicit memory.

Implicit memory also allows us to recognize distinct musical genres. Even if you've never heard a certain tune before, you can often pin down its genre from just a few bars because you have been exposed to genre structures so many times.

Implicit memory doesn't capture the specific content within a structure. That's why implicit memory and **declarative memory** work together in complementary and often powerful ways. For example, doctors in training deeply encode symptoms and diagnoses, but they see specific and individual cases of these same issues during their internships, building implicit memory and allowing them to make more confident diagnoses.

> **After experiencing a pattern over and over, our implicit memories help us interact in reasonable and expected ways.**

Script theory is the notion that we learn social behavior through this sort of implicit memory as well. Interpersonal interactions tend to unfold according to a regular pattern. After experiencing a pattern over and over, our implicit memories help us interact in reasonable and expected ways in similar situations. We learn the script.

A script not only tells us what we should be doing now; it also gives us a sense of how events will unfold in the near future. Implicit memory also helps you notice unexpected events that may warrant deeper consideration; it informs which events in an environment will attract your attention.

No matter what you do, or how you live, others will eventually develop a mental script of you specifically and of any category—parent, employee, teacher, stranger, and so forth—to which you belong. Fitting others' scripts will make you seem competent, but occasionally violating scripts will attract more attention and can make you even more effective.

You can learn the world's regularities in a more explicit manner. If you need your knowledge to be declarative—if, say, you are teaching grammar or music—declarative memory will help you communicate your knowledge to others. But if you are only concerned with your own behavior, implicit memory frees up your cognitive resources to focus on specific information, rather than its underlying structure. ■

Important Terms

declarative memory: Memory systems used deliberately to produce a clear, conscious answer to some query; these systems include episodic and semantic memory.

implicit memory: Memories encoded by repeated experience within some context but without a deliberate attempt at encoding; contrast with **rote memorization**.

script theory: The idea that social theory is learned via implicit memory.

Suggested Reading

Graf and Masson, *Implicit Memory*.

Lewandowsky, Dunn, and Kirsner, *Implicit Memory*.

Marsick and Watkins, *Informal and Incidental Learning in the Workplace*.

Reder, *Implicit Memory and Metacognition*.

Questions to Consider

1. Jim is learning to sing. In the hope that it will help, when he's not singing he plays background music that consists of other singers singing scales. Do you think this might actually help him? Why or why not?

2. Jim decides he'd also like to learn the principles of chemistry this way, so he plays lectures about chemistry in the background as he works. Will this help? Why or why not?

Think back to some recent event you have experienced and try to separate that event into content (things that happened) versus the structure underlying those happenings. For example, perhaps you are going to a movie, which requires you to go through a certain process both before and after the movie. Even the movie itself may tend to unfold in certain structured ways. Try to notice these background structures, which are the aspect of events we usually encode implicitly.

The Secret Passage—Implicit Memory
Lecture 8—Transcript

Most of the students who attend my classes seem to be listening carefully to what I'm saying. They're taking notes, and usually they're asking questions. However there is a completely different breed of students. Yeah, they show up for class all right. But once they are in class, they settle in, relax, and by all the available evidence they seem to be either asleep relaxing really deeply anyway.

In this situation sometimes, you wonder why they come to class at all? It seems like they believe that they might learn something by simply being in the context in which information is swirling around, almost like by osmosis that information will enter their body and they will learn what they want to learn without even trying. Let's assume for now that they do actually think they might learn something despite the fact that they have no intention of thinking deeply about anything I am saying. Could they be right? Can anyone learn anything without trying?

The system related to this kind of unintentional learning is called implicit memory. So far in this course I have been focusing on intentional encoding strategies, where people making a conscious effort to study information in a way that will later be remembered. Mnemonic strategies and rote memorization are both clear examples of intentional learning strategies. As we've discussed, the gateway for this sort of learning typically leads through working memory. It involves either mass repetition or efforts to organize the information and associate it with other information, especially information that might provide strong retrieval cues.

By contrast, implicit learning refers to memories that are encoded when people really are not trying to learn at all. The notion being that just repeated experience within some context can result in knowledge being acquired without any explicit attempt to learn that knowledge. A number of experiments have now clearly demonstrated that implicit leaning does indeed exist, and that it actually plays a major role in shaping appropriate human behavior.

Now, that doesn't mean that the student just relaxing in my class is on to something. That's because the kinds of information we can encode in such an unintentional manner are very different from the kinds that can be learned using intentional strategies. Intentional learning strategies are indeed the best if one wants to remember all sorts of specific content and information. So what's left to learn? What is there that's not specific content? Well, the things that we can learn unintentionally relate to the structure that underlies the information that we encounter in our lives.

The structure that underlies the information, what do I mean by that? Well, let me introduce the notion of regularities. The world that we live is indeed full of stimulation, and it's coming at us all the time, but this stimulation isn't random. Much of the information that comes our way is tied to some structure, some specific structure. For example, when people speak to us, they don't just piece together words randomly. Instead, the words and the way we put them together is what we call grammar. In English, for example, adjectives come before nouns. So we might talk about things like the red house. We don't hear people talking about things like the house red. Although, in other languages, the grammars are different. In French, it would be *la maison rouge*. But within any given language, the rules of grammar, the rules that govern how we put words together, tend to be relatively fixed.

So the rules of grammar represent the underlying structure, and that structure governs the role of each word in a sentence, and how those words interact. And we all learn this structure years before we ever set foot in a grammar class. And that's kind of the critical point here. Yes, there were times when teachers did try to explicitly teach us the rules of grammar but the truth is, most of us had already learned at least the basics of English grammar long before entering a class.

Perhaps we couldn't explain these rules, but we could use them. We knew how to put together sentences in meaningful ways, ways that the people around us could understand. We certainly did not run around talking about the "house red" until we were corrected by a teacher. As we'll see, that last point, the notion that we have learned the rules without really knowing the rules, that's critical. Unintentional learning typically results in an unconscious sort of knowledge, and it is that knowledge we refer to as implicit memory. That's why we're using the term "implicit." We learn how to basically mimic the regularities of some flow of information, but often we cannot specifically verbalize what those regularities even are. We use them, but we don't know them in a sense, at least not in an explicit sense.

So how did we first learn the rules of grammar then? Well, there is a debate over whether grammar is partly innate or not, but for purposes of understanding implicit memory, we can just ignore that debate for now. Clearly, most of what we learned about the rules of grammar came from simply being exposed to it over and over and over. From well before the time we can talk we are surrounded by this kind of exposure. For example, our parents talk to us, talk to their friends, talk to each other, and talk to our siblings. TV shows talk to us, and the characters on TV talk to each other. The radio talks to us. In virtually any situation we find ourselves in, speech is there. Sometimes it's directed at us specifically, and sometimes it's just there as context.

Of course, we learn speech not just by hearing it, but also by talking ourselves and getting feedback, and that does require tiny bursts of conscious effort. And when we are children, we receive lots of subtle, or less subtle, corrections: Things like, "No, Steve. It's not a weird foots, it's weird feet," and "the bird flew, it didn't flied." You remember things like that. If we said things properly, well then we were greeted by smiles, hugs, or maybe even just an appropriate response. "May I have a cookie?" "Yes, you may." That's a really nice reward for putting those words together well. So between the experience of hearing others using grammar, and the corrections we received ourselves as we began using it, we just learned it. We learned the regularities that were used by others without really putting any conscious effort into thinking about those irregularities. In fact, the most likely place where we do need the occasional burst of conscious effort was when there was a non-regularity. Just think about those examples I just mentioned again, "No, Steve. It's not weird foots, it's weird feet." Well, saying weird foots is actually the regularity of adding an "s" to make something a plural. And similarly, "The bird flew, it didn't flied." Well, "ed" is often added to do the past tense. We were in fact using a regularity. We only had to be corrected because in those cases proper grammar is actually an exception to the regularity.

By the way, this is also why immersion is often viewed as critical to developing a fluency in some language other than your mother tongue. Yes, you can pick up all the semantic knowledge relevant to that new language via intentional learning, but if you really want to become fluent you need to put yourself among native speakers, and preferably ones that are incapable of speaking your mother tongue. When immersed in their language in this manner, you will implicitly learn the nuances of the language, things that you would never learn in a classroom, These sorts of nuances would allow you to speak without an accent, as I mentioned in a previous lecture. But you might also learn things like the manner in which native speakers combine words with hand movements, a combination that often changes across languages.

For example, I have a good friend who spent time a lot of time in Brazil. In fact he married a Brazilian woman and learned to speak Portuguese. When he communicates in English, he kind of speaks like this. He comes across in sort of a low key way, very understated sort of guy. So that's the guy I came to know. And it would then amaze me when his Brazilian friends come over and speak Portuguese to him. It is as if his energy suddenly got boosted by three times. And his talking became very animated and very exaggerated. He became passionate, and his hands just came right to life. He didn't learn that from a book. He learned it by immersing himself in the culture, and absorbing the structure, both the verbal and the nonverbal structure, which comes together to define the way Brazilians communication.

So how does one study the processes of implicit memory specifically scientifically? Well, it might be nice to do studies where you just track learners of some new language from the very beginning until they are fluent, but that would take a very long time, and it would be very hard to control all the possible influences that could really come and affect the outcome of the study. A much simpler experiment is to create so-called artificial grammars and use them to study learning in that way.

For example, suppose we create a code or an artificial language that uses single letters in places of words. Then we make up rules for how those letters can go together. Certain letters can go together, and certain letters cannot. For example, maybe we decide that a "legal" string of letters will only begin with the letters *f* or *l*. If a string begins with *f*, then the string must be followed by either *w*, *d*, or *r*. But if it begins with *r*, then it must be followed by either *f*, *d*, *t*, or *l*. With enough rules about what's legal, the researchers can now create a set of strings that conform to these rules, and they can also create a set of so-called "illegal" letter strings, letter strings that somehow violate those rules and have letters occurring in combinations that are inconsistent with the rules that we set up.

In a typical experiment then, participants would be exposed to some of the illegal items. So let's say we have 40 legal items. We maybe show participants 20 of these items over and over and over again. So they've seen all these items, and they've seen them repeatedly. They are told to just look at these strings. Don't try to memorize them. But think of them as all members of the same family. Think of them as relatives and just try to get a sense of how they're similar.

Then in a second phase, we present another 20 legal strings, not the same ones, but ones that were created by the same rule. These new 20 legal strings presented along with 20 illegal strings. We mix them all up, randomize them, and present them one at a time to people, and we say, "Your task is just to say whether or not you think the one you are seeing now is a relative to the ones you saw earlier. You'll never see one exactly like what you saw, but you'll see ones that are relatives of them. And it seems kind of odd, but people say OK. They do that. They go through each string, and they say: Yes, I think that's a relative or, no, I don't think it is. They do that for the 40 strings. The first critical finding is that participants can indeed identify the relatives at high levels of accuracy. They are often in the 70 to 80 percent correct range. So they apparently do become sensitive to the structure that is common to the legal strings, and they can use that structure to identify other strings that seem to be created from the same structure.

What makes this form of learning and this form of memory interesting is that participants he structure of the rules created by the researchers without feeling like they've learned it at all. They'll often say they just feel like they are guessing. This latter finding is made especially clear via a follow-up study. In that follow-up study participants are explicitly told about the structure prior to the test. That is, the rules that were used to generate the legal strings is explained to them, and they are told they can use this new information now to distinguish relatives from nonrelatives.

They are then given the same test as before, but this time they do reliably worse. It is as if the conscious knowledge of that underlying structure made it harder for them to rely on implicit memory. So implicit memory is the secret passage to long-term memory. Working memory is the main gateway, and when information goes through that gateway then that specific information can be retrieved later, either with or without, the contextual details that were associated with the encoding episode. But when information enters long-term memory through the secret passage, through implicit learning, then something about the structure underlying the information is learned, but there is no explicit mastery of the information itself. This sort of implicit learning, in fact, is very common in our everyday lives.

Music is an area where implicit memory seems to play an enormous role, even in our ability to recognize musical genres as distinct. Musical genres are often defined by sets rules of rules that have been use to create those genres. And even thought we don't know those rules explicitly, we can still identify different genres from the structure of the music that we hear. So, for example, you've probably heard guitar solos, and some that occur, say, in blues music, and some that occur in other music, let's say, country. You may have no idea that there really is a structure that underlies how those different genres are put together.

For example, blues music tends to use notes that come from something called a pentatonic minor scale, and that gives them a sort of sad bluesy feel. Country solos tend to use notes that come from a major scale, often the pentatonic major, for example. And they tend to have a more bright or happy sound to them. So what I want to do for you now is kind of give you the sense that you in fact know about these scales, even though you probably don't know explicitly. So we're going to do that through a demonstration. I'm going to play for you two solos. One that's going to have a bit of a kind of country vive and one that's going to have a bit of a blues vive. I'm betting that you can kind of tell the difference.

Here's the first one: <short solo>. OK. That's one. Think about whether you think that sound was more country or bluesy. Here's another one: <short solo>. You've never heard either of those solos before. I know that because I just made them up. But did you sense the fact that the first one sounded a little more country, and the second one sounded a little bit more bluesy. Even if you're not a fan of either of those styles of music, you've still been around it. You've still heard it being played. And that's probably enough for you to have that sense.

While we're talking about music, let's stick with it a bit. Let me make a specific claim about what is and what is not being stored in implicit memory when you have music. If you had to define music, how would you define it by the way? Well, the oldest philosophical definition of music is actually very concise. Music is defined as "organized sound." Don't you love when something as complex as music can be captured in a two-word definition like that? Organized sound. Well, that's it. That's music.

But really, this is exactly what music is. It's a combination of rhythms, melodies, and lyrics that often repeat in some structured way. It's organized. You may think you don't know some of these structures, but you'd be amazed at how many you do. Let me just give you another little taste. Here's a structure that's in all sorts of blues music, in fact, it's called the 12-bar blues. It goes a little bit like this: <short 12 bar>. OK. That's the 12-bar blues. Again, you've probably heard that in a bunch of different songs without even really realizing it. But it's a structure that's very common, and that's the kind of thing implicit memory can capture. As suggested then, implicit memory and declarative memory can often work together, as they do in music, declarative memory being responsible for the lyrics, and implicit memory for the structure.

There are other powerful examples of this, by the way. One of them is medical diagnosis. Doctors, when they are in training, certainly engage in very deep effortful encoding to try to learn things, for example, the specific symptoms that are associated with various medical issues. And obviously that sort of deep learning aids their declarative memory. But they also do internships, and the purpose of those internships is to allow them to see many specific and individual cases of these same issues; it's a form of immersion. And that is the prime training ground for the formation of implicit memory.

As a result, many doctors will admit that while they have trouble sometimes giving a really explicit justification for their diagnosis, the sort of justification that they could get from their declarative memory, they nonetheless are confident basing some diagnosis on what they might call their "experience as a doctor." These experiences, seeing these various cases, have allowed them to recognize some medical issue, without necessarily giving them conscious access to the basis of that recognition. So don't get too upset when your doctor has trouble explaining why they think some course of action is appropriate. The examples I gave you so far are strongly related to rather specific domains: We've had language, we've had music, and most recently, medicine. But implicit memories are formed for a very wide range of stimuli that we experience. In fact, they are central to our being able to effectively function in our worlds.

So let's get a little more general, and I want introduce you to the notion of script theory. So you've been to sit down restaurants, and you've probably been to fast-food restaurants. If you thought about the sequence of events that occur within each context, and think about them sort of as a scene in a play, it is quite easy to specify a schema or script for what happens.

In a sit-down restaurant, for example, you walk in, you usually wait at some maitre de location. Then you follow the maitre d' to your seats. Waiter brings menus, and later returns to take your order, etc. Eventually the waiter brings your food and later comes by to ask, "Is everything OK?" Sometimes two or three times. When you finish, the staff clears your table, the waiter brings a bill, and you pay, and you leave.

The script, of course is very different for a fast-food restaurant. At a fast-food restaurant the very first thing you do is order and pay, and then you are given your food at some counter. You then bring the food to a table, where you can eat as soon as you sit down, and you clear your refuse when you're all done. The underlying structure or "grammar" of how these two types of restaurants work is usually called a schema or a script. It's part of our implicit memory. So you can think of it really as just like the rules of grammar, in the sense that grammar describes the structure underlying how words unfold in sentences. These regularities at these different types of restaurants describe general features of how events unfold (so in that sense it's a schema), and the role you play within these events (so in that sense it's a "script").

We learn these regularities, these scripts, and we learn them in the same way as we learn grammar, mostly just by being exposed to them repeatedly. As it was with grammar, there were probably a few corrections along the way from our parents, inappropriate behavior we displayed in one restaurant or another. But you can use these implicit scripts that you learned and function quite effectively. And you don't always have to learn them through direct experience either. You've probably seen restaurants on TV or in movies, or you've heard others describe events they themselves experienced. Regardless of the specifics of your learning experience, there is a structure underlying how things unfold, and you'll have a memory for that structure without ever intentionally encoding it. Your implicit memories of that structure help you interact in reasonable and expected ways when you enter either a sit-down or fast-food restaurant. Once the script is learned, it guides our behavior in ways that fit with the regularities of the context allows us to behave what we would call appropriately.

Of course, scripts aren't just about restaurants. We form scripts about the roles we play within classes, within movie theaters, airports, taxis, hotel check-in and check-out, shopping, really any context with some consistent underlying process, some regularity governing the way events unfold. When one takes the time to notice, you will notice that these sorts of regular processes are very common. Of course, we don't typically notice the regularities, we just learn them. And that's really the point. That's what implicit memory is doing for us.

There are two other points about scripts that add to our appreciation of implicit memory, in fact, memory in general. The first one is this. Once we have implicitly learned some script, that doesn't just tell us what we should be doing now. It also gives us a pretty clear sense of how events are going to unfold in the near future, which is really interesting because we often think of memory in a very retrospective way, something we use to revisit the past.

But implicit memory actually helps us to behave appropriately in the present, but also allows us to predict future events.

For example, let's say you invite a colleague to dinner, and your intent is to propose some new project or business venture. When do you actually bring up this proposition? Well, you'd like to pick a time when you can talk a little without being disturbed. So, you might wait until your order is taken and the waiter leaves, because you know that at that point, that it will then be a while before the food arrives. You may not even think about this explicitly; your implicit memory will may just guide you, and that just may be the time you find natural to bring up this proposition.

The second interesting point is that it can also help you to notice unexpected events, events that perhaps warrant deeper consideration given their unusual nature. So implicit memory is coding the normal chain of events, and sometimes things won't fit with that. And so when that happens, implicit memory can actually inform which events in your environment are worthy of your attention. In this way, scripts can really have direct implications for your life.

No matter what you do, or how you live, others will eventually develop a mental script of you in specific, and of any category to which you belong in general. For example, I am a professor, and we all have developed a schema of what a professor does, what my role is. However, by occasionally violating that professor schema, perhaps by playing guitar or by walking on desks—that's another thing I like to do when I'm trying to describe it to students—I can violate the schema and, in so doing, I attract more attention.

What is your profession? Is there a sense in which it too has a script? What about some other roles you play in life? Father? Mother? Grandparent? Neighbor? Whatever your role, and we all play many, it makes sense to both fit the script, but also occasionally to violate it. Fitting the script will make you seem competent, but occasionally violating it will attract more attention and can make you even more effective, more interesting. Thus the lesson here is that implicit memory is coming to represent the normal, the expected, and when things happen as expected all hums along just fine. Our implicit memory is, in essence, one step ahead of our experience and stays that way when everything fits. But implicit memory is also our advance warning system for the unexpected events.

None of what I have been telling you about implicit memory is meant to suggest that you couldn't also learn these same regularities in a much more explicit manner. The rules of grammar are taught in schools. The structure underlying music is taught in any good music theory class. And if one knew, for example, that they were going to an airport alone for the first time, they could do some research to find out the processes they'll be going through when they do.

So yes, the structure of information can be learned either by going through the "intentional" gateway of working memory or implicitly through the "secret passage" of unintentional learning. Which is better? Well, that depends on whether you ultimately will need declarative knowledge of that structure. Are you going to teach grammar or maybe teach music theory? Well then you'd better be able to communicate that structure to your students, which means you have to understand it in a much more explicit way yourself.

But if you just want to behave in a way that's consistent and appropriate with the structure, then you can just rely on your implicit memory to help you do so. So working memory can provide the detailed information, whereas implicit memory can provide the structure. As I speak to you now, your working memory, for example, can be working on what I'm saying and the meaning, and your implicit memory can worry about how I am saying it.

In this sense, then, there may even be a germ of truth in that old cliché that those who can't do, teach. That is, someone who is focused on the explicit knowledge of something from everyday life may not simultaneously be the person the same person who has the implicit knowledge of that same area of life. Those two things can be dissociated. Remember the absent-minded professor? I teach memory, but that doesn't mean I'm a master of memory in everyday life.

So to wrap up this lecture then, let's return to the student sleeping or just relaxing in my class. Is it worth his while to show up if all he isn't going to make any effort to learn at all? Well, not really, but not because he isn't learning anything. He actually may be learning something about me and about the structure of university classes in general. Perhaps I tend to begin and end classes in a certain manner. Maybe the lights drop a little as I begin to lecture, or maybe I introduce short videos or demos at certain points. Maybe I speak more quickly as I get near the end of a lecture, trying to get in what I want to say before the class ends.

He may ultimately gain a pretty good sense of what I might do when. He may also be developing his schema of professors in general. And if he gets a job working in the university administration, his implicit memories of professors may help him deal with them. Or if he tries a career as a stand-up comedian, his time in my class may have given him more raw material to work with.

But unfortunately, while he may be learning the structure of my lectures, he won't learn the content without doing effortful encoding and, of course, what we test in university is knowledge of content. You just can't learn content through the secret passage to memory I'm afraid. You must learn content through the main gateway of working memory, and that requires attention and cognitive effort. I thank you for yours.

From Procedural Memory to Habit
Lecture 9

Procedural memory, like implicit memory, is usually accessed without conscious thought. Even if a physical procedure is first explained by a teacher, it is only through practicing it that it truly enters procedural memory, and educators are trying new teaching strategies to take advantage of that fact. Particularly powerful procedural memories form the basis of habitual behavior.

When you begin learning a motor procedure, you rely heavily on your working memory to guide you through the necessary actions. While working memory is powerful, it isn't very graceful. By going through the procedure over and over, what begins as a graceless routine slowly transforms into a graceful orchestra of motor movements.

A well-encoded procedural memory can become so habitual that it is performed entirely without conscious intervention. Many of us, for example,

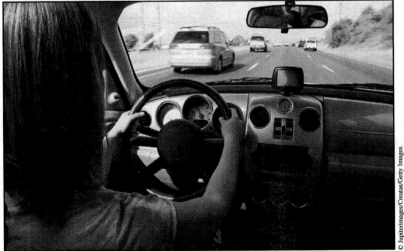

A complicated task like driving becomes smooth and nearly effortless with practice, thanks to procedural memory.

can drive without thinking about what we're doing. But no matter the skill, it's likely some teacher or book got you started by explaining the behaviors you need to perform, imposing some sort of structure on the learning process.

You might have come to understand the structure quite well that way, but understanding and performing are different things. Smooth performance only comes from practice.

Constructivist learning is the notion that a student better understands some structure when he or she must figure it

The environment simply triggers the procedure, even when it is inappropriate for the context.

out, rather than having it explained. Explicit instruction can be helpful in situations where there is a single right way do something. However, it can stifle creativity in situations where there are multiple ways to effectively combine processes. The principles of procedural memory hold just as true for cognitive processes, such as those underlying critical thinking, creativity, and effective composition—as physical processes.

Research from my own lab supports both the contentions of constructivist learning. Using an Internet-based software system called peerScholar, my colleagues and I have shown that when students are given repeated experience evaluating the work of their peers, they become better evaluators overall, and their ability to detect the quality of their own work is also enhanced.

Colloquially, we often refer to well-formed procedural memories as **habits**. Habits occur when you have practiced some procedure so much that you are no longer in control of it. The environment simply triggers the procedure, even when it is inappropriate for the context. In this sense, reading can be viewed as a habit, as demonstrated by the Stroop task. A person is asked to look at a list of color words printed in color ink, but the word and the color never match; for example, the word "red" is printed in blue ink. The person is asked go down the list and say the color of the ink; however, most people find this nearly impossible. Reading the word itself is such a strong habit, we cannot break it even when we want to.

By now, you should be seeing a clear distinction between memory systems used in a deliberate way to produce a clear, conscious answer to some query— that is, declarative memory—and memory systems used automatically, with little or no conscious mediation. These systems are called **nondeclarative memory**, and they include both procedural and implicit memory.

Recall that implicit memory encodes regularities in the environment and captures the underlying structure of things, which can then be used to guide behavior in the present. Procedural memory can do this too; the most famous examples of this are Pavlov's dogs, whose bodies went through the procedure of salivating when they heard a bell ring, even if the food that usually accompanied the bell was not present.

Through this process, which Pavlov called **classical conditioning**, we can subconsciously learn that certain stimuli predict certain other stimuli. As long as the predictable link between the stimuli is maintained, we will respond to the first stimulus as if the second were coming, even when we don't want to, even if we are aware that it isn't. Once created, habits are hard things to break. ■

Important Terms

constructivist learning: The principle that it is easier to learn structure through direct experience of the structure rather than by explanation.

classical conditioning: The encoding of procedural memory via the implicit memory system.

habit: A form of procedural memory that is so well formed the actor is no longer in control of whether or not he or she performs it.

nondeclarative memory: Memory systems used with little or no conscious mediation, such as procedural and implicit memory.

Suggested Reading

Covey, *The 7 Habits of Highly Effective People.*

Herbert, *On Second Thought.*

Tulving and Craik, *The Oxford Handbook of Memory.*

Questions to Consider

1. Imagine you are about to take a new job and you decide to use this as an opportunity to quit 2 habits: smoking and using a handheld device while driving. Which habit to you think might be harder to break and why?

2. Can a procedural memory form without our intention to form it? In the lecture I mentioned examples where a procedure was initially guided by working memory, but then control was eventually lost as the procedure became more automatic. But imagine the following: Out of sheer laziness, a person might toss dirty clothes on furniture or pile mail on a table. If this happens every day, it becomes a habit, one that can be hard to break. So does this imply that any motor behavior repeated often enough, for whatever reason, becomes automatized?

Exercise

Next time you are sitting at a table, put both hands on the table and tap the table with your left and right index fingers as follows: left, left (pause) right, right (pause) left, right, left, right, left, right (pause) right. Do this over and over, and try to go faster and faster without making mistakes. Through repetition, this simple procedural memory should get more accurate and faster. What you are experiencing are the rudiments of rhythm and how they become automatic with repetition. Virtually every musician must ultimately learn these rudiments to perform well, whether to explicitly provide rhythm as a drummer would or to attach melodies on top of a rhythm as a singer or other musician does.

From Procedural Memory to Habit
Lecture 9—Transcript

Today we're going to present the final type of memory we're going to be talking about in this lecture series. It's called procedural memory, and we'll move from there to talking about habit, which is very directly related. I want to start with a personal example.

By the time I was 16, I had saved up enough money to buy my very first car, the ultimate status symbol, of course, for a 16-year-old boy and, in my case, it was a bright yellow 1973 VW Super Beetle. Oh, and it had a standard transmission. At that point and time, I couldn't drive a standard transmission so I had to get my Dad to come with me to pick it up.

He drove us home in the car, and once in the driveway he looked at his watch and said, "Well. You have about two hours before you have to go to work. And I have a meeting I have to go to. So you've watched me shifting gears and stuff on the way home. Now you have two hours to figure it out. Have fun." Yeah. My Dad was a firm believer in the sink or swim approach.

When you begin learning a new motor procedure like this, you have to rely heavily on your working memory to guide you through the necessary actions and, while working memory is indeed very powerful, it really is not very graceful. Anyone learning to drive, when you're going through that process, you're doing something called creating a procedural memory. And the idea is pretty simple. Essentially, by going through some procedure over and over, the muscle movements that you need to perform that procedure become coordinated. What begins as a very non-graceful sort of attempt at getting something done slowly transforms into a graceful orchestra of motor movements.

In my case, my first week of driving would have been better described as a combination of jerks and stops, really. They were punctuated by occasionally smooth motion at least until it was time to shift gears again. As you may know from experience, if you release the clutch too quickly, or give it too much gas when the clutch is released, you jerk forward until you depress the clutch and hit the brakes in fear, at which time you stop quickly. That was my first week of driving a standard, a lot of that. However, with further practice, my ability to drive my car improved. After months of driving I was actually getting quite good at shifting gears and, in fact, could do so while doing other tasks simultaneously, like singing Bohemian Rhapsody in the way that was later ripped off in the *Wayne's World* movie. I hardly even had to think about what I was doing anymore. My hands and feet just did their thing.

Anyway, years went by and one day I found myself trying to teach my daughter how to drive a standard. Yes, I loved my Dad's approach, but I can't quite bring myself to mimic it. As we saw in the last lecture, even a little bit of explicit memory can sometimes go a long way. So instead tried to explain clearly and then demonstrate the steps involved in the smooth driving of a standard transmission to my daughter. To my surprise and embarrassment, I really couldn't do that without actually driving for a bit. I had to drive and pay attention to what my hands and feet were doing, making a mental note of it, so that I could then relay all this to her. My driving had become so automatic, so habitual, that it was happening completely without any sort of conscious intervention. I could literally drive without thinking about it at all and, apparently, I did so all the time.

You've likely encountered similar learning situations in your life. Perhaps you've tried to learn a musical instrument or to sing, after all, your voice is a musical instrument. Or perhaps you've taken up a martial art, or some sport, maybe you took dance lessons, or maybe some of you learned how to knit. No matter what the skill, some teacher or book likely got you started by explaining the behaviors you need to perform, trying hard to give you some sort of structure to the movements you ultimately need to learn.

So, unlike my Dad, who asked me to figure out the structure for myself, usually a teacher will try to give you a head start by explaining some structure to you, and then they'll ask you to "practice" within that structure. You may understand the structure quite well, but when it comes to the muscle movements, understanding and performing are two different things. Smooth performance only comes from practice. We all know that practice matters, but let me try to clarify what I mean by structure with an example.

When I was learning guitar, one of the first things my music teacher taught me was some scales. Scales are notes that sound OK together no matter what order you play them in. That's the structure, and you typically get that structure from a teacher. For example, my teacher taught me the pentatonic minor scale, and that was the scale I used in the last lecture when demonstrating a blues solo. But when he taught me that he taught me in the following way without a guitar. He said, I'm going to tell you some numbers. I want you to learn this sequence of numbers by repeating them over and over again. This may sound like explicit learning to you, and it certainly is. Here are the numbers. See if you can do it: 1-4, 1-3, 1-3, 1-3, 1-4, 1-4. I used my working memory: 1-4, 1-3, 1-3, 1-3, 1-4, 1-4. It didn't take me too long, and I had it. That's the structure, and I could get the structure down pretty quickly.

He then said now, take your guitar. Put your finger anywhere on the lowest string. So let's say I put it here. These are frets by the way. So he said let's think of that as No. 1. Now, this would be No. 4. And so now go through that structure that I just told you: 1-4, 1-3, 1-3, 1-3, 1-4, 1-4. But when you do it, every time you hit a No. 1, move to a higher string. <demo>. Of course I was very clunky at first. I was more like <demo>. You get the idea. Slow process. But through a heck of a lot of repetition over and over and over, often until your fingers are really sore. That notion of playing until your fingers bleed, is not just a term. It's a reality. You can get to a point where <demo> you get a lot faster.

I'm not fast. I've devoted probably 100 or more hours working on how to do things inside that structure. You don't always necessarily play the notes in that order. You fool around a little bit. So I've spent a lot of hours practicing, and yet if I ever go out and see somebody playing guitar, I get a really good sense of how basic my abilities are, how raw my own skills still are. It takes a lot of practice. That's the point.

If you were learning to sing, you might also have had to learn scales and how to sing them in this case. You probably had to practice the scales as well over and over. *Sound of Music*, anybody? I won't do that to you. I'll stick with my guitar.

If you took up a martial art, for example, you probably watched your instructor showing you certain movements or saw them in a book. In karate, for example, these are called "katas." If you joined a sport, you probably had a coach show you some things individually and maybe even worked with a team on sort of coordinated movements. If you took up knitting or something else, clearly there was a book that showed you the basics. These things are the structure. You learn the structure, and that's great. You can learn the structure very quickly. They give you a sense of the behavior that you're trying to learn, and that really helps to get started. But, as I highlighted in the last lecture, you might already know that structure at a sort of implicit level.

So for example, if you were taking dance lessons, and you saw somebody do the tango or the foxtrot, you could probably tell which was which. But it's different from being able recognize to being able to do. By having a teacher give you the explicit structure lets you know what structure it is. But now, to get to a fluid performance, knowledge of that structure isn't enough. Practice, practice, and practice is the only way to ever get fluid.

This is why so many of us often begin to learn something but then we give up. We see some behavior we'd like to learn. We take a few classes, and we become really hopeful as the structure of the behavior is revealed. It's like the curtain is being lifted to the magic. And we get really excited by that: I can see how it's done now. But then we suddenly realize that this structure is all that a class or an instructor can provide. And that structure alone will not make you fluid. You need to practice and to practice many, many more hours practicing more outside the class than you spend inside the class. Once many of us realize that, we are simply not willing to devote the energy to practice, and we give up. So the point of all this is that the structure is actually less important than the practice, and the teacher cannot just impart knowledge on you through words and demonstrations. The teacher is a guide not a provider.

Apparently my Dad knew that. That's why he didn't even worry too much about providing the structure at all. He figured instead that I'd figure out the structure for myself as I practiced. In fact, this approach is one that we now call constructivist learning. There's a notion out there that students learn better if they learn the structure, and they understand the structure better, when they have to figure it out for themselves rather than having it just told to them. Some educators, and I'm among them, argue that allowing learners to figure out the structure of a subject for themselves is a very powerful form of learning, and one that educational institutions should use a whole lot more.

The argument here is made more in terms of cognitive processes rather than physical processes. So if you're learning to dance some specific dance, it is clearly helpful to have someone literally walk you through the steps. The same could be said of driving a car, or most tasks that involve a pretty specific coordination of processes. But the cognitive processes we try to teach at university are often much more open ended in the sense that there is no single right way to perform them, and we like students to see this variety.

For example, in the book *Zen and the Art of Motorcycle Maintenance* the author, Robert Pirsig, describes his frustration with having students memorize the structure first when learning rhetoric, the art of arguing. Pirsig favored a process where students would begin by just producing an argument, any argument. Then, students would be exposed to each other's arguments, and their primary task would be to assess the quality of each and, in so doing, develop their own sense of what made a specific piece of rhetoric more powerful than another. In addition, they might also see that there are, in fact, different ways to produce strong arguments, not just a single way.

There are actually two points here. First, while explicit instruction can be very helpful in situations where there really is only a single right way to combine some set of processes, it can stifle creativity in situations where there are multiple ways to effectively combine processes. Second, while it is sometimes easier to discuss procedural memory in terms of physical processes, the very same principles also hold true for cognitive processes, the ones that underlie high level cognitive skills, things like critical thinking, creativity, and effective composition. These are skills that we value very highly in our society.

In fact, research from my own lab supports both of these contentions. Using an Internet-based software package called *peerScholar*, our lab has shown that when students are given repeated practice evaluating the work of their peers, that is, working in the same sort of constructivist manner, they become better evaluators. And not only has their ability to evaluate others improved so too does it improve their ability to evaluate their own work.

Their ability to think critically and to apply this cognitive process to their own work gets better with practice in a manner that mimics the same procedure as how to perform a motor task, that is procedural learning. So yes, even cognitive processes can be organized in ways that make them more fluid and effective, and constructivist- type learning experiences provides at least one way of supporting this development.

So now let's move a little further down the path of learning and assume that we've spent a lot of time practicing some procedure or skill. We often refer to a very well-formed procedural memory as a habit. The following example will probably resonate well with many of you. Do you remember what it was like when you found yourself driving a car with an automatic transmission? You likely did things like the following. As you increased your speed, you reached around for the gear shift, the one would use to change gears. And your left foot might have automatically moved toward the position where the clutch is on a standard car. Your foot might also have moved toward that imaginary clutch whenever you came to a stop. If someone were to ask you why your foot was moving, or why are you putting out your hand that way, you might have said something like, "Oh, that. That's just habit. Usually I have to press the clutch and my foot seems not to realize that I don't have to do that in this case."

The critical point here is that if we do practice some procedure enough, it reaches a point where we are no longer in control of it. The environment simply triggers certain procedures, and it can do so even when they are not really appropriate for the specific context you are in. So you begin learning some new procedure with a lot of conscious control and conscious guidance, that is, working memory, but eventually you lose control completely. A little like raising kids.

In fact we sometimes use the term "habit" to refer specifically to this automatic manner in which procedural memories can come to control our behavior. This control can actually be very strong at times as was demonstrated experimentally by John Ridley Stroop in 1935. So let's move away from driving and talk about another procedure that we have all practiced to the point where it has become automatic in just about everyone of us, the procedure of reading text.

You are now so good at it, that it may not seem like such a big deal to you, sort of like the way that driving a standard didn't seem like a big deal to my Dad. But reading text is difficult. Just ask any child who is struggling with the learning process. One has to learn how to first parse sentences into words, then to segment the words into phonemes, put these phonemes together and all the sound, and eventually get to meanings. Wow. That's a lot of work.

But you and I? Well, we've done this over and over and over, and we are now reading experts. We're like Michael Jordan's of reading. In fact, we're so good at it, we can't even control it, even when it messes with us. And that's the real lesson of the Stroop task.

Let me explain the Stroop task to you. It's actually quite straightforward. Words are presented in different colors of ink. So some words might be written in green ink, others in red, others in blue. A participant in a Stroop experiment would be shown a list of such words, and their task is pretty straightforward, simply name aloud the ink color of each word as quickly and accurately as possible. So ignore the word itself. Worry only about the color in which the word was written. and read those ink colors quickly going down the list of words as you go. Sounds easy, right? Not necessarily.

It's not easy when the word is fighting for control of your voice. That is, in the critical condition of the Stroop task, the words you are reading, themselves, spell colors, words like R-E-D, B-L-U-E, and G-R-E-E-N, etc. But these words are always presented in an ink color that does not match what the words say. So, for example, the word red might be presented in green or blue, and the word blue might be red or green.

When participants try to read these words, they tend to have some trouble. They find it difficult, and they're definitely much slower to read them than when the word was neutral, some neutral word or a symbol. Or especially if the word matches the ink color. The mismatch of the word, and what it suggests with the color is what produces the problems. So for example, let's say you have the word "red" presented in green ink. The right response is green. But what you'll often see is that subjects will actually say "red." When they don't say red, they often say something a little more entertaining. They'll say, "*R-r-r-r-r-r*-green." Obviously the brain is battling for control of the voice, and it's doing so because of the habit that's coming from procedural learning.

Again, we've learned to read words, and we are so good at it that we now do it automatically. It's out of our control. Put a word in front of our eyes, and we read it. It just happens. And it happens even if it annoys us, when it gets in the way of what we are really trying to do. If we're reading a list of incongruent Stroop stimuli, the automatic word reading is actually interfering with our ability to name ink colors. So it's suggesting an incorrect answer, and this habit is so automatic that we can't control it even when it messes with us.

By the way, marketing people are quite aware of the Stroop effect, and they sometimes use it to sell things, including marketing itself. A few years ago I was in a subway in Toronto, and I saw an otherwise plain white sign that said just something like the following in black ink. "Even if people don't want to read the text on a subway sign, they will. Advertise your product here."

The first time I saw that sign I thought it was kind of clever. By about the third or fourth time I was getting annoyed with myself for reading it even when I already knew what it said. By the eighth or ninth time well let's just say that the marketing company had made its point to me in a clear way. Reading and other procedures that we learn sufficiently can reach a point where they are completely beyond our ability to consciously control.

So procedural memory can produce habits, and I want to talk about habits more. But before doing so I think we need to be clear about the relation between procedural memory and implicit memory, the topic of last lecture. As you may have noticed yourself, we're beginning to form a clear distinction as I discuss these different memory systems. Some memory systems seem to be used in a very deliberate way, and they seem to produce a clear conscious answer to some query. I've previously described these systems as those supporting declarative memory, and they include both semantic and episodic memory and, of course, the system that works with them so much, working memory.

But when you drive a car, or when you read a word, you don't feel like you are querying your memory, and thus you don't feel really like you are getting any sort of conscious response to such a query. Instead, you are just trying to do something, and to the extent you have relevant past experiences, those experiences impact the fluency with which you can do it. Thus, procedural memories and implicit memory, together, reflect what we call non-declarative memory systems.

By non-declarative I mean to suggest that there is little in the way of conscious mediation of these systems. Implicit memory simply picks up on the regularities in the environment, and it uses those regularities to generate expectations and to guide behavior appropriately in accord with those expectations. Procedural memory coordinates physical or cognitive processes and allow them to organize into smooth procedures that can be executed without conscious intervention. Both have their effects without it feeling to us like we're using our memory at all. It is because of this lack of conscious intent that we sometimes refer to the effects of these systems as habitual.

I've described in some detail how procedural memory can give rise to habits, but I didn't emphasize the point when I discussed implicit memory. Recall that implicit memory encodes the regularities in the environment and captures the underlying structure of things. That structure can then be used to guide behavior in the present. With that in mind, I'll now describe how this can provide a different sort of habit, and I'll describe this in the context of one of psychology's most well-known figures, a Russian physiologist named Ivan Pavlov.

You've likely heard of Pavlov before, so I will make my rendition of his story brief and to the point. Pavlov was initially studying the canine digestive system. His primary interest was in how strongly the digestive system would respond to different kinds of food, once the food was placed in a dog's mouth. His experiments used a tube that was surgically inserted into the jaw, under the dog's mouth, and went into the dog's mouth. His tube collected saliva and measured its quantity; the more saliva, the stronger the digestive response. So by measuring by measuring the saliva, you could get a sense of how strong the digestive system was kicking in.

However, Pavlov's experiments ran into a snag very early in the process. All worked fine initially, so perhaps for the first day or two the experiments seemed to be OK. But once the dogs had repeatedly witnessed the steps that occurred prior to them getting the food, for example, the opening of some container or preparation of the food, that sort of thing, something surprising began to happen. The dogs began drooling, that is, saliva began to build up as soon as the food was prepared. The digestive system had kicked in before any food was even in the dog's mouth. But of course, this shouldn't be surprising. The dogs are merely showing evidence of implicit learning. They have picked up on regularities in the environment. Certain things consistently happen before they get food in their mouths. They use this structure, and they use it to guide their behavior by preparing for what is about to come. This is yet another example of memory preparing you for the future. Just like you warm up your car in the winter, they warm up their digestive system so that it is all ready when the food arrives.

Of course, if any of you have pets, you know this sort of behavior well. For example, we used to store our tea in the same cabinet as we stored Lola's and Layla's (those were our dogs) treats in that same cabinet. We had to eventually move our tea. Why? Well, because the dogs quickly learned that whenever they get a treat we first open that cupboard and, in no time, anytime we would open that cupboard door, they would be right there, looking up at us with a cute and thankful look on their face. Almost like they were saying, "Thanks in advance for that great treat you're about to give us."

Anyway, through a process that Pavlov called "classical conditioning," we ourselves, are able to learn that certain stimuli predict certain other stimuli. In those situations we begin reacting to the first stimulus almost as if it were the second stimulus, which gives us a bit of a head start on responding. As long as the predictable link between the stimuli is maintained, this can lead us to develop a habit of responding to the first stimulus in that way, even when we don't want to.

Here is a concrete example. Let's say you are the type of person who tends to go to bed at roughly the same time every night, and who wakes up to an alarm clock 5 days a week to go to work. Perhaps your alarm goes off at 6 am. Whether you realize it or not, there are consistencies in your sleeping environment that predict when your alarm will go off. Some of these consistencies might be external. For example, if have a heating or cooling system that is programmable, it may reliably turn on the furnace or air conditioning at a specific time each morning.

Other consistencies might be internal. Perhaps you like to have a glass of water before going to sleep. That water works its way through your system, and your bladder ends up full at some relatively consistent time, which causes a reliably timed internal sensation. Even your sleep cycles are regular, following something called a circadian rhythm, and thus your brainwaves and the chemicals floating around in your body and in your brain change in regular ways. All of these stimuli can give the brain a sense of what time it is and when the alarm is about to come on.

The result? You eventually acquire the habit of waking up slightly before your alarm goes off. On a work day this is fine. It means you tend to wake up feeling like you're ready to wake up. Maybe you missed a few moments of potential sleep, but mostly that's no big worry. But on weekends or days off, well, on those days you prefer to sleep in a little longer, and that is when the habit is annoying. Because even on those days when you actually remember to turn off your alarm, you may automatically wake up just before 6 habitually.

Well, you may not have noticed, but in telling you all about procedural memory and habits, I have actually been setting up a field of battle. You see, while habits do often help us to do things we want to do, things like driving a standard without paying much attention, or even arguing points in effective ways, there are times when we no longer want them controlling our behavior. However, once created, habits are very hard things to break, and in considering such contexts we will be learning what happens when declarative and nondeclarative memory systems do battle. That's right, it's time to turn this little story of memory into an action movie. To the battlefield, shall we?

When Memory Systems Battle—Habits vs. Goals
Lecture 10

> Breaking a bad habit or forming a good one involves a battle between our declarative and nondeclarative memory systems. Habits develop because the behavior is rewarding in some way, and they are reinforced by contextual clues that may not be under our control. The best way to break a bad habit is to replace it with a positive one, but this can be much harder than it sounds.

To defeat a bad habit, we have to remember our resolution to break it, which means loading an episodic memory into working memory whenever we are within the context where that habit might take control. Our declarative systems must take charge at the right time, or else the nondeclarative system will take control as usual. When declarative systems win this battle, we praise our own willpower; when nondeclarative systems win, we say willpower has failed. But memory is a more fruitful way to think about this age-old battle.

Battles between declarative and nondeclarative memory systems are a common aspect of our daily lives. The brain regions called **basal ganglia**, which are responsible for habits, require far less energy than the prefrontal cortex where goals are created and managed, and habits free the cortex up for complicated or unfamiliar tasks.

Nondeclarative systems exert control when all seems normal, and declarative systems step in when things are unusual. A **capture error** occurs when the declarative system seems to be working fine but still has difficulty taking control back from our habits. Capture errors can have dire results when they occur in contexts were errors are costly.

Capture errors are related to problems of prospective memory. When, for example, we try to add bringing a book to a friend to our usual morning ritual, we are breaking a habit. We have even more trouble avoiding capture errors when we must both remember to cue the goal at the right time and use that goal to take control of behavior.

When we want to take control of habit on a permanent basis or eliminate it entirely, the challenge is even greater. The original habit likely formed because there was something about it we found rewarding. Plus, throughout the development of our habit, our brains formed new connections among stimuli and between brain regions. Thus, our brains might be influencing us to complete the habitual behavior.

Stimuli related to habits are almost by definition regularly present in our life. For example, if you are trying to break the habit of computer gambling, just turning on the computer to do other work could stimulate you to visit a gambling site.

The original habit likely formed because there was something about it we found rewarding.

When we wish to permanently change a habit, we need to keep our goal of breaking the habit present in working memory every time we might engage in the unwanted behavior. We are virtually doomed to fail. When we do, the reward that helped form the habit originally will still be present, and each failure will strengthen the habit further.

Besides taking extraordinary steps to block stimuli for the old habit, it is sometimes useful to use working memory to support a new habit that competes with the current habit. To be effective, you must stick with the new habit for a long period of time; the folk belief that 2 weeks is enough time to form a habit is, unfortunately, an underestimate. Studies indicate you might need anywhere from 3 to 36 weeks to form the new habit, with 9 weeks being average.

When you form a new habit, at the brain level you are forming and shaping new connections. The hope is that with enough consistency, you can make these new connections stronger than the old ones. The best time to try to change a habit is in the context of more general change.

Evidence suggests the existence of a continuum from weak memories to stronger memories all the way to habits. Therefore, it is best not to start bad habits in the first place, but if you have to have a bad habit, then the best bad habit is a weak bad habit. ∎

Important Terms

basal ganglia: A group of brain regions associated with motor control, both voluntary and involuntary.

capture error: A situation in which we are consciously trying to not perform a strong procedural memory (i.e., a habit) but are unable to stop.

Suggested Reading

Eichenbaum and Cohen, *From Conditioning to Conscious Recollection*.

Forgas, Williams, and Laham, *Social Motivation*.

Vanderwolf, *The Evolving Brain*.

Questions to Consider

1. Why do we sometimes put our milk in the microwave when we mean to put it in the fridge? From what you know now, could you devise a potential explanation?

2. Brain injury often has its biggest effects on declarative memory systems. How do you think this tends to affect the behavior of the injured patients? Do you think they would have a harder or easier time escaping habitual behaviors?

Exercise

Pick some very regular habit and try to avoid it for a day, or even for a few hours. When do you most feel it trying to control your behavior? Is it when you are around cues associated with that habit? For example, if you tend to chew your nails, do you tend to do so in a specific context? How much conscious control (i.e., working memory) does it take to avoid the behavior? Would this activity be harder if you were tired?

When Memory Systems Battle—Habits vs. Goals
Lecture 10—Transcript

"What have I done? I've created a monster." Ah, the famous words of Dr. Frankenstein when he realizes that the entity he so lovingly brought to life has turned against him. It's a theme that is central to many a good horror story, but it is also a theme that plays out between our declarative and nondeclarative memory systems over and over. With the best intentions, we cultivated some habit, or at least allowed it to develop. But then the habit grows strong, stronger than our ability to control, and if we suddenly decide we don't like what it's doing well let's say we understand Dr. Frankenstein's perspective a little bit better.

In fact, once a year we have an interesting ritual that puts us even more directly in Dr. Frankenstein's position. Each New Years Eve we make resolutions, mostly resolutions with respect to behavioral change. So we've been behaving in some way, probably for a long time, so long that either implicit memory or procedural memory are now controlling the behavior; some behavior has become a habit controlled by our nondeclarative memory systems, a habit that we have allowed to persist until this fateful day. But today we decide that habit is a nuisance, and we want it to stop exerting its influence.

To defeat this habit we are going to have to remember our resolution, which will require episodic memory, and we will have to load that memory into our working memory whenever we are within the context where that habit might take control. Thus our declarative systems must take charge at the right time, or else the nondeclarative system will take control of the behavior, as usually happens. Friendly cooperation between our systems of memory now becomes conflict, a battlefield, to control that specific behavior.

More concretely then, the next time we pass by that donut shop and feel the habitual pull that brings us to the cashier, we need an episodic memory to remember our resolution, and we need working memory because working memory must wrestle control of our muscles away from procedural memory in order for us to walk past the store, feeling proud of ourselves for doing so. When declarative systems win this battle, we praise our "will power" for succeeding, when nondeclarative systems win, we say will power has failed. But memory is actually a more fruitful way to think about this age-old battle.

We've already visited one experimental version of such a battlefield. Remember the Stroop effect I mentioned in the last lecture? The task was to name colors, but sometimes the colors were used to write out the words, words that were in fact mismatching color, so in fact the word "red" written in green ink. The actual ink color and the habit of reading words came into conflict, and naming the ink colors was harder, slower, and more error prone. This is the classic experiment situation in which the highly developed habit—reading–can interfere with some other goal, reading the ink color.

These sorts of battles between declarative and nondeclarative systems don't just occur in the lab. They are actually a very common aspect of our daily lives. Have you ever intended to go somewhere you've only been once or twice, only to suddenly find yourself driving towards work or some other common destination instead? This usually happens when the two routes are similar; there's some level of overlap. Somewhere along the way our minds become distracted, that is, our working memory turns to some other thoughts, and habits take over.

These sorts of situations are called "capture errors." They occur in contexts where well-practiced habits are supporting some behavior that goes against current goals and the habits win. In fact, the term "capture error" is meant to describe a situation in which behavior is captured by habit when it should be controlled by the current goals we have instead. In terms of the brain, what's happening is that the basal ganglia responsible for habits require far less energy than the high-energy prefrontal cortex, and that's where goals are created and managed.

Of course, one of the real challenges is that these same habits can often be quite helpful. In the case of both the Stroop experiments and the case of driving to work or the store, the habit is generally a good thing. It's not that we wish we suddenly didn't know how to read, or that we want to take control of every action that we make in our car. Your prefrontal cortex is thrilled by the fact that some other memory system is taking care of a lot of these mundane things. It's OK usually to have these things handled by habit.

Let's stick with the example of driving to work for a moment to flesh out the orchestrated manner in which these declarative and nondeclarative systems normally interact. The first important point is this. When I discussed procedural memory in the context of driving before, I focused on memory for how to operate the car. However, if you repeatedly drive your car along a familiar route, even the higher level aspects of driving will also become habitual.

So for example, at certain points you merge into lanes or take certain turns. You speed up when you go onto a highway, and you slow down when you're not. Generally speaking you navigate your way along some path in an appropriate. All of these decisions that you make along the way are consistent, and they tend to be associated with very specific environmental stimuli. You turn left at this intersection, right at that one. Given this level of consistency, your implicit system encodes this structure, and your procedural systems takes control of your behavior accordingly. Thus, your nondeclarative memory systems begin to function almost as a sort of autopilot.

That's a way of describing how we feel like we can drive to work without thinking; often we can. We only need to think when something arises that is out of the ordinary, something that does not fit with the consistent events that occur and that our nondeclarative memory is based on. For example, maybe construction prevents us from taking our ordinary route, or perhaps some emergency happens that requires different patterns of braking or acceleration, or maybe weather conditions require us to slow down and be more cautious than we normal would. Or heck, maybe some pedestrian runs out in front of our path. In these situations our declarative memory systems, working memory especially, must flip off the autopilot and take control.

Given this depiction of driving, consider what happens when one drives when intoxicated or, the new variant, driving while talking on a cell phone. You might have wondered why anyone ever drives while distracted or drunk. Distractions or drunkenness certainly are bad for reasons you can now name explicitly. They interfere with sensory memory, they interfere with working memory, and they even interfere with muscle memory. However, it's also true that when one is driving a familiar route and everything about the driving is routine, nondeclarative memory can get somebody where they are going, and it can even give them the illusion that their driving is not being impacted at all.

Of course, the problems occur when those contexts, where working memory would normally be required and would step in, when those things arise. That's why we hear terms like, "Alcohol was a contributing factor." Accidents don't generally happen because of alcohol, they happen because something out of the ordinary occurred, and the drunk or distracted person was simply not able to react as quickly and accurately as they normally would have.

The larger point then is this: Non-declarative memory systems learn our regular tendencies, and slowly take control. This control is very often helpful, but the behaviors supported by the nondeclarative memory system are not flexible. So typically nondeclarative and declarative systems will interact in a way that allows the nondeclarative systems to exert control when everything is normal, with declarative systems stepping in when things are unusual.

So let's now return to the notion of capture errors. In the case of capture errors, it is not the case the declarative memory systems are impaired or less able to respond to new circumstances. Rather, capture errors reflect situations in which declarative systems seem to be working fine but still has difficulty taking control back from habits.

And capture errors, by the way, can have some very dire consequences. For example, one study that has drawn attention from researchers is an issue related to air traffic control. Here is the scenario, and this scenario was first described in the 1990s. Apparently it is common for airports to have two inbound runways that are usually both available to use. So the air traffic controllers will typically cue inbound planes into two lines, one corresponding to each runway.

Occasionally one of the runways is shut down, perhaps for maintenance or for some other reason. In those conditions the air traffic controller must control their usual habit of creating two lines of incoming arrivals and instead cue all planes into a single line. The interesting thing is the following: During busy times, busy periods, having only one runway for landings can create delays for passengers, but the air traffic controllers apparently handle the crowded new pattern with very few problems: That's because the radar shows a single line of planes to the air traffic controller, providing a very strong perceptual stimulus of the goal that is relevant to the current situation.

However, accidents have occurred when the air traffic is light, and here's why. In that case, there are no lines of planes on the radar, and if the air traffic controller does not think about the closed runway when an inbound flight approaches, the controller might fall prey to habit and assign one of the inbound planes to the runway that's supposed to be closed, perhaps even directing a plane into a maintenance crew.

This example actually highlights two relevant points. First, it clearly shows that capture errors are not just annoyances, but rather they can have very dire results when they occur in contexts where the errors are very costly, like in the one I just described to you. Secondly, it begins to give us a clearer sense of the factors relevant to our ability to control habits. Remember when I highlighted the fragility of working memory? I said that it was theoretically possible to, say, hold 3 words in working memory for a very long time, theoretically possible, but in practice it's nearly impossible. Stimulation, both external stimulation and internal stimulation, tends to grab our attention. When our attention is pulled to something, that something becomes represented in our working memory. We begin to think about it, and whatever was in working memory before is lost. It falls off the conveyor belt I told you about.

So now imagine yourself as an air traffic controller. You've been told that runway 2 is closed today for maintenance. Don't use runway 2. Of course when you are told that you put it in your working memory, and you likely try to keep remembering that fact throughout the day. This may be rather easy to do when that information is continually relevant as is the case when there are many inbound planes. What's more, when things are busy, the environment also provides you with a really nice visual cue to help you remember the single line of planes waiting to land.

But when things are not busy, your mind may wander. What's worse, the radar does not provide a nice visual cue anymore. Perhaps your mind is just clear or wandering until a plane shows up. That is when you'd be most prone to a capture error. You'd step out of your reverie a little, but perhaps not far. After all, you've landed planes over and over. The habit is in place. You can land planes even without thinking. And of course that's true. It's true as long as the conditions now match the conditions back when the habit was formed. And they do not.

The importance of working memory with respect to the prevention of capture errors has been demonstrated in the lab. Capture errors can take over even when a habit is just our tendency to pay attention to something new that happens. Remember those rapid glances I told you about, "saccades"? They usually allow us to construct those sensory memories of a visual scene. In a sense, these saccades can be thought of as a habit we have. When something appears in our environment, we saccade to it.

However, the experiment I'm going to tell you about, we're going to ask people not to do that. It's the so-called anti-saccade task. It works as follows. You are told to look at a small x located at the middle of a computer screen. After some random time passes, a stimulus is flashed either to the right or to the left of where you are looking. You are told to move your eyes in the direction that is opposite to the side where the stimulus appears. So if it appears to your right, you should look left, and if it appears on your left, you should look to your right.

Of course, this is really an unnatural thing to do, and that is precisely the point. Our natural habit is to look at things that suddenly appear, not to look away from them. However, as unnatural as it may be, people are able to do this task. Well, they can look to the opposite. Well, they can as long as they are able to keep the instructions in their working memory. If instead you ask them to use their working memory for something else while doing this task, then capture errors occur. For example, remember our friend the "count backwards by 3s task? We used this one to occupy working memory when we were trying to remember lists of words. Well, you can use that in this context as well by giving the participants a number, and then insisting that they keep counting backwards when the stimulus is shown. When you do this or something like that, their eyes will go towards the stimulus not away from it.

By the way, this discussion of capture errors is also relevant to our previous discussion of the problems that humans encounter when they try to remember to do something in the future, so-called prospective memory. I gave the example of remembering to bring a book for a colleague to work. Well, we all have our morning rituals, and those rituals are actually habits as well.

Remembering to find a book and bring it with us as we leave for work— that's not part of our normal ritual. So that would require us to take control of our normal habit at some point. The capture errors we've been discussing so far are only part of the challenge for prospective memory. Capture errors arise even when a current goal has been cued up. But we have even more trouble avoiding capture errors when we must both remember to cue the goal at the right time and use that goal to take control of behavior at the same time. It's a small wonder we are so poor when it comes to our prospective memory abilities.

Well, capture errors can be as dramatic, embarrassing, or fateful, as the additional challenges of prospective memory that can make them even worse. But all that still doesn't really capture why New Year's resolutions are even more challenging to keep. There, we don't just want to take control of a habit, not just some temporary control. We actually want to eliminate that habit because we want to control that habit on a permanent basis. We really want it completely gone.

So maybe we have the habit of online gambling. Maybe it started out as fun, but now we find we are actually losing a fair amount of money, much more than we are comfortable with. So we make a resolution, New Years or otherwise: We're going to quit.

Well, let's first appreciate the challenge. The computers that we have used for online gambling are computers that we likely use to do other things as well. We have developed the habit of sitting in front of that computer, opening a web-browser, and going to some online gambling site. One important thing to note is that the original habit likely formed because there was something about doing this that we found rewarding. Each time we engaged in that habit in the past, the reward of doing so strengthened the habit.

Remember when we discussed neural plasticity and learning. Well, throughout the development of our habit, our brains are forming connections, connections among the stimuli related to that habit, and relating this stimuli to parts of our brains, those parts of the brain that initiate action for example. Quite literally then, when we find ourselves sitting at the computer, our brains might be influencing us to complete the habitual behavior, that is, to open the browser and go to the gambling site.

So now, some more intelligent part of us, our working memory specifically, figures out that this is a problem. And this revelation probably came when we realized that the habit was no longer under our control. It had become like reading, a behavior that just happens when the right stimulus is there. In the case of a destructive behavior, that can be really quite scary, perhaps even scary enough to make us want to stop altogether. If we manage to encode that thought into long-term memory, that might become literally the solution.

Now, of course, the problem is that stimuli related to the habits of our life are almost by definition present in our life. For example, it is hard to get through life these days without ever opening a browser on a computer. But in performing those actions, perhaps for some other good reason, they can trigger the habit and suddenly we find ourselves gambling. Worse yet, at some level, you will probably feel rewarded for that behavior, just as you were originally did and, therefore, the habit will be further strengthened.

So let's consider this in light of what I discussed previously in the context of capture errors. In that case I suggested that in order to avoid making a capture error, one had to have their goal represented within their working memory. If their mind was distracted or occupied by anything other than the goal, then the error would occur.

When we extend this to habits we wish to permanently change, we need this level of focus to be present every time we have the potential of engaging in the unwanted behavior. That's a very tall order. If capture errors reflect problems we have overcoming a habit just once, or during just some small temporal interval, these problems are magnified many times if we wish this control to become permanent. We are virtually doomed to fail at some point in time.

Of course when we do fail, the rewarding aspect that helped to form the habit originally will still be present, and each failure will strengthen the habit further, and this is working directly against our goal to overcome that habit. This is when the interactions of declarative and nondeclarative memories are really like that battlefield I described.

After a few failures, one might just give up. They may just feel that habit is completely beyond our control. They may be right. Trying to stop a habit that is already very well formed may be extremely difficult, and doing so may require extraordinary measures. So for example in the case of online gambling, the only solution might be to find ways to block access to all gambling sites from any computer you use. Besides taking these extraordinary steps to block stimuli for the old habit, another approach that is sometimes available is to use one's working memory to support a new habit, a new habit that competes with the current habit.

So let's return to the online gambling habit, and pretend that it is my habit. Here is the process I might go through. First I might ask myself, when do I tend to engage in that habit? If it happens to be something I do at a consistent time, let's say it's something I do just after supper each day, I might try to pick up a different habit that is inconsistent with the gambling habit. I might try to find something else I also find rewarding. So let's say that I love to swim, and let's say I can find a swim club that meets each evening from 7 to 9 pm, I can't be gambling at the same time.

Of course, I must be very firm with myself and insist that I stick with this habit every evening for some rather long period of time. You may have heard the notion that it takes 3 weeks of doing something consistently to form a habit. Really there is no reason why all habits should take the same amount of time to form, so I'm a little dubious about the 3 weeks.

In fact, a 2009 study at University College London found that people volunteering to change a specific habit in either their eating, drinking, or activity, ranged very widely in terms of how long it took for the new habit to feel like a habit. Their range was anything from as quickly as 18 days to 254 days, two-thirds of a year for the new habit to feel automatic. The average, however, was 66 days. So, hoping for a new habit to take root in only 3 weeks may be a bit optimistic for all but the easiest new habits. The practical conclusion from this is if you want a habit to feel like a habit, look ahead to a period of at least 2 months of literally controlling that habit and insisting to yourself that you engage in it.

So let's suppose we go swimming for 66 days . If we're swimming, we can't be gambling, and hopefully by the time we arrive home we are tired enough to go straight to sleep without touching the computer. At the brain level we are forming new connections yet again or, really, we're shaping them. We are taking the time-based cues from our environment that used to push us to the computer and are instead associating them with a different activity. The hope is that with enough consistency we can make these new connections stronger than the ones currently in place, and if we can keep up the consistency, the new connections should eventually become stronger than the old ones.

Of course, if we fail along the way, we will be re-strengthening the old connections instead, and if this failure convinces us that it's hopeless, well, then it will be hopeless. However, one good piece of preliminary news from that 2009 study was that those participants who missed their new habit for a single day still did OK. So missing just one day didn't really affect their ability to form a new habit. That is good news: you need to be habitual to create a new habit, but you don't have to be perfect.

By the way, the next time that you try to change a habit, there are some times that are better to do that than others. If you can ever change a habit in the context of a more general change, that's a really good time to pick. You see habits, as I described, become linked to stimuli, stimuli that are present in your home, in your social situation, or in your work environment, so if any of these are going to change anyway (perhaps you have a new job or you're moving), that's a great time to change habits, since you will be escaping a lot of the stimuli that triggered those habits, and it will be easier to link your new stimuli with new habits.

Still, creating a new habit and setting aside an old habit at the same time is really one of the biggest memory challenges of all. One recent survey suggests that 92 percent of New Year's resolutions are not kept, and now you likely have a better sense of why. Once nondeclarative memory systems are controlling some behavior, it can be very hard to wrestle them back.

When it comes to eliminating some habit, not only do you need declarative memory to step in at the right time, but in order to actually change your existing habit you need to unlearn it, which means declarative memory must repeatedly and consistently step in. A few failures along the way and one might stop trying, giving control back to the nondeclarative memory systems. Suppose you've been smoking 20 times a day in a very regular way: same times and same places every day. If you can resist 5 of those times and places, then you are indeed eliminating that part of the habit, at least in those five places. That's one mindset to have when you're in that situation. That's progress; it doesn't always have to be all or nothing.

Another perspective we can take is from the advice we get from the story of Dr. Frankenstein and that story. Be careful of the beasts that you nurture, because they will only get stronger and stronger. If you know that certain behaviors have caused misery for others, don't assume they won't also for you. Procedural memories become stronger the more they are practiced, and at some points they become so strong they become habits. So this suggests a continuum from weaker memories to stronger memories all the way to habits. But the stronger procedural memories get, the more difficult they are for declarative systems to control. So it's best to never let a bad habit get started, but if you have, the best bad habit is a weak bad habit.

So we have talked about capture errors, which represent our attempts to control behavior at a single point in time, and we've talked about trying to eliminate habits altogether. But much like Frankenstein's monster himself, this may give you the sense that habits are bad things. But for every bad habit you have, you also have many good habits that allow you live life more fluently and more effectively. Frankenstein's monster was actually a nice monster; he was just misunderstood. The same is often true of habits.

Sleep and the Consolidation of Memories
Lecture 11

Encoding is important to getting information into memory, but it is not the whole story. Sleep seems to play a role in consolidating the memories we encode during the day, and different stages of sleep consolidate different kinds of memory. Slow-wave sleep seems critical to the consolidation of declarative memories, and rapid eye movement sleep is critical to the consolidation of nondeclarative memories.

Perhaps the most basic debate with respect to sleep is whether it serves any sort of critical function at all. Experimental evidence now suggests that sleep plays a role in reinforcing and reorganizing our memory systems to make the memories of recent events stronger, a process termed consolidation.

It has been suggested that sleep's only purpose is to conserve energy during the hours of darkness, when human senses are inadequate for hunting and gathering. But experiments have shown that sleep is critical for survival; extreme sleep deprivation may even be fatal.

There are 5 stages of sleep, each of which may be relevant to the consolidation of different sorts of memory. Scientists distinguish between types of sleep by the different patterns of electrical activity each produces in the brain. In general, the sleep stages can be divided into **rapid eye movement (REM) sleep** and non-REM sleep. We cycle through the stages several times during the night.

The deepest stage of non-REM sleep is stage 3, called **slow-wave sleep**. During stage 3, our brains receive very little input from our external environment. If you are awakened during stage 3, you would feel extremely tired and sluggish. One function of slow-wave sleep may be the repair and maintenance of our bodies. REM sleep is the stage of sleep when we dream. During REM sleep, our glands stop releasing several neurochemicals that send signals to our motor neurons. This produces a paralysis called **REM atonia** that keeps us from acting out our dreams. Early in our night's sleep, we tend to spend most of our time in slow-wave sleep. As the cycles repeat, we reduce the time in slow-wave sleep and increase the time in REM sleep.

When we dream, the electrical activity of our brain looks extremely similar to how it looks when we are awake and alert. We think, solve problems, and do all sorts of real-world things in REM sleep, but the stimuli come from inside our brains and not from the external world. Evidence suggests dreams are replays of critical events from our recent past, making our memory of those events more stable. In shock-avoidance tests performed on rats, it was found that rats being trained to avoid shocks (that is, those forming nondeclarative memories) spent 25 percent more time in REM sleep than did control (unshocked) rats. This suggests that dreaming allows us to consolidate new motor behaviors without physical practice.

In contrast, slow-wave sleep seems to improve declarative memory consolidation. Among human test participants, humans who spent more time in slow-wave sleep were much better at memorizing lists than those spending more time in REM sleep. The hippocampus, which we know is critical for the transition of memories from working memory to episodic memory, is very active during slow-wave sleep. Some researchers speculate that the hippocampus is a conductor of sorts: It connects activity in different brain regions to form a meaningful overall pattern, then brings back that pattern by stimulating brain areas to fire the way they did when the episode occurred. Maybe it is performing these sorts of functions as we sleep as well.

Working memory seems to be online during REM sleep, which is why we

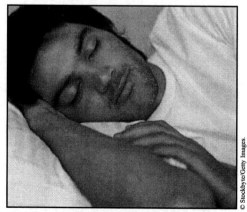

© Stockbyte/Getty Images.

Scientists have long debated the purpose of sleep, but evidence now suggests it plays an important role in the consolidation of memory.

are conscious of our dreams. Working memory is not online during slow-wave sleep.

Infants have been shown to spend 50 percent or more of their sleep in a REM state, whereas time spent in REM sleep declines as we age and in some older adults may be missing altogether. Slow-wave sleep also declines as we age. This suggests that memory consolidation in general may be less important as we age, when we are not trying to learn as many new skills. ∎

Important Terms

rapid eye movement (REM) sleep: The sleep state during which dreaming occurs.

REM atonia: The temporary state of paralysis that occurs during REM sleep that prevents us from acting out our dreams.

slow-wave sleep: The deepest stage of sleep, in which memory consolidation occurs.

Suggested Reading

Medina, *Brain Rules*.

Plihal, *Differential Effects of Early and Late Nocturnal Sleep*.

Weingartner and Parker, *Memory Consolidation*.

Questions to Consider

1. Often when people suffer concussions, they are never able to remember the events that occurred just prior to their injury. What does this suggest about the link between head trauma and processes of consolidation?

2. Some people claim they never dream. This is likely untrue, but some people dream much less than average. What sort of learning tasks would you expect these people to have trouble with?

The next time you wake up and can remember a dream you were having, think about the activities you were performing in that dream. Are they at all similar to activities you have been recently performing in life? We know that memories are strengthened with practice, and the lecture discussed a link with procedural memory, but the data suggests that dreaming does not strengthen episodic memories. Does this mean that we never dream about an episode we remember? Think about your own dreams and see whether they ever include entire episodes from conscious memory—that is, not Edgar Allen Poe's "dream within a dream," and not fragments from your day, but intact instances of episodic memory within a dream.

Sleep and the Consolidation of Memories
Lecture 11—Transcript

There is a movie called *50 First Dates*. The premise of the movie is the following: Boy meets girl, has a great day and a great evening with her, and a great first date. But then they go to sleep, and when the woman awakes she has no memory of the previous day, and no memory of the man that she spent it with. The notion that's implied is that without right kind of sleep, certain memories might not form and, because her sleep was impaired in this way, the events of the previous day were never stored in her memory. So every day she awakes with no memory of the previous day. Thus, the man in the movie must court her anew each day, and does so 50 days, 50 first dates.

While this makes for a really fun premise for a romantic comedy, it is not the case that without the right kind of sleep we could forget an entire day's events. However, there is a germ of truth to the movie in the sense that sleep may indeed help to strengthen certain kinds of memory. That is, while good encoding is very important for getting information into long-term memory, some psychologists believe sleep actually consolidates those memories. The suggestion is that during sleep we may somehow reinforce or reorganize our memory systems in some manner in a way that makes the memories of recent events stronger, and that process is termed "consolidation."

There's actually a good deal of debate within the scientific community about the importance of sleep with respect to memory. In fact, there is debate about the relevance of sleep in general. These debates are primarily due to the fact that it can be really difficult to scientifically assess the effects of sleep on cognition. But that is part of what makes sleep so interesting and so mysterious.

Given this intrigue then, the current lecture will focus entirely on sleep and on its potential effects on memory. That's right. In the first lecture I told you that memory was a party. Well we're going to make it a slumber party. We'll discuss sleep in general for a bit, and then I will highlight why it is such a difficult topic to study in an empirical way. We'll then discuss some of the suggestive research, research that purports to show the importance of sleep with respect to the consolidation of memory and, more specifically, the importance of different kinds of sleep to different kinds of memory. Let's get started.

Perhaps the most basic debate with respect to sleep is whether it serves any sort of critical function at all. We spend almost a third of our lives asleep, typically lying somewhere in a relatively prone and defenseless manner. Some say that based on this fact alone, it obviously must be critical, otherwise why wouldn't we have evolved to sleep less and maybe not at all.

But others argue that sleep may not really be so important. Humans rely primarily on vision as their primary sensory system. And we use that for hunting or escaping predation, but that system is not so good during the night. When the light levels are not sufficient to support vision, then really we cannot hunt, and we cannot gather. This means that we cannot acquire sources of energy during that time. If we remained awake and active we would be consuming large amounts of energy, so the idea is that perhaps sleep is simply a mode of energy conservation. We find some safe place, and then we go to sleep in order to not burn energy, and maybe that's all there is to it.

One way to assess whether or not sleep plays some important role is to simply prevent it. In one extreme experiment a group of rats was prevented from sleeping by simply waking them up each time they fell asleep. After 32 days of this, all the rats were dead, despite having full access to food, water, and anything else needed to fulfill their normal biological needs. Researchers still don't agree on the precise cause of death. It may have been hypothermia because there was an observed decrease in core body temperature the longer the animal went without sleep. Or it could have been due to a failure in their immune system that left them open to germs that normally they would have been able to fight any significant health issue. In fact, those animals that died did have sores on their bodies and lost hair, and so that fits with the immune system story. At the very least, though, these experiments make one thing clear, at a very gross level at least, sleep is critical for survival.

But is sleep really relevant to memory? To answer that question we first need to consider sleep more specifically because, like memory itself, sleep is not a single thing. Instead there appear to be distinct stages of sleep, and different stages may be relevant to the consolidation of different kinds of memory. We know about these stages of sleep thanks to studies that utilize an electroencephalograph, or EEG system. You've probably seen pictures of people in sleep studies, people with electrodes on their heads. These electrodes measure the electrical activity in the brain. If this electrical activity was converted into an auditory signal, it would sound a little like the static you hear when a radio is tuned to a frequency that nobody is broadcasting on, a sort of white noise.

The specific quality of this electrical signal changes as we sleep. Sometimes the wavelengths that are generated are closer together, and sometimes they are further apart. This would correspond to the frequency of the white noise we'd hear, if we could actually hear it. In addition, sometimes the amplitude of the waves is small, and sometimes it's quite large, and this would correspond to the loudness of the white noise. Luckily, people are actually able to sleep with these electrodes stuck to their heads so that we can measure the electricity as they sleep. Some of the very earliest studies of sleep simply examined these changes in this electrical activity over the course of an evening.

The findings of these studies were truly fascinating. Researchers were able to identify 4 distinct patterns of electrical activity, patterns that correspond to five different stages of sleep. At a more general level, these stages can be divided into two kinds of sleep, non-REM sleep and REM sleep. The term "REM" corresponds to rapid eye movement, the sort of movement one can see and measure when we dream, and only when we dream. So w hen we say REM sleep, we're actually talking about sleep for dreaming. And non-REM sleep is sleep when we are not dreaming.

More specifically then, the stages of sleep proceed as follows. Stage 1 is a transition stage from wakefulness to your first true sleep stage. Stage 1 sleep is characterized by drowsiness. Stage 2 reflects the onset of sleep proper, and once you are within that our brainwaves continue to slow down, but they increase in amplitude until we hit stage 3. And stage 3 is going to be one of the stars of today's lecture. It's called slow-wave sleep. And it is the deepest sleep we achieve.

If someone wanted to awaken us during stage 3 sleep, they would find it very difficult to do so, and that's because our brains receive very little input from our external environment when we are in this kind of sleep. If they did succeed in waking us up, we would feel extremely tired and sluggish, and it would take us a long time to feel awake. When people sleepwalk they typically do so while they're in slow-wave sleep. By the way, while we are in slow-wave sleep our body also releases growth hormones, and these growth hormones seem very important for repairing tissue and perhaps reinvigorating our immune system. So one function of slow-wave sleep may be some form of physical maintenance necessary to keep our bodies functioning well, and this could be the reason why many rats die when they are deprived of this kind of sleep.

Eventually we emerge out of slow-wave sleep and into REM sleep. A few truly amazing things happen at this point. For example, just prior to entering REM sleep our glands stop releasing the neurochemicals called norepinephrine, serotonin, and histamine and, as a result, motor neurons can no longer send their signals. This produces a literal paralysis called "REM atonia." This temporary paralysis is the only thing that keeps us from acting out our dreams.

For some people this paralysis does not always occur, and their sleeping partners often complain about being hit or kicked as they slept. That shows us how important this paralysis can be, a very useful thing to have happen. By the way, if you've ever dreamt about being tied up, or held down, or felt you just couldn't move very quickly in a dream, it is likely that your paralysis is somehow finding its way into your dream content. At some level your body notices that it cannot move, and that feeling enters into your dream in some other form.

So we move from stage 1 to REM sleep. Then what? Well, first of all, one whole cycle from stage 1 to the end of REM sleep takes anywhere from about 75 to 105 minutes, and when we finish, we repeat the cycle again. However as we repeat it, we don't spend the same amount of time in the various stages. Early in our night's sleep we spend quite a bit of our time in slow-wave sleep, maybe as much as 70 to 90 minutes worth and only very little time in REM sleep. However, as the night progresses and these cycles repeat, we gradually reduce the amount of time we spend in slow-wave sleep, and we increase the amount of time we spend in REM sleep. And that's why we often when we awaken in the morning, we have dreams in our mind, of course, only to feel them slip away.

When we dream, the electrical activity of our brain looks almost identical to how it looks when we are awake and alert. In a sense it looks like we are awake and alert, but just cut off from the external world. We think, we solve problems, and we do all sorts of real-world things, but the content of our thoughts comes from our brain and not from the external world. In fact, it is probably completely correct to think of this as working memory online and doing it's thing as it always does, but the information it has to work with comes entirely from internal sources.

In fact this may be why dreams tend to be so unstable in terms of their content. One minute we are in one place interacting with one person, and the next we're somewhere else with someone else. The claim here is that because the real world is bound by the physical reality of it, it has a certain stability, stability in terms of time and stability in terms of place. So when it is feeding into our thoughts, we gain that stability from it, and it keeps our thoughts stable. But when the real world is not providing the input, then the source of the stability is lost. Internal input need not be so stable; thoughts can jump, and the dreams jump around with it. But do they jump with some purpose, or are we just experiencing some sort of random brain activity that we somehow weave into a semi-meaningful chain of events—the story that plays out in our minds? That's really the critical question.

In fact, this is a good place to visit one notion sometimes put forward with respect to sleep and memory. In Aldous Huxley's novel *Brave New World*, written in 1932, children were conditioned as they slept. The suggestion here is that perhaps we can learn new information while we are sleeping, and many companies still market products that claim to do just that. Is this sort of sleep learning possible? Well, probably not. The problem is, once we make the transition from wakefulness to stage 2, our brains perceive very little of the information entering our senses, and so the window during which our brains are actually alert enough to hear is very small. So perhaps as we are drifting off, we might be capable of some sort of unintentional learning, something like what I talked about in the implicit memory lecture. If we exposed ourselves to stimuli that contained some regular patterns then, perhaps maybe a foreign language, the learning episode would be brief, and we'd actually likely learn it much better if we exposed ourselves to the same material while we were fully awake. So it's a cool idea, but not one that really has any scientific backing.

However, there's a different notion about sleep and dreaming, and that is that in some way it reflects a sort of replaying of critical events that have happened to us in the recent past, and that this replaying actually makes our memory of those events more stable. That is, sleep and dreams consolidate memories. It's another fascinating idea if it's true, but how do we test it? As you'll see, testing theories related to sleep can be quite complex. One very simple approach is the following: We can first present participants with some task to learn. If we are interested in memory, maybe we give them a list of words to try to remember. We then break our participants into two groups. One group is allowed to sleep; the other must remain awake. Eight hours or so later, we test their memory. What do we find? Well, invariably we will find that the group that slept will perform better than the group that did not, and this seems to imply that sleep is indeed aiding memory in some manner. But does it really demand that explanation?

Remember when I discussed theories of forgetting? I mentioned that one of the notions of forgetting is that if you learn something, and then you go on to learn other things, the things that you learn after may make it harder to remember the things you learned earlier. Remember the clothes on the floor notion? So maybe it isn't the case that sleep really benefits memory. Maybe it's the case that those participants who stayed awake had experiences while they were awake, and those experiences made it harder for them to remember the word list. The sleeping participants did not have those experiences, and hence found it easier to remember the list. Or maybe the group that stayed awake is just more exhausted and that's why they perform worse.

In general, that's the problem with sleep studies. No matter how clever the researcher is when designing an experiment to test some prediction, it's really very difficult to manipulate some aspect of sleep without also changing other variables, including a lot of variables that might be relevant. Because of this, most of the data we have about the effects of sleep are more suggestive than definitive. But, with that caveat in place, some of the suggestive findings are actually really fascinating. So let's discuss them a little along with some of the experiments used to support them.

Do dreams serve to consolidate memory and, if so, what kind of memory? Let's consider REM sleep first, dream sleep. In one study rats were taught what researchers described as a skill of shock avoidance. Specifically, two groups of rats were tested. Both were placed in a box that had two chambers with a metallic grate floor. For the experimental group, the following events would occur: A light would turn on and a tone would sound (these things would happen together). Five seconds later a small electrical current would pass through the floor of the chamber that the rat was in. If the rat left the chamber, the current was turned off. In fact, if the rat left the chamber anytime during the 5 seconds between when the light and tone sounded and the floor was electrified, the electrification would never happen. Over a number of trials of this, these rats would learn to simply move whenever the light and tone came on, and this behavior is assumed to reflect nondeclarative memory systems; implicit memory learning the experimental contingencies, the regularities of the environment, and procedural memory, learning the appropriate behavioral response: move.

The control group experienced the same events, but nothing they did would prevent the current from coming on. In both cases, when the current was turned on, it was always terminated after 5 seconds. So what do we have? We have one group of rats that are forming these new nondeclarative memories, and we have another group that is not because nothing they did will prevent the shock. If you now look at the sleep cycles of these rats, after they experience these experimental events, you see something interesting. The group of rats who were learning this new nondeclarative memory, they ended up spending a lot more time in REM sleep than did the control rats, in fact, over 25 percent more time. The researchers argue that this is because REM sleep allows for the consolidation of new nondeclarative memories. The rats were reliving the experiment in their dreams and were consolidating their memories as they did so.

Of course it's impossible to know what is going on in the rats' minds as they dream, but when I first heard about these studies, they did make some sense to me. As a teenager I flipped burgers at a local fast-food restaurant. Flipping burgers is a pretty mind-numbing task, and I did this only so I could afford gas for my prized 1973 Super Beetle that I told you about earlier. So you can imagine I would find it quite annoying when I would return to my workplace in my dreams, flipping burgers over and over, all night long.

More recently I have been learning to play guitar. It's another task with a strong nondeclarative procedural component. Again, whenever I am learning some new fingering or riff, I often notice that I dream about it. I repeat the behavior over and over, sometimes to the point where I badly wish I could dream about something else, anything else. So maybe this makes some sense. Maybe the neurons we use when we're learning some new motor behaviors somehow reactivate when we dream, and that essentially allows us to learn better, at least at the level of the relevant brain connections.

If we go back to that evolutionary story I mentioned at the beginning of this lecture than we could add the following. Yes, maybe we sleep as a way to conserve energy, and maybe we do that specifically during times when we can't be hunting or gathering. But if we could both conserve energy and also improve our skills at hunting and gathering that would be even better, right? Perhaps that's exactly what we do.

But what about slow-wave sleep? Does that have anything to do with memory consolidation? Well again, if we're willing to accept the imprecision that comes with most studies of sleep, the answer appears to be yes. Here is how a typical study of slow-wave sleep is performed. Once again we require at least two groups of participants. One group might be allowed to sleep for 3 hours prior to seeing some list of items to recall; the other group has to stay awake for those same 3 hours. Both groups are shown a list of items, and then both groups are allowed to sleep for 3 hours before a memory test. Note then, that in this case, we are going to test their episodic memory, their declarative memory.

Now here's the critical point of these studies. Remember when I said that the amount of time that we spend in each stage of sleep changes the longer that we sleep throughout the night. Well, that fact is critical for the logic of these studies. Specifically, the group that we allowed to sleep for 3 hours had already spent a lot of time in slow-wave sleep, so now, after they see the items and go back to sleep, they won't spend that much time in slow-wave sleep. Instead they'll spend a lot of time in REM sleep. However the group that we had stay awake for 3 hours, awake right up until they heard the list, will just be getting their first sleep after hearing the list, and this sleep would be dominated with slow-wave sleep.

So we have one group that is mostly in REM sleep, and another that is mostly in slow-wave sleep. Who remembers the list of items better? Well, despite sleeping only 3 hours, the group that was forced to stay awake and therefore the group that spent most of their sleep in slow-wave sleep remembers the list better. So slow-wave sleep seems to consolidate declarative memory and, in this case, episodic memory.

By the way, if you repeat the procedure I just described, but instead of learning a list of words, you ask participants to learn some sort of motor skill, then the group that was mostly in REM sleep performs better. This provides further confirmation that REM sleep seems important for the consolidation of nondeclarative memories. That's pretty cool. Different stages of sleep seem critical for the consolidation of different forms of memory. When we think about this, we can maybe get a sense of how dreaming might consolidate a procedural memory. I mean if we are essentially reliving the relevant motor sequence, we can imagine that the brain areas relevant to that are getting trained up. But how does slow-wave sleep consolidate episodic memories? One clue might come from the following: When we are in slow-wave sleep that part of our brain called the hippocampus becomes active. We know that the hippocampus is critical for the transition of memories from working memory to episodic memory, and when people are performing deep levels of encoding, the hippocampus is also very active. What is it doing?

Some researchers speculate that the hippocampus is like a conductor of an orchestra that somehow glues together activity in different brain regions to form a meaningful overall pattern, a pattern of brain activity. And it may do so in both a receptive and a productive sort of way. That is, during encoding, the various areas of the brain relevant to perception of some external event are activated by the event itself, and deep encoding of that event may involve some sort of gluing together of these different areas. And the hippocampus may be involved in that gluing together.

The hippocampus can then subsequently bring back that memory by stimulating those same brain areas. And so if it can stimulate them to fire in a manner similar to the way they were activated when the actual event occurred, that may reflect our conscious reliving of that event, episodic memory. The fact that the hippocampus is active during slow-wave sleep suggests that maybe it is performing these sorts of functions as we sleep, reactivating and perhaps strengthening the episodic memories and, in fact, declarative memory more generally. Any of these memories related to recent events may actually be reactivated stronger.

Procedural events, events that require some sort of sequential unfolding of muscle movements get replayed while we are in REM sleep, when our muscles are paralyzed. However, episodic events, things that we saw or heard, might be replayed during slow-wave sleep. In both cases the replaying might make the relevant memory systems more stable, more consolidated, and perhaps this division of labor is based specifically on the fact that muscles are paralyzed during REM sleep.

Of course they are also distinguished by another difference. Working memory seems to be online during REM sleep, which is why we feel like we consciously experience our dreams. In contrast, working memory is not online during slow-wave sleep. If we awaken somebody during slow- wave sleep, again, a very difficult thing to do, but typically they will report no sense of having been dreaming. We only seem to sense dreaming during REM sleep.

There is one interesting addition to all this. If we consider the stages of sleep across our life span, we see the following. We spend the most time in REM sleep as infants. Infants have been shown to spend 50 percent or more of their sleep in a REM state. This makes some sense given all of the new motor behaviors they're learning.

REM sleep, though, declines as we age and, in some older adults, it can be missing altogether. Perhaps this is why, as we like to say, it is hard to teach an old dog new tricks. Slow-wave sleep also declines as we age. In fact, older people spend more time in those transition stages than do young people. So it takes them longer to get to slow-wave sleep, and they often sleep less overall, so their total slow-wave sleep and REM sleep is often much less than it is for younger people.

This may simply reflect what I like to think of as coasting later in life. Early in life we need to learn a lot, and learning brings with it all sorts of new experiences. As we age we can increasingly coast on our prior learning. It may be less important to keep learning new things. Memory consolidation in general, then, may be less important as we age. We're going to return to this issue when we talk specifically about aging and memory later in this course, but this link to sleep may be part of the story.

So the main point to take away from this slumber party of memory is the following: While encoding is clearly very important to getting information into memory, it's not the whole story. Processes during sleep seem to play a role in further strengthening these memories, that is consolidating these memories we encode during the day, and perhaps even just days previous. What's more, the distinct stages of sleep differentially consolidate different kinds of memory. Slow-wave sleep seems critical for the consolidation of declarative memories, and REM sleep is critical to the consolidation of nondeclarative memories.

Of course, the age when we sleep most of all is during infancy, when we sleep more than half of every day and continue sleeping almost as much as that during early childhood. As we'll see in the next lecture, all this sleeping corresponds to a vast leap in the development of memory during early life.

Infant and Early Childhood Memory
Lecture 12

Babies spend much of their time learning the regularities of their environment and developing procedural memories. Between the ages of 2 and 5, the brain structures underlying working memory and episodic memory slowly mature. By about 5 years old, all memory systems are online and functioning. The memories we form thereafter can be retained long-term, and we begin piecing those memories together to create an ongoing sense of self.

Most people have no memories before the age of 3. Our inability to remember events from before that age is so pervasive that it's called **childhood amnesia**. But this amnesia only refers to episodic memory; not all memory systems take this long to develop.

At birth, our brains contain most or all of the brain cells we will ever have, about 100 billion. What's missing is connectivity. As babies interact with the world, connections form between neurons. This neural plasticity allows the brain to wire itself based on early sensory and motor experiences. Infant brains form connections more quickly, and may also form more connections overall, when exposed to lots of variable stimulation.

Developing the light reflex—pupil constriction when exposed to light—is the first step in developing iconic memory, whereas hearing, and possibly echoic memory, seems to be present before birth. Most other behaviors are acquired gradually as brain connections develop.

By about 3 days of age, babies can mimic facial expressions; this is called **modeling**, and it is evidence that a baby's procedural memory system is functioning and growing. By 3 months, most babies have learned that their behaviors can affect their environment—for example, shaking a rattle to make a noise. The baby is forming simple semantic memories. At 5 months, many babies begin acting uncomfortable around strangers. What begins as attraction to the familiar develops into an avoidance of the unfamiliar. This suggests the development of links between perceptions of familiarity and emotional systems.

Babies begin to babble at 5 months, begin imitating vocal units at 8 months, and begin mimicking animal sounds by 1 year. The sounds they make are derived from their environments, an indication that their implicit memory systems are functioning well.

Experiments show that babies remember for longer periods of time the older they get. The increasing memory skills correspond to behavioral leaps and bounds over the first 2 years of life, particularly the acquisition of language.

Before the age of 2, a baby's implicit learning and procedural memory development reign supreme; infants also get a lot more REM sleep than children and adults, supporting the suggestion that dreams consolidate procedural memories. On the other hand, most of us do not form episodic memories before the age of 2. The hippocampus and the prefrontal cortex are slow to develop, neither reaching maturity until 3 or 4 years of age.

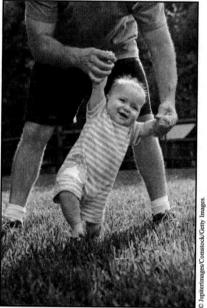

Between the ages of 2 and 5 years old, children display a powerful ability to learn the regularities of language, which may reflect implicit memory, but once language is learned, it allows us to learn things in a way that can lead to semantic and episodic memories.

As early as 18 months of age, most children have learned their own name; at this same time, the first

Babies don't form episodic memories of their first steps, but they don't need to. Thus their brains are wired for forming procedural memories.

struggles for independence also emerge. At about 3 years of age, children can describe their dreams; this is important because dreams share certain tendencies with autobiographical memory. The year between 3 and 4 years old might be especially important for the development of a sense of self. In this period, behaviors like cooperation, self-consciousness, and negotiation appear. By the age of 5, children are not only able to play games that involve rules, they can and do cheat—evidence of a strong working memory.

Once all memory systems are in place at around the age of 5, the clouds of childhood amnesia dissipate for good. However, during periods of intense brain development, there is also evidence of **synaptic pruning**, the removal of weak brain connections to make space for more new connections. This happens during infant development, but it also occurs during adolescence. ∎

Important Terms

childhood amnesia: The human inability to encode episodic memories before about the age of 3.

modeling: Learning by imitation; specifically, an infant's mimicry of others' facial expressions.

synaptic pruning: The removal of weak brain cell connections to make way for new ones that occurs at least twice in normal, healthy humans: once in infancy and once in adolescence.

Suggested Reading

Bauer, *Varieties of Early Experience*.

Markowitsch and Welzer, *The Development of Autobiographical Memory*.

Nelson, *Memory and Affect in Development*.

1. What is your earliest childhood memory? Are you sure what you remember is the event itself, or could it be based on later retellings of the event? How would you know for sure? How might a study of the memory of adopted children be interesting? After all, adopted children are unlikely to hear stories about their life prior to adoption. What might you expect such research to show?

2. At various points in the course, I have made dramatic claims about how important memory is with respect to functioning smoothly in our lives. Perhaps this claim seems especially valid as we consider the ways that our various memory systems support the development of a growing child. Can you imagine how this development process would be different if the child's implicit memory system were less efficient than normal? What if it took 2 years for implicit memory to be fully functional? What implications would that have for the child and caregiver?

Exercise

Ask yourself and a few of your friends the following questions: Do you know how old you were when you first walked? Do you know how old you were at the time of your first retrievable episodic memory? Do you see any relationship and, if so, why might that be?

Lecture 12: Infant and Early Childhood Memory

Infant and Early Childhood Memory
Lecture 12—Transcript

What is your very earliest childhood memory? Can you figure out how old you were you at the time? I suspect for most of you it's no younger than 3 years old because the range for most people is from 2 to 5 years. Does that mean that your memory system takes 3 or more years to develop, or is that just your episodic memory system? In this lecture we will address the origins and early development of memory. Along the way, we'll also look at suggestions for enhancing the memory abilities and cognitive abilities in general of any infants you may be interacting with.

For me, the earliest memory involved meeting a man with a camel on a family trip we took to Cypress. The man was willing to let me and my 3 older sisters ride the camel, one at a time of course. All my sisters took their turn, but when it was my turn I chickened out. I really wanted to ride the camel, but it looked kind of mean, and I didn't like how it stood up. It scared me, and when Dad forced the issue a little bit, I essentially had a temper tantrum. As we drove away I vividly remember perhaps the first time I really felt regret. The only camel I had ever had a chance to ride was literally disappearing into the horizon.

But now here is question that might not have occurred to you: Is that memory real? I wonder because I have another memory that makes me worry. The memory is of a picture in our family album of our family posing beside a man with a camel in Cypress, a picture that was revisited repeatedly, along with the story of me refusing to ride the camel. Given all that I now know about memory, that makes me question my memory of that camel. Was it a true memory of the original incident, or is this all a memory created by the retellings of that incident in the context of the picture?

Most scientific studies of memory for childhood events suggest that very few children have valid memories for events that occurred within the first 30 months of life. Our inability to remember events from before that age is so pervasive that we call it childhood amnesia. And often, the effective period of childhood amnesia can extend to 3 or 4 years old at least. That's probably about the age I was when I passed up my opportunity to ride a camel.

Of course, when we talk about this sort of childhood amnesia we are really talking about what you and I now know as episodic memory, our ability to replay some past experience in our mind. In fact, it does seem as though the processes and the brain structures that we need to lay down those sort of durable episodic memories do take a while to develop, perhaps as long as two or three years maybe even a little longer.

But that doesn't mean that all memory systems take this long to develop, as you'll definitely see, that's definitely not the case. So what we're going to do is follow the development of a typical infant, both in terms of its behaviors and in terms of brain systems. And we're going to see the story it tells about the development of memory. By noting the developmental milestones, we can make inferences about the cognitive development that is going on. Already by the time of birth, our infant brain already contains most, if not all, of the brain cells it will ever have. That number is about 100 billion by the way. In fact, during the very early stages of pregnancy the brain cells are being produced at a startling rate, literally at about a quarter of a million per minute. Wow.

However, what babies lack is connectivity between these brain cells. Literally as the babies interact with the world, these connections are formed. These connections are formed between neurons, and these connections allow the brain to perform ever more impressive feats. Remember our discussion of neural plasticity? Well, a baby's brain is incredibly plastic. The brain essentially wires itself in a way that's consistent with its early sensory and motor experiences. In a sense, the brain ultimately fits the world into which it is born. For example, if a baby was born with just one hand, the brain tissue that would have been used to control the missing hand is used for something else instead, perhaps, for example, it may allow this baby to get more effective use of his feet as manipulators. This is why it is so valuable to expose infants to a range of sights, sounds, touches, smells, and tastes, any sensory stimulation when they are very young. The infant brains ends up forming connections more quickly, and may also form more connections overall, when the infant is exposed to lots of stimulation.

After all, at birth, babies are essentially blind. They're not just squinting because it's so bright outside the womb. They initially cannot see. They have to learn to see, and their visual system develops as a function of stimulation. The first step in the development of vision requires babies to learn something called the light reflex. The light reflex refers to the pupils constricting when they're exposed to light. If a baby is intentionally exposed to intermittent periods of bright and dark, this reflex can be trained to occur in that way. And in that way, it will occur in weeks or months before it would if we just left the eyes up to random acts than polite stimulation.

Developing the light reflex is the beginning of that sensory memory that we've been talking about, and it's so important for vision. So by intentionally training this reflex, the baby really gets a big head start in processing visual input, and that could have beneficial cascade effects for other cognitive development. Although vision almost starts right from scratch after birth, other senses are better developed. Auditory stimuli are present long before birth. But regardless where each of the senses begins at birth, variable stimulation across all the senses can only be a good thing. In fact, virtually all of the typical behavioral milestones that an infant reaches have something to say about the development of memory systems, of course, the memory systems we've been talking about throughout this course.

But there are a couple of early exceptions where some behaviors have a basis in genetics and that are present right from birth. For example, a newborn will automatically root for a nipple and will automatically suck it. Another possible example is turning toward faces, despite the very poor vision alluded to before. Even just minutes after birth, a baby will show a preference to look at faces rather than other objects. Given how little newborns can actually see, this preference for looking at faces may well be genetic, and not completely unlike rooting for a nipple. Babies forming a bond with a primary care-giver as quickly as possible may be the single strongest factor that can ensure survival for that baby. So turning toward faces may have evolutionary advantages, even though a newborn doesn't yet have a visual system capable of seeing in any developed way.

In any case, most other behaviors gradually become acquired as muscles and brain connections develop. And of course these things develop in an almost orchestral manner as muscles become stronger and more refined and as the brain areas that support them become more interconnected and organized, new behaviors become possible. For instance, development of hearing gets underway well before birth. Newborns will already show a distinct preference for their mother's voice over all others, and let's think about what this means. The infant has heard that voice within the mother's womb. It was exposed to those frequencies of sound very frequently and had plenty of time to encode the regularities of that sound. Those regularities could result in preference. This recognition of the mother's voice provides the first clear indication of memory. And in this case it's implicit memory of a mother's vocal characteristics and, of course, an identification of that memory as something familiar and comforting.

It is not surprising that the processes controlling implicit memory are given priority. The baby is being born into a complex world full of all sorts of regularities. For example, some faces and voices come and go, others are much more consistent, and some are linked to events that really enhance the baby's comfort. These are the sorts of things that a baby needs to figure out, and the sooner the baby figures it out, the better.

So let's move on a little bit. Let's move on to 3 days of age. Many babies, by this point, are mimicking some of the facial characteristics of their parents. One of the ways we learn to do things is by watching others and doing what they do. This is called modeling. By 3 days of age a baby's procedural memory system is functioning, and it is learning links between certain muscle movements and stimuli in the environment. In a sense it is learning how it can interact with the environment into which it was born.

Many developmental psychologists stress the relevance of the cognitive stage within which babies learn that their behaviors have effects on the environment. To some extent this can be viewed as the baby forming a very basic foundation for semantic memory. If our semantic memory is our knowledge of the world around us, perhaps it is based on us seeing ourselves as one who is distinct from, but yet can still interact with the world.

To study this, psychologists have come up with some very clever ways of measuring the development of semantic memory, sometimes measuring procedural memory at the same time. Let me give you an example. In a study conducted by Carolyn Rovee-Collier, a ribbon was tied to the foot of infants as they were laid on their backs in a crib. If the baby kicked a certain way, and if they kicked with enough force, then a colorful mobile above their face would move in a way that the babies found entertaining. The study showed that by 3 months of age, babies could learn the link, and they would soon learn to kick their legs whenever the mobile stopped. This demonstrates semantic memory. The fact that babies learned to do the kicking at all is a further example of developing procedural memory. So the procedural memory system that is capable of doing simple modeling after 3 days has already grasped its ability to interact with the world through its actions by 3 months. Procedural memory and semantic memory are already working together.

And as a further example of the social nature of this development, most infants will laugh aloud by 4 months of age. Of course infant laughter tends to cause all sorts of lavish attention being paid to the baby, and the baby learns this fact; laughter is simply another sort of ribbon that allows the baby to get what it likes from the world, just in a different way.

Let's move to 5 months of age. By 5 months of age, babies begin acting uncomfortable around strange people. This is an interesting extension to that notion of feeling more comfortable around, and preferring, the familiar, like that mother's voice I told you about earlier. That is, what begins as a mere attraction to the familiar develops into an avoidance of the unfamiliar. This suggests the development of linkages between memory, the sort of memory systems that allow for perceptions of familiar with emotional circuits that are linked to fear. We're going to discuss these links further in a future lecture that will really focus on the links between emotion and memory. But clearly, the basis for emotional memories, and for the emotional enhancement of memory, begins already at about this stage.

Also at about 5 months, babies will begin to babble. Critically, while they are not speaking any specific language at this point, they are actually babbling in the language that surrounds them. North American babies babble differently than do Chinese or Russian or French babies. The sounds that they make when they babble are derived from the language they have been exposed to. This is another clear indication that their implicit memory system is functioning well. By about 8 months of age a baby will begin imitating vocal units, like mama or dada. By a year, they will begin mimicking the sounds of animals. So this suggests that the linguistic parts of their brain is listening and mimicking, but the system is still pretty basic.

Muscle memory may be more of a constraint here than semantic memory. Some studies are showing that babies can begin using sign language from about the same age that they start to babble, but their ability to communicate and to be understood in sign language during those early months is typically greater than their ability to form understandable words with their mouths. In general, infants given a nonverbal way to communicate will demonstrate memory for stimuli and events far more than was realized.

A very clever experiment has shown that babies remember for longer periods of time the older they get. Remember that ribbon experiment with the mobiles? Well, babies only 2 months old might remember how to move the mobile for about a day, while 3 month olds might remember for 3 to 4 days, 6 month olds about 2 weeks, and 9-month-old babies might remember for about 6 weeks. So as they age their memories are getting more longer term.

The increasing skills in memory correspond to a series of incredible behavioral leaps and bounds as well, sometimes quite literally. If we kind of think about the first few years of life, for example. By 2 months, they can hold their head up. By 4 months they can sit with support, and by 7 months they can sit alone. By 10 months they can crawl, by 11 they can stand alone, and by the end of their first year many babies can walk.

Let's get back to memory. By 18 months babies can point to objects when they are named, thus they have clearly linked words and objects. By 21 months they usually remember their first 10 to 20 words. By 2 years they begin forming two-word sentences, short sentences like "you come," or "doggie barks." It is at around this point where their language skills can suddenly really take off.

By the way, here's a tip. Psychologists suggest that when you are interacting with an infant who's experimenting with language, it is best to listen very carefully to the infant, look like you're listening, and be patient and wait for a response when one is asked for. Be enthusiastic if the infant does try to communicate verbally, and assign meanings to any sound it utters. Also use real words when talking to babies. You should not speak to an infant in baby talk no matter how tempting that might be. And you should never ask a question but then not wait for a reply. And you should not imitate or make fun of sounds he or she makes. Essentially, the more you treat the baby like a grown up, and the more you encourage the baby to speak with both your attention and your reinforcement, the more quickly the language skills will develop. Once again, helping an infant to develop language sooner may give that infant a real head start with respect to the development of any other abilities that depend on language.

Let's take stock for a moment. We've made it to about age 2, and again, that's a time that few of us have any episodic memory of, a time that lies within those clouds of childhood amnesia. As described, this seems to be a period during which implicit learning and the development of procedural memories are reigning supreme. During the first months after birth, infants are getting far more sleep than at any other time in their lives, and the main differences seem to be that they are getting far more REM sleep. Well, more REM sleep fits with that earlier suggestion that the dreams are consolidating procedural memories. So everything is fitting together.

Semantic memory is developing, too, of course, especially in the sense that the baby must learn the facts about the world in which it finds itself, and it must learn how to interact with that world via both movement and communication. These seem to be the priorities of the developing brain and body during this time. However, again, it seems that enduring episodic memories are not formed. Why not? Well, for one thing it seems as though the brain areas that we need to store such memories take about 2 or more years to form. Specifically, the hippocampus and the prefrontal cortex are among the slowest brain regions to develop, neither reaching maturity until about 3 or 4 years of age. Given the relation of these structures to both working memory and the ability to form episodic memories (a relation we're going to visit in depth in later lectures), it is reasonable to think of the maturation of these structures as reflecting essentially a second bi00rth birth. It's the birth of conscious thought and all that comes with it. Luckily this second birth is a little less painful for the mothers.

Of course, the further development of language is also part of the story. Language learning highlights a very important aspect of cognitive development, a notion called critical periods. As children learn any cognitive skill, their brain is literally reorganizing itself as a function of experience with that skill. There are certain periods in development when the brain seems optimally able to reorganize itself if it has exposure to a certain kind of information. Language is like this. When a child is between the ages of 2 and 5 years, the child displays a very powerful ability to learn the regularities of language. A child at this age can learn multiple languages if necessary and with very little effort. However, if the child has not had experience with language before age 5, then they will find it much more difficult to learn. Similarly, those of us who are above age 5, also find it quite difficult to learn a new language.

The ability to learn the regularities of language may reflect implicit memory, but once language is learned it can allow us to learn things in a way that ultimately can lead to both semantic and episodic memories. After all, words represent concepts, knowledge. To use words well, one must have an understanding of the underlying concepts. A baby's vocabulary provides at least a crude reflection of how much they know, and this vocabulary grows at just an astonishing rate during the years from 2 to 5. Semantic memory seems to be developing very well during this time. This is perhaps most apparent in the fourth or fifth year when the child's favorite question is, "Why?"

Just think about that innocent little question. It's not just a word, why. Really it is a request for knowledge, for understanding. It is a direct plea from a system that wants to understand the world better. When you provide an answer, you are feeding the child's semantic memory. So as the semantic memory develops between the ages of 2 and 5, and as the hippocampus and prefrontal cortex mature, we begin to see evidence of some developments that are intuitively linked to the potential to form episodic memories.

Let's talk about those a little bit. As early as 18 months of age most children learn their own name and, at this time, the first indications of struggles for independence also emerge. For example, a child at this age may begin to defy his or her parents by refusing to do things they ask, and they may struggle if they are forced to do something that they really don't want to do.

At about 3years of age, children can describe their dreams. This is important because dreams share certain tendencies with autobiographical memory. That is, they often feature the child within some mentally created world in which events occur. This, of course, suggests that working memory is able to perform the sort of mental simulations that are associated with episodic memory. The year between 3 and 4 years old might be especially important for the development of a sense of self. At about 3 and a half years, children begin to play cooperatively with others, and that suggests some level of empathy or mental modeling, the sort of thing we would expect working memory to underlie.

At this age, children also show the first signs of being self conscious. For example, children will get angry at this stage when they are laughed at or otherwise made fun of. By 4 and a half years of age, children will begin to negotiate with other children, and that literally implies their ability to weigh the relative advantages and disadvantages of some course of action for themselves. By about 5 years, children can play games that involve rules, but they very much like to win these games, and they quite typically are willing to cheat to do so.

Of course the tendency to try cheating is relevant because deception is generally viewed by psychologists as a high-level ability, an ability that some animals never reach. If you do it right, cheating can allow one to gain benefits for oneself without the cost of social consequences. But of course, doing it right is key. And a strong ability to create a mental world that includes the consequences in the minds of others, well that's what you need to deceive well. Clearly children of about 5 to 6 years of age are beginning to play with these sorts of cognitive abilities. Fortunately, we don't have to rely totally on developmental milestones to understand the development of a sense of one's self, because this is actually an area where some relevant experiments have been performed.

A very important procedure that's used at this age is something called the rouge test. The rouge test works as follows. As children are playing or are otherwise distracted, a small patch of rouge, rouge makeup, is put on their face. One can almost imagine a mother coming over, as they do pretending to lick their hands, and clean something off the child's face. But what they are really doing is applying a little bit of rouge, and then they leave the child alone.

Later the children are exposed to a mirror, and the question of interest is how they react to their reflection in the mirror. Less than one year of age, all children treat the mirror reflections as another social playmate. They think it's another child. They do not recognize the reflection as themselves. Of course, they do not try to touch the rouge. However, by about 18 months of age, half of the babies do touch the rouge mark, and I mean the rouge mark on their own face. So when they are confronted with their reflection, it seems that they know that that's them that they are looking at. That number, by the way, climbs to about 65 percent by two years of age, at least according to classical studies. More recent studies suggest the proportion ma climb even higher. So by 2, the rouge test suggests that they have some sense of their self. At about the same time, again as I mentioned, babies are learning their own names, and they're beginning to exert independence, and the rouge test suggests they are also gaining a sense of themselves and what they look like in a mirror.

Interestingly, there is a period from about 14 to 20 months of age where many babies will actively avoid their own reflections in mirrors. It is as though they are learning that the reflection is not another baby to play with, but they have not yet figured out what it is. So the reflection takes on some alien quality that they would rather just avoid. However, once they recognize the reflection as themselves, they sometimes become quite enamored with the mirror. Some of us never lose that.

So we've now formed a pretty clear story of the development of memory systems, one it's one that explains the phenomenon of childhood amnesia. For the first 2 years of life the brains of babies spend much of their time learning the regularities of the environment, and they do this using implicit learning processes that seem to be in place right at birth. Procedural memories also develop at an astonishing rate during this time, and they allow the baby to develop an ever increasing behavioral repertoire.

Between years 2 and 5 years old the brain structures underlying working memory and episodic memory slowly mature. As they do, language skills and an understanding of the self and self-identity develop along with it. Our first childhood memories occur somewhere within this range as we get a sense of who we are and are we embed that sense of "self" within other events we can describe and remember. By about 5 years old, all of the relevant memory systems appear to be online and functioning. In fact, part of functioning well may even involve the pruning of some of the earliest memories, which might also contribute further to childhood amnesia. But once these memory systems are finally in place, the clouds of amnesia finally dissipate for good. The memories we form thereafter can be retained long-term, and we begin piecing those memories together to create an ongoing sense of self.

There is one interesting caveat to this story of development. Throughout I've been focusing on how connections are formed between nerve cells in reaction to stimulation, and these connections support the development of memory. However, there is another equally fascinating aspect of brain plasticity that is part of development.

During periods of intense brain development there is also evidence of so-called synaptic pruning, and that's a removal of weak brain connections to make space for more new connections. This sort of pruning is also happening during infant development, and it goes hand in hand with the creation of new connections. Brain biology giveth, and brain biology taketh away.

By the way, this sort of pruning also occurs during the teenage years, and apparently that's allowing the brain a final burst of learning before it settles into a form that is less plastic in adulthood. And that's a good thing. After all, once we're all free from the challenges of drastic internal transformation, we can at last take on more fully the challenges of external life.

In the next lecture, we're going to take a break of sorts, as we put the development of human memory into a really broader perspective. We're going to look at surprising features of memory across the animal kingdom.

Animal Cognition and Memory
Lecture 13

The available evidence suggests (but does not prove) that apes, elephants, birds, and even octopuses possess all of the same memory systems as humans and therefore may possess a sense of self. The specifics of how these systems function, however, could be quite different. Researchers face 2 challenges: how to test animal memory without the help of language and the ethical implications of self-awareness in animals.

They say an elephant never forgets, and chimps have proven themselves surprisingly adept at simple memory games—often more adept than humans. These studies are not only interesting but also raise questions about what is and is not uniquely human.

Our memory is critical to our sense of self; imagine not remembering anything that had happened in your life prior to this moment. Our memories give us a sense of a continuing self that exists across time and space. A catastrophic loss of memory results in a catastrophic loss of self, as seen in advanced cases of Alzheimer's disease.

While some animals possess something like language, none use it the rich way humans do. They would not have anything like the phonological loop but may have something like the visual-spatial scratchpad, or even a type of working memory based on smell instead.

Researcher Gordon Gallup tested for self-awareness in animals using mirrors. When confronted with a mirror, most animal species were initially afraid of this "other" animal. Some became **habituated** to the image once they realize it is not a threat. Some animals, including chimpanzees, used the mirror to inspect themselves. When subjected to a rouge test—having their faces marked with rouge without their knowledge—chimps react much like human babies do, curiously poking and prodding the colored spot. This implies awareness that the self has changed and, by extension, that chimps have a sense of self.

Gallup's experiments have suggested an ever-growing list of animals that pass the rouge test: nearly all of the great apes; dolphins and killer whales; elephants; and some bird species. Animals clearly have procedural memory (e.g., you can train a dog to fetch) and something like semantic memory (e.g., your cat knows that the sound of the can opener means food). The memory systems in doubt are working memory and episodic memory.

A wide range of demonstrations have implied that animals do have episodic memory. "What-where-when" memory has been demonstrated for a number of bird species and in lab rats as well. Scrub jays appear to be able to worry and anticipate future events, just the sort of planning humans use their working memory for. Furthermore, lab rats with damaged hippocampi seem unable to form episodic memories, just like humans.

Perhaps most startling of all, planning and deception—the hallmark of cognitive development in human children—have been discovered in an octopus housed at the Seaquarium in Miami, Florida. It not only waited until its room was dark and quiet to sneak out of its tank and steal lobsters

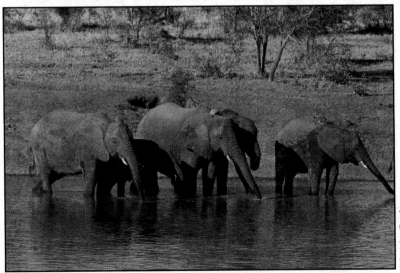

© iStockphoto/Getty Images.

Elephants seem to have excellent memories, particularly a herd matriarch, who seems to serve as a repository for generational memory.

from another tank nearby, it actually hid the shells, as if trying to cover up its crime.

The cliché about elephants is true; they have especially impressive memories. The matriarch of an elephant clan must lead her clan to good water sources year after year, season after season. What is more, elephant matriarchs are able to adapt this process to different weather patterns. The brains of elephants are actually more densely packed with neurons than human brains and have more folding, so they can store more information.

What are the larger implications of this evidence? First of all, if animals have a sense of self, they are more like us than we have previously believed, and this may have broad ethical implications for their use and treatment by humans. Scientifically, the fact that the same sorts of memory systems operate within so many different species points to the importance of these systems for survival. ∎

Important Term

habituation: An acquired tolerance for a stimulus in an environment.

Suggested Reading

Hiby and Weintraub, *Conversations with Animals.*

Kendrick, Rilling, and Denny, *Theories of Animal Memory.*

Spear and Miller, *Information Processing in Animals.*

Questions to Consider

1. If you have or know someone with a dog, does the dog seem to hold a grudge if it is, say, left alone for a while? The dog might not be pleased at the time, but does it hold a grudge when the family returns? If not, do you think that means dogs forgive because they so easily forget?

2. The elephant with the best memory is the matriarch of the herd. Unfortunately, this matriarch also tends to have the best tusks. As a result, ivory poachers often go after the matriarch. If you think of this at the herd level, what are the consequences for the long-term memory of the herd? In what ways do human families experience analogous losses?

Exercise

If you have a nonhuman animal of any sort in your home, place a mirror in front of it and see how it reacts to the reflection. Based on its reaction, try to understand what sorts of memory processes might be occurring. If you have contact with young children, especially those younger than 3 or 4 years old, try the same thing. How are the reactions different? How easy or hard is it to make inferences about memory based on these reactions?

Animal Cognition and Memory
Lecture 13—Transcript

An elephant never forgets. That's what they say. Do you know why they say that? Apparently it has a lot to do with elephants that destroy villages that had encroached on their lands, or elephants that specifically target individuals who had caused death to their family. These acts of revenge apparently occurred sometime after the act and gave rise to the retaliation, hence the saying. Do elephants really have such strong and emotionally charged memories? Well, we'll get back to elephants, but let's begin with an interesting study of chimpanzees.

In a Japanese study, chimps were pitted against humans in a game of memory. To understand the study, it's first important to know that chimps can learn the numbers 1 through 9, and they can learn how to press them in order, even if those numbers are presented at random locations on a computer screen. Actually, they can get really good at it. With that clear, here's how the game works.

In the first part, the numbers 1 through 9 are presented at random locations on a computer screen. They are presented very briefly before they're covered up by solid squares. The task is to remember the location of the numbers, and then to show this memory by touching each square in the right order. So you press the square that corresponded to the 1, then the 2, then the 3, then the 4, etc., up to 9. Can the chimps do it? You bet they can do it. They do it very well. They seem to have no problem whatsoever in knowing where each number was. And they can do it really fast, too. Kind of like this. [Professor whispers a beat.] And the numbers come up, and they just go.

Now how about humans? Well, they don't do it nearly as well. Usually humans can get up to about the numbers 5, 6, or 7. That sound familiar? Yes. Seven plus or minus 2, and not getting to that "plus 2" most of the time either. Very seldom can humans get all 9 in order like the chimps can. In fact, the chimps are even more impressive in the second part of the game. This time only some of the numbers are shown like, for example, 2, 4, 5, 7, and 9. The numbers are once again covered over by squares, and the task is to touch each square in the order of the numbers that had been presented, starting with the lowest and going up. Once again, the chimps do very well. And the humans do only OK. And we're not just talking about one bright chimp either. There were a number of chimps involved in the study.

In fact, if you were to see video of this game in progress and, by the way, such videos are available online, the really amazing thing is the fluency with which the chimps perform the game. When the squares appear, the chimps respond immediately and with a seemingly sure confidence, just bang, bang, bang, bang. The humans? Not so fluent; not so confident. It really seems that in this game we cannot claim any kind of superiority.

Obviously such studies are interesting. In fact, they are fascinating. And they make us think about animals a little differently, and sometimes they make us think about ourselves a little differently. And sometimes they make us think of ourselves a little differently. Heck, we all love it when the underdog wins and, when it comes to animal species, any species that betters us intellectually, well that sure has the feeling like an underdog winning.

But from a scientific perspective, these sorts of studies are interesting for two other reasons. First, whenever we study any cognitive ability like memory, we are always interested in the extent to which that ability is or is not uniquely human. In the case of memory, this is an especially interesting question given that some of the memory systems we have been talking about—working memory and episodic memory especially, have links to our subjective impressions of our self and to consciousness of self. Could animals have a sense of self, and do they also have the subjective sense of being conscious?

These questions are linked to the second reason why these studies are interesting. Our society very often makes distinctions based on whether an organism is or is not human. Even within science itself, we will conduct certain research procedures on animals that we would never conduct on humans. Is this double standard justified? To the extent that animals share our cognitive experiences, especially the very high-level experiences like the sense of self and an experience of consciousness, our understanding of such issues at least becomes much more informed.

Within this framework then, let's use what we know about memory and use it as a window to better understand animal cognition. Do they have the sense of self that is clearly such a big part of autobiographical memory and many of the experiences we have with working memory? Do they show evidence of episodic memories? If so, what does this all mean?

Let's begin with our human sense of self. Clearly, our memory is critical to that sense of self. Imagine not remembering anything that had happened in your life prior to this very moment. You don't remember your name, where you live, who you know, what you do for a living. You have no idea of the skills you have or the things you like, and you have no memories of past experiences. Do you think you would be the same person?

To a very large extent these are the things that define our own sense of self. Without them, we would feel like an empty human being, like a shell. Our memories are what fill that shell and give the entity within us some sense of a continuing self that exists across time and space. If you have any doubts about the importance of memory to our sense of self, consider what happens to patients suffering from Alzheimer's disease. Initially Alzheimer's patients suffer brief bouts during which they forget who they are, where they live, and what they were doing. However, as the disease progresses, the memory failures become worse and worse.

In fact, patients in the latter stages can no longer recognize family members and, eventually, they cannot even recognize themselves. They have been known to literally looking behind the mirrors to see the person who is looking back at them. A catastrophic loss of memory results in a catastrophic loss of self. We will return to a full consideration of Alzheimer's disease in a few lectures from now.

So let's return to this question then. Do animals have the sort of sense of self that would be necessary for any kind of autobiographical memory? Of course, while some animals possess what could be considered basic languages, none use language in anything like the rich way that we humans do. So we can't just ask them. Note that this also means they would not have anything like the phonological loop that we use when we verbally rehearse items in working memory. If they have any sort of subjective experience, it is more likely visual, like the sort of phenomenon we have described in terms of the visual-spatial scratchpad. How could we know if they have some sort of visual sense of themselves and who they are?

Well, remember that rouge test that I mentioned in a previous lecture? That test was originally created by Gordon Gallup, a researcher from the State University of New York, to test for self-awareness in animals. Gallup created the rouge test after a student of his decided to hang mirrors in all of the cages of a wide range of animals that were housed in their animal research facility. The student reasoned that animals aren't used to seeing their own reflection, and he was curious how they would react. Initially virtually all of the animals reacted to that reflected image as though it was a newly introduced member of its own species. So they might be aggressive. They might be curious, really, whatever would be normal for them if one of their species was introduced into their environment. Some animals continued to always react this way, but most didn't. Most changed the way they reacted in one of two ways.

Some animals, dogs are one example, eventually realized that the reflection was not another dog and, further, that the reflection was essentially irrelevant. It didn't cause trouble, but it also didn't bring anything new and interesting to the context. So over time, dogs simply began to ignore the reflection completely. This is how most dogs react to mirrors they are familiar with. If you have a dog and you have a mirror in your home, you've probably seen this. The process of learning, that process that kind of makes us ignore stimuli, is something called habituation. And it's very much tied to that notion that I mentioned, that the stimuli results in no good consequences or no bad consequences: It makes them just largely irrelevant.

By the way, humans also habituate to stimuli. If you've ever been in an unfamiliar house, you may have, the first time you were there, heard all sorts of creaking. It may be hot water heaters or floorboards or maybe stairs as people were walking on them, all sorts of noises that every house makes. But if you stay in that house for any length of time, those noises would just seem to disappear. They would no longer disturb your sleep. They would just be gone. Again, you've learned that those noises produce no consequences: Nothing positive follows them; nothing negative follows them. And when that happens, our brains essentially learn to just shut out the stimulation all together. It's irrelevant. So this is one way that many animals, dogs included, eventually react to a mirror. It's like the reflection doesn't even exist. In fact, it can be very hard to even get them to look at it. It's like it isn't there.

Other animals, though, changed their behavior in a different way. Chimpanzees, for example, start to use the mirrors as a tool. They started inspecting themselves in ways that are not possible without a mirror. For example, they might look inside their mouths, or they might turn their bodies so they could look at their butts. A funny image, but, hey, you're not kidding anyone if you want me to believe that you haven't done the exact same thing. Anyway, this behavior seems to suggest that the chimps did indeed have a sense of self, and wanted to get to know themselves better.

Gallop formalized this process, and he turned it into something called the rouge test. Let me give you a clearer sense of how the test was employed. In the case of animals he would first familiarize some species with its reflection by hanging a mirror in its cage for a while. So let's say this camera in front of me is a mirror, and I'm a chimp. And I've had this mirror in my cage for quite a while, and I've been allowed to kind of experience my reflection, do whatever I want to do with the mirror. It's there.

Now, if there's some time when the animal, that's me, if I had to be anesthetized for some reason, let's say dental surgery. Well, when I was unconscious, Gallup would place a red mark over one eye and on one earlobe. So let me show you what that might be like. I'm anesthetized, while having these marks put on me, but I don't. I was out cold. And Gallup was very careful to make sure these marks didn't have any dyes that any animal could feel or any scent that they would smell and did not produce any sort of sensation at all.

The anesthetized animal would then be returned to its cage, and its behavior would be recorded once it awoke. The question is how do chimps behave when they wake up? Well, OK. I wake up, and I'm looking around. I see my reflection, and this is the important point. What happens? Well, what happens is this. They become very curious. They approach the mirror, and they begin to touch the dyed spots. In fact, what makes this a nice scientific experiment is you can compare how often they touch these spots to a pair of controlled spots, that is, the unmarked eye and the unmarked ear lobe. And what you will see is that they touch these spots a whole lot more. It is as if they are saying, "What the heck is on my face?" In order to do that you have to have a sense of "my face," and that requires a sense of self. (OK. I'll remove my marks.)

Experiments since those conducted by Gallup have now suggested an ever-growing list of animals that pass this rouge test. This list includes nearly all of the great apes, including bonobos and orangutans and, recently, some lower primates have also passed. It also includes aquatic animals like dolphins and killer whales. Now the test is more complicated in that case. Those animals can't just touch their face like I did, but they turn to the mirror, and they seem to be trying to self inspect in ways that, again, suggests that they're trying to see what it is that's on their bodies, in that case.

By the way, elephants pass, and some bird species passed. If you accept Gallup's test as a valid test of self-awareness, then it seems we certainly are not alone in the sense of knowing ourselves. I should also point out that not all scientists view these results as definitive. Some come up with alternate explanations, but they are certainly fascinating, and they are, at the least, very strongly suggestive of a sense of self.

If some animals do have a sense of self, then they also have the potential for some forms of conscious memory, and that includes episodic memory. I should step back for a moment here to highlight the following. Animals clearly have procedural memory. I mean all you have to do is watch a well-trained dog to know that it can learn new behaviors and execute them appropriately, just as the stimulus context demands. If you go to Sea World, you'll see dolphins jumping through hoops. They learned those new procedural memories. Those weren't even natural behaviors for them. They can even learn unnatural behaviors.

Animals also show clear evidence of something like semantic memory. So my dogs, Lola and Layla the Wonder Dogs, certainly know where their treats are stored, as I mentioned earlier. They know that when we put their seat belts on they are going in the car, and they know that when we sleep in rather than wake up to the alarm, we will be going on a hike. This is knowledge of the world, is it not?

So the main memory systems then in doubt are working memory, which is a whole lot like consciousness and episodic memory, which almost always includes a representation of the self. That is why the quest for evidence of episodic memory in animals is the primary question of interest, and is primarily what we've been talking about. All right. Well, we've talked about the self, but let's talk about episodic memory more specifically. Animals possess episodic memory. Just as was true with Gallup's work, the available evidence is not airtight, but there have been a wide range of demonstrations that do show animals behaving in ways that seem to imply episodic memory. Let me tell you about some of those.

A researcher named Nicola Clayton has recently described some truly fascinating studies of scrub jays. Scrub jays are one of many birds that cache food. A lot of birds do this. When they find food, they hide it. Anytime, when there's a lot of food in the environment, they find what's available, and they hide as much of it as possible. And that of course means they have to remember where they've stored their food so they can retrieve it later.

In one experiment, Clayton provided jays with both nuts and juicy dead worms to store them both. And they did so. Then on subsequent days they first preferentially retrieved the worms, but then after a few days, they switched to the nuts, even though there was still some worms left. The implication is that the jays could remember what had been stored where and when it had been stored. If the worms had been stored for too long, they weren't worth going after.

That sort of "what-where-when" memory has now been demonstrated in a number of bird species, and while researchers are often guarded. They'll call it "episodic-like" memory, it definitely bears all the hallmarks of human episodic memory. Of course, we can't be sure that the jays are experiencing real episodic memory because they simply cannot tell us that they are subjectively experiencing some sort of "movie in their minds," the kind of thing humans associate with episodic memory. That's the sort of thing that we suspect they would need working memory for. However, remember when

I said that working memory is used for all sorts of things other than episodic memory. It's also used for planning and for worrying. I gave you a whole list. Well, let me also tell you this about scrub jays.

Sometime they live in areas where other birds will steal the foods they cache. If they are given food in such an area, then they will look around for thieves. They'll look, in fact, very carefully before hiding any food. This is only behavior you'd see when they are in one of these areas. Again, we can't know what is going on in their little bird brains, but given they do this only when they are in the areas that thieves are, it sure seems that they are making sure that they are not being watched, and that implies that they can also anticipate future events that will occur if they are not careful, if they just stash the food without thoroughly checking for thieves first. That's just the same sort of planning that humans use working memory for.

So many great apes, elephants, and aquatic mammals show behavior suggestive of a sense of self, and birds that cache their food show behavior consistent with episodic-like memory and working memory. Maybe this finding with birds surprised you a little, but actually it turns out that birds are much more intelligent than many of us give them credit for. Some parrots have displayed amazing cognitive feats and are known to be deeply emotional. That term we like to just throw around, "bird-brain," is really not giving birds the credit they deserve once we realized the potential intelligence of birds. Then, to some extent, this may seem like we arrived at the expected list of guests. We talked about the animals that we might most expect to be more cognitively advanced. So maybe some animals have episodic-like or human-like, I should say, memory systems, but just the most advanced. Just the usual suspects.

Well, this is where the story takes an interesting turn. If you will, welcome to center stage, the lowly lab rat. For many humans the rat is sort of the epitome of the nonhuman species, and it certainly is the species we seem most willing to conduct even very invasive research procedures on. Surely the rats have nothing like a conscious memory system, right? Not so fast.

Let me tell you about a couple of experiments. First of all, there's this device that you can use to probe the memory of rats. It's something called a radial arm maze. And it looks like the following. There's an area in the middle, and then outside of that area there's arms that kind of go off. So kind of think of a sun pattern. And there may be 6 to 8 arms radiating from this middle platform. If you put little bits of cheese at the end of each arm, and then you take a perfectly healthy rat and put him in the middle, this is what he does. He'll first go down one arm, and he will eat the cheese. Then he has to come back to the middle. And then he'll go down a different arm, different being the operative word. Every time he comes back, he chooses an arm that he has not yet been down. He does not tend to revisit an arm that he just recently visited, almost as if the rat knows that if, well, there was cheese down there, I already ate it. So no sense going back down that arm. That sounds like episodic memory. That can seem like a strong claim. Perhaps you think I stretched pretty far on that one.

Well, step 2. Remember the following. Remember when I talked about Clive, Clive Wearing, that English musician and conductor? I told you that one of the areas that was damaged in Clive was his hippocampus. It's the structure in the very middle of the brain. As a result of that damage he could no longer form new episodic memories. Data from Clive and from many others provide strong evidence that the hippocampus is critical for forming strong episodic memories.

So, let's go back to our typical lab rat. Let's say we take this rat, and now we intentionally damage his hippocampus, and now we repeat the experiment with the radial arm maze. What do you think happens now? Well, I'll tell you. Start the rat in the middle. He goes down an arm. He eats the cheese. He goes back to the middle. Then what? Well, he goes down another arm, but critically, he makes his choice in a seemingly random way this time. That is, he seems just as likely to visit a recently visited arm as he is to follow a new arm. It's as if he now has no memory of which arms he has visited and which he hasn't. Essentially, by damaging the same brain area that we know is damaged in Clive Wearing, a brain area that we know is crucial for the formation of episodic memories, we have created a rat version of Clive Wearing. Interesting. The lowly lab rat.

Now let's take one step even further afield. All of the animals we have been discussing so far are what are called vertebrates, that is, they all have internal skeletons. On its own that fact need not make them especially impressive but, generally speaking, animals with internal skeletons are often seen as more advanced than those who lack internal skeletons, like worms and snails for example.

But there's one invertebrate that really seems to defy this rule in a way that makes us wonder just how many forms of memory systems can reside within. The animal I am alluding to is the absolutely alien, and absolutely fascinating, octopus. An octopus is truly unlike any other life form. In fact, it can change its color in seconds to match any background, becoming virtually invisible. Even a very large octopus can push its entire body through a very thin tube. Sometimes, having no backbone, can come in pretty handy, and it moves using jet propulsion. But perhaps the most fascinating thing about octopi is that they can be extremely sneaky in a very intentional seeming way.

I mentioned previously that this ability to behave in sneaky and deceptive ways is often seen as a hallmark of cognitive development. I know something about that kind of seems wrong, but if you consider it in terms of working memory, it makes sense. Working memory is the system that allows us to solve problems, to essentially get what we want. Sometimes we want things we're not really supposed to get unless, of course, we can come up with a clever enough plan to both get what we want and get away with it. That would mark a highly complex sort of problem solving.

We know some apes use deception. For example, in a typical monkey troop, different monkeys have different jobs. One job is to scout ahead for food sources and to let the troop know when they are found. Another job is to look out for predators, and really all of the monkeys are really supposed to be alert to predators, and they're supposed to alert the troop when they are seen. Researchers have noticed the following. If you take some stash of food, and you leave it out for the apes to find, most of them (if they find it) will give the "food" call. But some apes will actually sound the "predator" alarm, that is, they will walk up to the food. They will see the food. And then they will signal that a predator is in the area. While all of their troop mates run and hide, these monkeys eat the food. Pretty clever.

Now let's return to our octopus and a very mysterious fish tale. In the Seaquarium in Miami, Florida, lobsters were mysteriously disappearing. The night watchman, himself, was one of the suspects, so he was really determined to clear his name. And yet night after night, under his watch, lobsters went missing, and the night watchman saw nothing. One night he decided to do his rounds especially quickly, much more quickly than normal, and then he took up a position close to the tank close to the tank where the lobsters were.

At some point he thought he saw some movement in the tank, something that didn't look right. So he flipped on the lights. What he saw amazed him. The octopus, that lived a few tanks over, had come out of his tank, walked over the catwalk, and was reaching in and scooping out a lobster. He grabbed that lobster, and he brought the lobster back to his tank. The watchman was amazed.

When they then checked the octopus's tank afterwards, they found a whole bunch of lobster shells, but not just left in the open. The lobster shells were hidden away, out of sight. Everyone who saw this was absolutely sure this octopus knew what it was doing, that it was trying to cover up its crime. Heck, it succeeded for quite a quite a few good meals.

And elephants, let's return to elephants. They are indeed especially impressive. The head matriarch of an elephant clan can have an especially strong memory, as she is in charge of leading the entire clan to good water sources, something she does in a different, effective way depending on the weather patterns. How? Well, the claim is that between her own experiences, typically about 40 years worth, and the things she learned from the matriarch of her own clan, she has learned to remember how different locations react to different weather patterns, so she can effectively steer the clan even in years of drought that could have been decades apart. She remembers the previous drought and steers the clan accordingly. Yes, it is indeed the case that elephants have strong memories. In fact, the brains of elephants are actually more densely packed than human brains, and elephant brains have more foldings so they can store more information. Given how little we know about human memory, it's safe to say that new discoveries about the memory of elephants will be made in the future.

So what are we to take from all this? Well, if one limits the question to one of memory systems, then the available evidence may not prove that animals possess all of the same memory systems that we do, but it is certainly not inconsistent with that notion. In fact, to all but the most critical, it seems likely that animals do possess the same memory systems we do. Rats may even possess episodic memory, and octopi clearly have an ability for deep and calculated thought.

It's important to emphasize that the specifics of their memory systems could be quite different. For example, we rely very heavily on our phonological loop, and we are constantly talking to ourselves within our minds. It is very unlikely that animals do the same. Their working memories are likely more dominated by visual representations, and maybe even other sorts that we don't even have. For example dogs have a very superior sense of smell than we do. Do they remember scents? Do they think in terms of scents? Could they perhaps show self-awareness if the test involved them reacting to their own scent, instead of their own reflection? It's certainly possible. The point here is that by using a test that emphasizes vision, the primary sense used by humans, we may be even underestimating the cognitive abilities of animals.

What about the larger implications of this sort of work? Rene Descartes famously described animals in purely mechanical terms. He thought of them as simple machines, whereas humans were machines driven by souls. For example, centuries of scientific research has been conducted on animals without even using anesthetic. The protestations of the animals were seen as analogous to the squealing tires on a hard-braking car. Sure, it may sound like the car is in pain, but it's really just the sound of rubber under high friction. The car feels no pain and neither do animals. Well, in terms of memory abilities and memory systems, evidence continues to accumulate suggesting that animals actually do have many of the abilities that we have, as well as others that we may not. At a more general level, the fact that the same sorts of memory systems operate within so many different species points strongly to the importance of these systems for survival. And of course, all of these memory systems stem from brains, animal brains and human brains. We've drawn links to the brain at a number of points in this lecture series, but now it's time to go visit the brain more directly. That's our next stop on this tour of memory: the human brain.

Mapping Memory in the Brain
Lecture 14

Thanks to functional magnetic resonance imaging, neuroscientists are creating a map of the brain showing which areas are responsible for which functions. It seems that we use the same brain regions to recall a memory as we used during the original experience; for example, the phonological loop occurs in our language center. The more we learn about brain function, the more support we find for cognitive psychology's theories of memory.

The human brain weighs only 3 pounds but contains about 100 billion neurons, about the same as the number of stars in our galaxy. Although it accounts for only 2 percent of body weight, it consumes about 20 percent of the body's energy. Obviously, it is doing a lot of work.

The branch of psychology concerning the link between cognitive processes and the brain is called cognitive neuroscience. Over the past 10 to 20 years, we have gained some powerful tools allowing us to study these links. The most powerful of these tools is **functional magnetic resonance imaging (fMRI)**.

fMRI is a method for watching blood flow through an active brain. A regular MRI is a common procedure for body imaging; it works much like an X-ray but can show distinctions between different tissue densities, not just between soft tissue and bone, and produces a 3-dimensional image instead of a flat one.

The "functional" in fMRI means that the patient performs some function during the scan. Brain tissue works much like muscle tissue; when an area of the brain is active, blood flow to that area increases. So an fMRI detects where the blood is going as people perform various tasks. Neuroscientists and psychologists have used such fMRI images to create a map of the brain.

The brain can be subdivided into 5 regions: the primitive midbrain and the 4 lobes of the **cortex**.

- The occipital lobe, at the back of the head, is home to the primary visual cortex, the part likely associated with iconic memory.

- The temporal lobe, just above each ear, is where the primary auditory cortex resides; this is the part likely associated with echoic memory.

- The very top of the brain is the **parietal lobe**, and it is especially active when we are processing input from our bodies or spatial information.

- The front of the brain, or **frontal lobe**, is activated during decision making and intentional action.

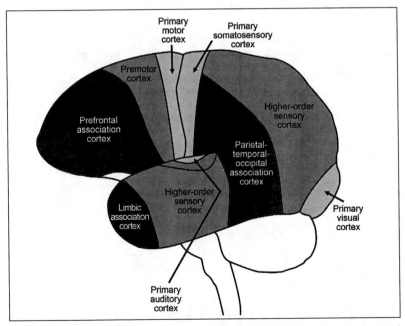

The primary sensory and motor cortex (light areas), higher-order sensory and motor cortex (gray areas), and the 3 association areas of the cortex (dark areas) are co-activated during complex memory retrieval.

The phonological loop, part of our working memory, allows subvocal articulation (talking to ourselves) and subvocal reception (replaying others' speech). fMRI studies reveal that these processes occur in **Broca's area** and **Wernicke's area**, the exact same areas used to produce and understand speech. Another part of working memory, the visual-spatial scratchpad, produces a lot of blood flow in the occipital cortex, which is also used to process visual stimuli.

Using working memory to solve problems involves a more complex process. Scans of people involved in deep encoding show activity in a subarea of the frontal lobes called the **dorsolateral prefrontal cortex** and in the hippocampus, as well as activity in the areas corresponding to what the person is trying to remember. Current theory suggests that the frontal lobes are activating the other regions but that the hippocampus creates the episodic memory by binding the regions together.

Brain tissue works much like muscle tissue; when an area of the brain is active, blood flow to that area increases.

Retrieving episodic memory involves a similar process. For example, if someone asks you where you went on vacation last year, Wernicke's area receives the question and activates the working memory in the dorsolateral prefrontal cortex, which activates the hippocampus. It is not clear whether the hippocampus is activated to retrieve the information, to re-encode it after retrieval, or both. Finally, the areas where the relevant information is stored are activated.

Retrieving semantic memories doesn't involve the co-activation associated with episodic memory retrieval. Instead, areas called the association cortices in each lobe of your brain are activated. These areas are encoded with abstract concepts rather than specific incidents.

Procedural memory resides in a strip of cortex that runs over the top of your head from ear to ear called the motor cortex. Signals originating in the motor cortex are sent through the cerebellum, which refines the information. So the motor cortex controls raw movement, and the cerebellum makes that movement graceful.

One of the most encouraging aspects of all these findings is the extent to which the neuroscientific findings match up with findings from cognitive psychology experiments. The theory of memory emerging from both disciplines seems to be on the right track. ■

Important Terms

Broca's area: The brain region involved in speech production.

cortex: The outer mantle of the cerebrum.

dorsolateral prefrontal cortex: The area of the frontal lobe where current theory indicates that working memory resides.

frontal lobe: The lobe at the front of the cortex involved in decision making, impulse control, and long-term planning.

functional magnetic resonance imaging (fMRI): An imaging process that uses magnets to create detailed images of which areas of the brain are active during certain tasks by showing the blood flow to each region.

parietal lobe: The lobe at the top of the cortex that contains areas for processing sensory and spatial information.

Wernicke's area: The brain region involved in language recognition.

Suggested Reading

Eichenbaum, *The Cognitive Neuroscience of Memory*.

Matthews and McQuain, *The Bard on the Brain*.

Schacter, *Searching For Memory*.

1. Based on what you now know about the brain and about fMRI, if I was scanning your brain while you were imagining seeing a rainbow, which brain lobe would show the most blood flow? If the rainbow then reminded you of the perfect rainbow you remember seeing on that trip you took to Hawaii with a special someone, which areas of the brain would then show increased blood flow?

2. In the movies, mummies always walk in a very clunky and graceless manner. It seems that one part of their brain, at least, does not survive the resurrection intact. Which parts of a stereotypical mummy's brain seem least intact and why?

Exercise

Do some push-ups, climb some stairs, or do some other exercise, and pay attention to how the muscles feel as you work them. Now spend a while thinking about and speaking aloud all the words you can think of that begin with the letter *r*. You're using Broca's area to do this, an area located just above your left ear. Does that part of your brain start to feel sore, like your muscles did when you worked them out? Probably not. What do you think the difference is? When you work muscles, muscle tissue breaks down; then it is built back up stronger than it was before. But when you use brain tissue, you just use it. Brain parts do not get "bigger and stronger" with work; instead, they strengthen by forming new connections, as was the case for hippocampi of London cabbies. So brain tissue is like muscle tissue in some ways, but not in others.

Incidentally, at one point in history people thought brain tissue was exactly like muscle tissue and thus that you could tell which parts of the brain a person used a lot by feeling the bumps on their heads (apparently caused by pressure from the bulging brain tissue). Thus, instead of having your palm read, you could have your head read. If you'd like to learn more about this misconception, look for the term "phrenology" on the Internet.

Mapping Memory in the Brain
Lecture 14—Transcript

Now that we know a lot about our memory systems, how about we go visit the place where they live. It's that really extraordinary place we call the brain. By the way, it's about 6 and a half inches long, about 5 and a half inches wide, and about 3 and a half inches tall, and it weighs about 3 pounds. But the number of cells in the brain is about 100 billion; that's about the same number of stars in our galaxy.

And although our brain just makes up only about 2 percent of our total body weight, it consumes about 20 percent of our bodies' energy. Just transporting all this energy around takes about 3 soda cans worth of blood flowing through our brain every minute. In just one minute, the brain will consume about a fifth of a cup of oxygen from that blood, and almost all of that oxygen, 94 percent to be precise, is consumed by the brain cells in what we call the gray area, and they're the ones who do all the hard thinking work. Something must be going on up there.

Of course, the something we are most interested in during this series is memory, and in this lecture we'll be examining the links between the brain and memory in detail. By the way, the kind of psychology that tries to understand the links between cognitive processes and the brain is called cognitive neuroscience, and it is perhaps the hottest area in psychology research today, the area that is most dramatically increasing our understanding of human behavior.

Why is it having the impact it is, and why now? Well, sometimes scientific progress is a function of the tools that are available to the scientist, and over the last 10 to 20 years, we have gained some new and very powerful tools that allow us to directly watch the brain as conscious participants are performing, really, any task we may ask of them. Moreover, we can do this without having to remove the participants' skulls or in any other manner compromising their well being. Obviously, that provides a definite advantage.

So, I have two goals in this lecture. First I want to describe the tool that has had the largest impact to date in cognitive neuroscience, and that's a tool called functional magnetic resonance imaging. Once you understand how the tool works, I then want to highlight the things that it has helped us to learn about the neural basis of the various memory systems we have been discussing. So, let's jump in.

Functional magnetic resonance imaging, which is often simply labeled fMRI, is a method for watching blood flow through an active brain. fMRI machines combine two powerful technologies. The first is often used all on its own, and is called magnetic resonance imaging. You may have heard of sports figures going for an MRI when a shoulder or some other body part feels sore. Essentially, an MRI is like an X-ray, but with a whole lot more resolution and a whole lot more power. In the case of an X-ray, radiant light is sent through your body, and the light that makes it through is detected on a photosensitive plate on the other side of your body. This light can easily pass through sparse tissue like fat and skin, but it does not pass through denser tissue as well. So the dense tissue, bones for example, leave a shadow on the photosensitive plate. Those shadows clearly show the structure of your bones and allow a doctor to detect fractures or other structural abnormalities.

X-rays only provide 2-dimensional pictures, and that's because light is sent from just one location and measured at another, so there is only one path of light, one image. MRIs differ from X-rays in two different ways. First, they use magnetic resonance as opposed to radiant light. The difference that makes is this. The images obtained from MRIs are much more detailed. Much more subtle differences in densities can be detected. So MRI images not only reveal stark density, like bone versus fat, but can also detect and represent even small differences in densities, like the difference between harder and softer bone, for example.

The second difference is that MRIs use a rotating set of sensors and emitters that ultimately provide many different images from many different angles. This large set of high resolution images is then sent to a powerful computer, and that computer is able to combine these images into a full 3-dimensional model of whatever it is being scanned. When MRI scans are performed on a person's head then it's possible to obtain a similarly detailed 3-D model of that person's brain. So the computer will display the brain exactly as it is, almost as if the brain had been removed, and you were looking at it from any angle you would like.

In fact, you can virtually dissect the brain to look at the structures inside of it, essentially slicing it and seeing what it would look like if you had sliced and looked at it from that perspective. It is truly amazing to be able to look inside the skull with this level of detail without harming the individual in any manner. But it doesn't stop there. What I've described so far is the MRI part of an fMRI. The f stands for functional, and this is the part that allows us to watch the brain in action. Now to really understand this, let's move to the gym.

OK. I have some barbells here. Why? Well it's always nice to dual tasking. Why not work out and do a lecture at the same time? But seriously, if I do arm curls as I am doing now, my biceps are working, and as they are working, as they flex and unflex, the muscle tissue that underlies them burns oxygen. That's why you can feel your muscles burn, and if I were to do this long enough, you would see me start to breathe a little bit more heavily. Why is my breathing increasing when I work so hard? Well, my lungs are pumping oxygen into my blood stream, and my heart is delivering this oxygen-rich blood to my biceps to keep them fed. This is not something I do consciously. Working the bicep just makes it happen.

Here is the fascinating part. Brain tissue works in exactly the same way as muscle tissue does. Remember those statistics I mentioned at the beginning of this lecture with respect to blood flow and oxygen consumption? Well, if we work a certain part of our brain, it also demands oxygen and nutrients to compensate for what is being used. What's more, if we inject a bit of radioactive isotope into the bloodstream, we can detect this radiation and therefore follow the blood. This is the fMRI machine in action. It can literally detect where the blood is going as people perform various tasks. So when we combine these two, an fMRI machine can both provide a very detailed structural model of a person's brain, and it can show you which parts of that brain are demanding oxygen when the person performs various tasks. This literally shows you the part of the brain involved in performing that task. I know I've said this before, but that's pretty freaking cool.

It costs a lot of money to do experiments using an fMRI machine but as their potential became obvious more and more psychologists began using these machines to perform what some label as "brain mapping." That is, they would ask questions like the following. If I ask my participants to silently speak to themselves as we perform an fMRI scan, which part of the brain is demanding more oxygen compared to a situation where I ask them to just relax and think about nothing. Once they find an area or areas they then conclude that this area must be the part of the brain that is critical for silent speech, so silent speech happens here in the brain, hence, the brain mapping.

If this sounds like a bit of a simplification of how the brain performs various tasks, well, to some extent it certainly is. It doesn't really highlight the complexity of what is likely going on, and it really doesn't tell you much about the processes of producing silent speech. But still, it does give you a good sense of which parts of the brain are relevant for various tasks, and that's a really good start for understanding the link between the brain and cognition.

And we have indeed learned a great deal from these brain-mapping adventures. Given that this course is about memory, let's focus on some of the memory systems we've been discussing to see which parts of the brain seem related to them. I'd love to begin by telling you where sensory memory happens, I can't, not definitively at least, because as amazing as fMRI machines are, they have limitations. Their biggest limitation is in terms of their temporal resolution. What that means as that while they can indeed provide models of the brain that have fantastic spatial resolution, that is, very detailed images, it takes the device about 10 to 20 seconds to do so.

So for the functional part to work the participant has to be experiencing the relevant psychological state during that entire period. If you recall, iconic memory lasts about a second, and echoic memory, about five seconds, tops. Neither lasts long enough to be detected by fMRI. Now with that said, we do know that when people are looking at some image versus not looking at an image, the area at the very back of their skull, an area that we call primary visual cortex, is active. So this is probably where iconic memory resides as well. Similarly, when we hear sounds, an area of the brain just above our ears, an area called primary auditory cortex. That's the part that becomes active. Echoic memory likely resides there as well. So although we can't be certain that these are the relevant areas, there is every reason to believe they are.

So what about working memory? Well to explain working memory properly, let me step back a second and give you a general sense of brain structure. Often when psychologists talk about brains they begin by kind of subdividing the brain into five areas. The most primitive brain regions are in the very center of the brain, in the middle of the brain and, in terms of evolutionary development, these are probably the oldest brain areas that we have. They are literally referred to as midbrain. And the midbrain is then surrounded by the cortex. The cortex itself tends to be divided into four lobes when we talk about it.

The occipital lobe I already introduced you to. It's at the very back of the head, and it's especially active when visual input is being processed. So again, this is where primary visual cortex lies, and this is the part likely associated with iconic memory. The temporal lobe lies just above each ear, and it's especially active when an auditory input is being processed. This is the lobe where primary auditory cortex resides and the part likely associated with echoic memory.

The very top part of the brain, and a little to the back, is the parietal lobe, and it's especially active when we are processing input from our bodies, so-called profile perception, or when we are processing spatial information about the world around us. Finally, the very front part of our brain is called the frontal lobe. Whereas those other three parts are really important for processing information that comes from the external environment, the frontal lobe seems more relevant to decision making and to action. This is the lobe that controls our intentional behaviors. Each of these lobes is sometimes further divided when focusing on more specific functions, and you'll see examples of that in a minute.

So back to working memory. Remember that working memory is actually a very powerful memory system, and we use it for all sorts of tasks. Its main component is what I previously described as a virtual reality simulator, some sort of mental workspace where we can combine information usually to solve some novel problem. But we also highlighted two other systems it can call upon, one being the phonological loop, and the other being the visual-spatial scratchpad. Let's begin with these two subsystems and then build our way up to a more complete picture of the structures relevant to working memory.

So we use the phonological loop to essentially speak to ourselves within our mind, and that's a process that is sometimes called sub-vocal articulation. Note that when we talk to ourselves, we also listen to ourselves—at least usually we do. So really there are two processes involved, sub-vocal articulation and what could be called sub-vocal reception. It turns out that the brain areas relevant to these processes are the exact same areas that we use when we're actually producing speech or receiving speech.

With respect to production then, there is an area in the cortex called Broca's area. It is named after Paul Broca, a physician in the late 1800s. At that time Broca came across a number of patients who could show clear understanding of language, but they could not produce speech themselves. So if you asked them to, say, go pick up that vase over there, they would pick it up, just as you asked. Clearly they understood that. But if you then said, "Tell me to go pick up the vase," they could not do so. They would utter words, but the words would make no sense.

Broca did not live in the days of fMRI, so to understand what brain area might be involved with this deficit, he used a much slower technique. That is, he waited for his patients to die. Once they did, he opened their skull and looked at the brains, and each one showed evidence of damage to the area that now bear's Broca's name. This is the part of the brain that we use to produce speech and also the part used when we speak silently to ourselves.

Following Broca's lead, another doctor named Wernicke noticed that some patients also showed the reverse problem. They could speak just fine, but they couldn't understand speech. When these patients died and when their brains were examined, the damage was close to the same area, close to Broca's area, but a little further back in the head. This area is what we now call Wernicke's area, and it's the part of the brain we use to understand speech.

The approach used by both Broca and Wernicke for studying brain damaged individuals is something called neuropsychology. And we're going to talk about neuropsychology in detail in a couple of lectures from now. For current purposes though it's heartening to know that when we now perform fMRI studies on people as they silently speak and listen to themselves, blood is clearly flowing in both Broca's and Wernicke's area. Thus the phonological loop that seems to be involved in the coordinated activity of these parts of the temporal lobe seems to be exactly what underlies that sub-vocal articulation that we've been discussing.

Now let's move onto the visual-spatial scratchpad. Just to remind you, earlier in the course I asked you to do things like imagine some house or a house-like place that you know well and to count how many windows it has. This brought an image to mind, one you could virtually move around as you counted. This is the visual-spatial scratchpad in action. Perhaps not surprisingly, when people do such tasks as we scan their brains, we see lots of blood flow in the occipital cortex, that part of the brain that is at the very back of the head, the part that also lights up when we experience a visual stimulus.

You're likely sensing a trend here, whenever we are internally creating or manipulating something that has a real world analogue, things like speech or vision, we use the same parts of the brain as we would when we're experiencing the real-world version of the same stimulus. The story gets a little more complex when we deal with the manner in which we use working memory to solve various goals. For example, in an earlier lecture I described working memory as a gateway that will allow information into the episodic memory. In general, the notion was that if you think about some experience deeply enough just after it occurs, for example if you organize it, visualize it, associate it with other concepts, then you will be able to increase the chance of that information later being retrieved as episodic memory. So what's going on at the level of the brain in this sort of situation?

Well, it seems that anytime you ask participants to do this sort of encoding while you scan their brain, you see a lot of blood flow in the frontal lobes, especially a sub-area known as the dorsolateral prefrontal cortex. Remember I said that the frontal lobes, that area in the front of the brain where decisions are made and where actions are initiated, is where we do our conscious thinking and problem solving, so really it should be no surprise that it is related to working memory. However, it does not work alone. When encoding information deeply you also see blood flow in areas of the midbrain, especially the hippocampus. You see blood flow in other areas, too, that seem to depend on what it is you are trying to remember. So for example, if you're trying to remember words you may see blood flow in Broca's area and Wernicke's area and maybe even in the visual areas of the occipital lobe, and that would be especially true when people are forming images of the words like I did when demonstrated the method of loci to you.

Current theory suggests that the frontal lobes are essentially activating the brain areas that represent information that working memory is working with. For example, if you are thinking about something we just saw, the parts of the brain stimulated by that experience may be active, but so too may be other areas that working memory is associating with that experience. The hippocampus apparently binds these active areas together and does so in a way that allows them to become reactivated, together, in the future.

Thus, the frontal lobes are creating the experience, but the hippocampus is committing this experience to memory by strengthening connections between active areas. Remember when we said that slow-wave sleep may be important for the consolidation of declarative memory, and that this consolidation process seems linked to activity in the hippocampus. The suggestion from this work is that the hippocampus doesn't just bind areas right after we have some experience but that this process of binding may continue as we sleep and may be orchestrated by the hippocampus.

This brings us to episodic memory. In some sense retrieving an episodic memory reflects the very same processes as those involved in encoding, though with the processes working a little differently. Let's say I ask you where you last went on vacation. This query would be represented by the relevant language processing areas, in this case Wernicke's area, and an answer would be sought by activating working memory, which again seems to be located in the dorsolateral prefrontal cortex. Any connections between the linguistic area and other areas related to that query, for example any areas that the hippocampus had previously linked to "last vacation," could become active and could result in other related information becoming active.

At the same time, the dorsolateral prefrontal cortex also activates the hippocampus. It is not entirely clear what role the hippocampus then plays. Does it somehow help to activate other areas related to those becoming active already? It may, and in so doing, it may aid in the retrieval process. Or perhaps it is active in preparation for again encoding the active information for the future. That is, if some experience becomes relevant, some past experience, maybe this is an experience that is more likely to be relevant on a repeated basis, so maybe we should give it another shot of encoding.

It may also be the case that it is doing both: aiding retrieval by somehow promoting appropriate co-activation of brain areas while also strengthening the links between those areas as they become active. At any rate, the result of all this is that the information in the query becomes a seed that then activates other information previously associated with it. So you think, hmmm, last vacation. And maybe that brings an image of you and a friend on a beach in Mexico, which would likely be reflected, by the way, as activation in the occipital lobe because it's an image. Maybe you also remember doing the limbo. You can almost feel yourself dancing. That would likely be reflected by activation in the sensory cortex in the parietal lobe. Perhaps you also hear the music, the music that was playing as you were dancing the limbo. The music would be reflected by activation in your right temporal lobe.

All of these activations together give rise to your episodic memory of that specific event in your life, and as they become active they form a sort of complex reliving of the experience in your dorsolateral prefrontal cortex, that is, episodic memory. Of course, that may activate Broca's area in your left temporal lobe, to allow you to respond, "Mexico. My last vacation was in Mexico. I remember."

So what about semantic memory? Well, let's imagine that you've taken, in fact, a number of trips to Mexico, let's say 20 or more. Each time you were there, you've noted things about the language, the currency, the music, the culture, the food. So you encode strong links between Mexico and these things, but each time you do, the links each form to other more specific experiences, things like that time when you decided to bury your friend in the sand, for example. They're not so strong.

So if I now ask you to name three ingredients common to most Mexican foods, you might quickly think (that is, you might activate the representations) of tomatoes, lettuce, and some form of corn-based bread wrapper. But because both the concept of Mexico and the concept of Mexican food have been associated with so many other more specific events from specific episodes, there would be no convergence of activation from these concepts to a single specific episode. Instead, you would get the answer without all of the co-activation associated with a specific episode coming to mind.

So to some extent then, semantic memories are actually represented as brain areas activated by association. I sometimes think of it as a convergence sort of process. If I asked you about typical foods of Mexico, then you would activate the concept of "food," then the concept of "Mexico," each of which might then activate other concepts that they are associated with. The concepts that are both associated with would gain double activation, and that might be enough to make them stand out as potential answers to the query.

Suddenly I'm talking about concepts being represented and associated with other concepts. Notice first of all that concepts are different from raw sensory experiences. When I use the word "concept" I am actually referring to the generalized notion of some object or some idea.

For example, imagine a candle. If you see a candle, the actual visual attributes of it, for example the fact that it's cylindrical and has a bright pointy tip, that would stimulate the primary visual cortex, allowing you to "see" those attributes. But after you've seen a number of specific candles from a number of specific angles across a number of specific contexts, your brain is able to represent some general notion of what a candle is and what it is used for. That is, in a sense, your semantic memory of a candle.

Where is that represented? Well, within each lobe of your brain there are areas referred to as association cortex, and we think the role of these areas are to learn these abstract concepts, these generalized notions of things we have experienced. So this, then, would be where semantic memories are.

This is an issue we will return to when we discuss brain injuries and the memory problems that can result. So let's leave it there for now, but I assure you we will come back to this issue.

This brings us, though, to our last stop on our mapping-memory-of-the-brain tour, and that would be procedural memory. Remember, procedural memory is all about coordinating muscle movements. Two brain areas seem especially relevant to procedural memory. First, there is a strip of cortex that runs over the top of your head (if you had headphones on, [it's] where the strip of the headphones would be). This area is called motor cortex, and when any behavior is initiated, this part of cortex seems to be the source of that behavior. It's activated first. So if you decide to move your arm, for example, it seems that your frontal lobes stimulate a specific part of your motor cortex, that part associated with your arm, and that part of motor cortex sends the signal onwards towards your arm.

Now, if that was the whole story, then all of our movements would be very crude, kind of like how we imagine zombies, or mummies, or our friend Frankenstein, who we were talking about earlier. However, the signal is sent through the cerebellum, and the cerebellum is the part of our brain that makes our movements graceful, located at the very back and bottom of the brain, under the brain, near the back.

Maybe some of us are more graceful than others, but we are all actually pretty graceful in our movements. Stubbed toes and things like that are really exceptions to the rule. This seems to be the job of the cerebellum to orchestrate very fine motor movements, and thereby, allow us to move our muscles in a way that's both smooth and effective. So when we are learning some new procedure, like dancing for example, maybe we want to dance the waltz. It's likely our cerebellum is doing most of the fine tuning as we practice.

Wow, we really covered a lot of ground in this lecture. I have turned you all into cognitive neuroscientists. But one thing that is really cool about all these new findings is the extent to which the neuroscientific findings match up with the theories and ideas that came from cognitive psychology experiments.

Cognitive psychologists were not particularly interested in the brain when performing these experiments. Instead they were interested in the processes of thought and, through empirical research, they were able to identify specific components of memory. The fact that these components map so well onto specific brain areas is really quite encouraging, and that suggests that the story of memory that is emerging from both seems to be on the right track.

Our understanding of these basic memory processes seems sound, and being able to link processes onto brain structures makes that understanding even more complete. In the next lecture, we'll look at the rise of efforts to model this complexity of the brain and get at the processes and how they interact more fully.

Neural Network Models
Lecture 15

Cognitive neuroscientists have created biologically inspired neural networks—computer models of the brain—to tease out the complexities of human brain functions in general and memory in particular. These models indicate that no single neuron is particularly important to cognition; it is the relationships among them that matter.

Neurons, or nerve cells, are covered in branches, through which they send and receive signals from many other neurons. These signals may be excitatory (on) signals or inhibitory (off) signals; when the number of excitatory signals received outweighs the number of inhibitory signals received, the neuron fires—that is, it sends a signal out. The entire complexity of cognition arises as a result of interconnected networks of these very simple signals.

Early psychologists tried to emulate and predict the behavior of the brain through mathematical modeling, but the mathematics became far too complex. Now, biologically inspired **neural network** models attempt to imitate this behavior through the interaction of neuron-like processing elements.

Neural network models, and cognitive models in general, are computer-based models that not only try to simulate the intelligent behavior of humans, they model the physical brain systems underlying that behavior. The basic building blocks of these models are artificial neurons called **nodes**. Real neurons operate by sending electrochemical signals—on and off, positive and negative. Nodes signal via electricity rather than chemicals.

Neural network models contain input nodes that create the signals and output nodes that respond to them. When input nodes are on, we assign them a value of 1, and when they are off, we assign them a value of 0. Each signal the output node receives is then given a weight. The output node sums the number of 1s and 0s it receives from all the input nodes, multiplies them by the weight, and compares the result to a threshold value. If the total weighted input is greater than the threshold value, the node fires. If less, it does not fire.

The first neural network models hit a snag when trying to model the "exclusive or" function—making an output node fire when just one of the inputs was active but not both. This problem stopped neural network models in their tracks for almost 30 years, until scientists began building larger networks. In a large network, no single node is especially critical; it is the overall pattern of firing that matters. This is called **parallel distributed processing**.

> **In a large network, no single node is especially critical; it is the overall pattern of firing that matters.**

Scientists are reasonably certain that the brain represents concepts in a distributed manner for 2 reasons: First, an fMRI typically shows many different brain areas activated when a person tries to perceive or remember an event or concept. Second, when people suffer brain damage or the brain ages, they do not lose concepts; instead, these people show a pattern of memory loss termed graceful degradation, a general impairment of memory not specific to any one concept.

Via connections between nodes, initial input to a neural network causes changes to the states of other nodes within the network in a feed-forward structure. Virtually all neural network models therefore use parallel processing: Nodes are not considered one at a time; the input to all the nodes in the network is considered simultaneously. The nodes all change their activations—or don't—together. In comparison, the chip in your computer or cell phone likely uses serial processing, making changes to one node at a time.

Neural network models all need to be trained before they work effectively. Input is given to the network; then the difference between the output produced and the output the scientists wanted is determined. The scientists adjust the connection weights accordingly and run the text again, repeating the process until the error is reduced or eliminated. Because these are parallel distributed networks, a change to one node changes all other nodes, so the training process can be very complex, just like the human learning process.

Models that integrate slow learning systems and fast learning systems re-create the relationship between the association cortex and the hippocampus. Therefore, they can produce output that models our semantic and episodic memory systems, respectively.

All of these models are still just theories for the most part, but we can use them to run tests that advance our understanding of memory systems. ∎

Important Terms

neural network: A system of on/off switches interconnected in such a way as to imitate the structure of the brain or a region of the brain.

node: A switch in a neural network that stands in for a neuron.

parallel distributed processing: A form of neural network processing where the overall pattern of ons and offs is more important than the on/off state of any one node.

Suggested Reading

Gurney, *An Introduction to Neural Networks*.

Haykin, *Neural Networks and Learning Machines*.

Konar, *Artificial Intelligence and Soft Computing*.

Questions to Consider

1. Imagine a simple network with 2 input nodes and 1 output node. Can you come up with values for the weights and for the output node's threshold that would allow the network to solve an "or" problem, meaning that the output node should fire any time the first or the second input node is on?

2. Many students are interested in psychology because it seems more human and real than, say, chemistry or physics. These students go on to become professors of psychology. Can you see why this tendency might work against a widespread use of computational approaches to understanding the mind?

Exercise

The next time you are in a room with about a half-dozen friends, bring up some issues that people can either be for or against, then ask people to raise their hands when they are for a given issue. Notice that there are some people who you will often agree with, others who you will often not agree with, and still others that you are as likely to agree with as not. If you imagine the amount of agreement between you and another as a link between you, that link is kind of like the weight between 2 nodes in a neural network; sometimes this link is positive, sometimes negative, and sometimes it is almost zero. When thought of this way, can you see how weights affect the amount of influence one node might have on another?

Neural Network Models
Lecture 15—Transcript

Imagine I am a neuron. I have many arms that reach out like limbs of a tree. And I use these arms to get signals from other neurons. At any given point in time, a number of those neurons are sending me excitatory signals, and others are sending me inhibitory signals. I essentially listen to those signals and integrate them. I add them up, and if at any time the number of excitatory signals outweigh the number of inhibitory signals by enough of an amount, then I will fire.

What that means is that I will then send a signal to other neurons that I'm connected to. Depending on the sort of neuron I am, I may be sending an excitatory signal or an inhibitory signal. Somehow, the entire complexity of cognition arises from a network of these sort of interconnected neurons sending these very simple signals to each other. Amazing.

In the previous lecture I described recent research that links many of the memory systems we have been discussing with the brain areas associated with each, and that research identifies the what we call the neural basis for cognition. In the current lecture I want to highlight how findings within cognitive neuroscience have supported the development of a brand new way of theorizing within psychology, one that relies heavily on what are called biologically inspired neural networks.

These models try to computationally emulate the interaction of neuron-like processing elements in an attempt to use such models to account for memory phenomena. This work represents the cutting edge of current memory research, and our discussion of it will highlight how it brings together issues of brain processes and issues of brain structure in an attempt to provide a powerful and comprehensive theoretical framework for understanding memory.

The embracing of neural network models in psychology is similar in some ways to phenomenon that happen in many of the older sciences. So for example, in their infancy, many sciences began by testing hypotheses that are based on what we call simple verbal theories. A verbal theory is a theory that is so straightforward, one can state it in a sentence or two, and the predictions of that theory are so obvious that they follow naturally from that verbal description.

Simple theories are great, as far as they go, but as scientists continue to learn more about virtually any topic, they tend to realize that verbal theories can't do everything. For example, when trying to understand the movements of heavenly bodies, Galileo felt that verbal theories would not suffice, and he began relying on mathematics to describe the complex motions he was observing. Galileo was actually criticized for relying as heavily as he did on mathematical theorizing. Many of his colleagues felt that the language of math was too elitist, too academic, and as such it would take the study of the universe too far away from the abilities of common the people to understand.

In the scientific study of memory, we saw that this turn to mathematics was there right from the very beginning. Remember that Ebbinghaus not only conducted experiments, but he also came up with a mathematical formula to summarize the results in his famous forgetting curve, for example. Moreover, memory phenomena are so complex that the kind of mathematics needed to address most topics might be far more complex than even what Ebbinghaus had in mind. As our tour of the brain and its relation to memory showed us last time, the behavior of our memory systems results from complex interactions of brain systems.

In fact, I was actually simplifying these interactions, when I presented the primary players involved in various memory phenomena one by one. In reality, anytime we ask people to use their memory, we see a number of different brain areas becoming active at the same time; the story we developed last time highlighted only the most prominent player for each memory systems we've studied so far.

The universe inside our heads is every bit as complex as the universe beyond our atmosphere. If we really want to understand the complex links between brain and memory systems, then, we may also need to embrace new theoretical tools capable of capturing this complexity. Mathematics may be important, but more than simple formulas, it may be computer-based simulations that are helpful.

This is where neural network models, and cognitive modeling more generally, come into play. These models represent current approaches to a field that many know of as "artificial intelligence." That is, they describe computer-based models that not only try to simulate some sort of "intelligent" behavior that humans are capable of, but they do so in a way that also simulates both the structures and the processes that underlie human cognition.

The goal, then, is to predict and account for human behavior, but the approach is to do so by building a model of the brain systems that's assumed to underlie the behavior. Thus, these models become simplified versions of the brain systems that inspire them, and they aim to reproduce the critical aspects of those brain systems in a manner that produces an overall theory of cognitive processing. It's for this reason that we often use the term "biologically plausible" in conjunction with these neural network models. They are not verbal theories; they are not even mathematical theories, not of the type that Ebbinghaus had in mind. But rather they are computer-based models of the structures and processes that occur in the brain. Somewhat like an artificial heart is a model of real heart, these models are assumed to be models of our brain systems.

Of course, don't expect to order an artificial brain anytime soon. I would love to say that psychology as a whole is moving in this direction. But if I imply that it would be inaccurate. To model brain systems in this manner, a scientist needs to understand biology, psychology, computers, and mathematics. That's a tall order and, as a result, the scientists that perform this work make up a relatively small but determined group who are literally pushing the envelope of research on memory in this way. Their successes will likely be critical to making this sort of approach more common in the future of psychological research.

So, let's enter their world and let's get a sense of what they do and how it can provide a better understanding of memory systems. As you might expect, if I try to get too detailed, things are going to get messy fast. That is, to use these systems in a research context, one needs to start using math, and sometimes rather complex math at that. Rather than turn this into a lecture about mathematics and computers, my goal is to give you a general sense of cognitive modeling. Those of you who find this area interesting and would like to learn more, I direct you to the additional readings listed in the booklet that came with this lecture series.

So where do we start then? Well, if we are going to model the brain, what is the basic building block of these models going to be? As I highlighted in the beginning of this lecture, the most basic computational system in the brain is the neuron. Neurons, or nerve cells as they are sometimes called, receive their input from other neurons and, based on their analysis of that input, they either send information along themselves or they don't. When a neuron sends information to another then the first neuron is said to have "fired."

The information they receive and send is actually very simple. Essentially it all boils down to one of two chemical signals: One neuron can either send a signal that encourages the next neuron to fire, or it can send a signal that discourages the next neuron from firing. That first kind of signal is called excitatory, the second inhibitory. When these excitatory and inhibitory signals are sent in appropriate ways, the magic of cognitive processing happens.

It follows then that if we want to model this amazing feat, we want our models to be based on some sort of neuron-like processing elements. In this point, it's important to highlight the distinction between the terms "biologically plausible" and "biology." Neurons in the brain are actually little sacks of chemicals that survive in a sea of other chemicals, and they always separated only by thin semi-permeable membranes. The separation of positively and negatively charged chemicals results in things called chemical and electrical gradients. When I speak of signals being sent from one neuron to another, they are sent by releasing chemicals that produce changes in these gradients in highly complex ways.

When we model these neurons, we model the process, but not necessarily the specifics that give rise to the process. Neural network models, for example, do not try to replicate the electrochemical basis of real neurons. Instead they model the neurons in a manner in which information is received and subsequently transmitted. They typically do so by passing along positive or negative numbers, rather than positively or negatively charged chemical elements.

Thus the building blocks of these models are neuron-like elements, often referred to as nodes, and they are considered "biologically plausible" because they model the processes that neurons accomplish, while not modeling the specifics of the biochemical system underlying these processes. Let me give you a taste of how one can combine these simple nodes to produce a system that makes simple decisions. Imagine two input nodes that might, at any given time, be on or off. When they are on, we assign them a value of 1; when they are off we assign them a value of 0. Both input nodes are connected to an output node, and the connections between the input nodes and the output node are given a weight. Let's say that the connection weight between each input node and the output node is set at 0.5. At any time, the input coming to the output node will equal the sum of the state of each node multiplied by the weight between it and the output node.

So let's say now we want this little network to perform what is called the "and" function. What that means is that we want the output node to "fire" only when both node 1 "and" node 2, the input nodes, that is, are both on or firing. All we need for this to work is to set the threshold of the output node to some number bigger than 0.5 but less than 1. So let's say my threshold number is 0.8. Now, when both input nodes fire, the total activation coming to the output node will be 1 x .5 (the weight for each node). So when we sum, .5 plus .5, we get a total of 1. Given that 1 is bigger than the threshold of 0.8, the output node will also fire, indicating that both input nodes are on.

If only 1 input node was on, the summed input would be just 0.5. The other would be 0.0 x 0.5, and that would be zero. So that would not be enough to raise above the threshold, and it would not be enough to make the output node to fire. That's the general idea of how these computations are done. Weights are multiplied by activations, and then these weighted activations are summed across the input units, and this sum is compared to a threshold that we are modeling, and basically if it sees the threshold then some very simple decision can be made or not. These sorts of very simple simulations were first carried out actually in the late 1950s, and the networks created at that time were something they called perceptrons. By the way, perceptrons hit a snag when trying to model something called the exclusive-or function. That is—and you can try to do this yourself and see if you can set up numbers— how do you set up weights to make an output node fire when just one of the inputs is active but not both so that the input node must fire whether input node 1 is on and 2 is off, or vice versa, but not fire if they are both off or both on. It turns out it's impossible to set up a type of mathematics that will do that, and the problem stopped neural network models in their tracks for almost 30 years.

The solution came about when people began to build larger networks. We can connect sets of nodes together to model brain systems, and then we can connect up these brain systems to model performance. For example, one of the models that rejuvenated interest in neural network models was a model of reading development that was originally proposed by Mark Seidenberg and Jay McClelland in the 1980s.

That model contained a set of nodes assumed to represent the spelling of words, that is, their visual features. Another set was assumed to represent the sound of those words, that is, their phonological features. The challenge of the model they were investigating was to see if they could somehow train it to provide a proper sound representation for both regular words (like "pill") and exception words (like "yacht"). By exception I mean the sound, not just the sounded out version of the spelling that would by y-a-ch-t. They wanted to say the right sound, yacht. They wanted to trace the development of that ability within their model and, ultimately, they wanted to relate their findings back to the development seen in childhood reading skills.

The spelling of a word was represented as a very specific pattern of neural firing across the so-called "spelling" nodes. These nodes would be seen as analogous to the neural tissue that might exist in the occipital lobe, the lobe that deals with visual input. Thus, when representing a given word, some of these nodes would be on analogous to a neuron firing, and some would be off.

No single node is especially critical. It's the overall pattern of firing that matters. In Seidenberg and McClelland's model, there were 105 nodes used to represent the spelling of just short of 3000 monosyllabic words, 30 of which represented the onset of the word, 27 represented the vowel, and 48 represented the ending sound, or what is sometimes called the coda. Thus a given word was represented by 3 nodes firing, one that represented the onset, one that represented the vowel, and one that represented the coda. ke-aa-t: "cat."

The concept of a distributed representation can seem a little complex at first, but when we think about it a little it a little, it's really not such a foreign idea. For example, if when you watch TV, how are concepts represented? Well, they are represented across a fixed number of so-called pixels or little points of light. Many high-definition televisions use a grid of 1920 by 1080 pixels, a total of just over 2 million pixels in all. Each pixel lights up with some mix of 3 colors, a combination of red, green, and blue. But here's the really important point. No single pixel tells you anything about what is being shown on the screen at any given time. The image that you see is determined by the pattern of light across the entire set of pixels.

Scientists are reasonably certain that the brain represents the concepts in a similarly distributed manner, and they are convinces of that for a couple of reasons. First of all, when people see some event or remember some event, it's typical to see many different brain areas activated as they perceive or remember. So if they see an apple, for example, that does not cause a single neuron to fire; it causes a whole distributed pattern of neurons to fire.

Second, when people suffer damage to their brain or when their brain ages and neurons die, for example, we do not see them losing particular specific concepts. They don't suddenly forget what a tree is or what a car is. They don't have that part of semantic knowledge just suddenly gone forever. Instead they tend to show a pattern of memory loss that's termed "graceful degradation," a general impairment to memory that is not specific to any concept.

Now think back to your TV. Imagine that your TV somehow suffered damage to its pixels. Let's imagine that 1 out of every 10 pixels suddenly stops working, and that these defective pixels are randomly broken. What would be the result? Well, the picture would not be as good as it was. It would be somewhat degraded. But it would be a very general degradation. Your TV certainly would not have lost the ability to display certain concepts. Instead you could still see what is being shown fine. Every concept would be a little degraded, but none would be lost. This is what is meant by graceful degradation, and it is a general characteristic of distributed representations, one that seems to mimic the effects of damage on human memory.

So now we have models that represent information in a brain-like manner across a set of brain-like nodes. Where does cognition come in? Well, cognition is often described as information processing, the altering of information into different forms as it is processed in a cognitive system. So if we return to Seidenberg and McClelland's model, for example, that model would begin with a representation of the letters of a word and then via connections between the nodes, that initial representation would cause changes to the states of other nodes within the network.

Specifically, this particular network had three layers of nodes that were organized into what is sometimes called a "feed-forward" structure. The bottom layer contained the nodes that represented the spelling of the words. And as I mentioned before, there were 105 nodes in this layer. Every node in that layer was connected to each of a 100 nodes in a middle layer. They are sometimes called a hidden units. That layer was not associated with a specific kind of representation. Instead it performs more of a re-mapping function. These hidden units are very important. The nodes in this middle layer, the hidden units, are then connected to each of 61 nodes in the third, or so-called output layer, a layer of nodes assumed to represent the sound of the word. A word could be represented at the letter level, the pattern associated with that word would pass activation to the middle layer, the so-called hidden units, via connections that weight those activations. Based on the input that each node in the middle layer receives, it may or may not then pass activation on to the sound layer, with that activation again being weighted by the connections between nodes.

Based on the activations they received, nodes in the sound layer would either become active or not, and the overall pattern of active and non-active nodes would represent the sound that the model produced when presented with that specific letter pattern. If this sounds like the description I gave you earlier of neurons receiving input and then either sending output to other neurons, or not, well great. That's the idea. That's what we mean by biological plausibility.

Two things to now note about all of this. The first is the character of the processing. Virtually all of these models use what is termed parallel processing. What we mean by that is that the nodes are not considered one at a time, with each one being changed or not at a single given point in time. Instead, the input to all of the nodes is considered simultaneously. And based on the state of the nodes in the layer before them, and then the nodes, they get that state, the activations of all the nodes in a given layer changed together, or don't change. Again, depending on the input they receive.

So we have a mass changing of a number of nodes at once. That's what's called parallel processing, and that's yet another example of mimicking the sort of processing that we believe to be true of the brain. Most computers that we use are serial devices. They make changes to information in a one-at-a-time manner, and this is basically true even when they have two or more parallel processors. The brain, though, is a parallel computing device. It changes lots of information at once in a single step. So once again, the models are trying to simulate the kind of processing that occurs in the brain. So there are distributed representations, and there is parallel processing, and that's why these models are often referred to as parallel distributed processing, or PDP, models.

On to the second noteworthy point. I described information flowing from the word nodes to hidden units in the middle, to the sound nodes. But how does the network know how to produce the right sound for a given word? This is really where the hard work comes in with respect to these models. The models all need to be trained before they can work effectively. In the case of the model I described, training would mean presenting a word and initially letting the model produce any sound it wished. So it produce a sound in a rather arbitrary way. But then we compute the difference between the pattern that it produced and the pattern that we wanted it to produce, and the difference is a quantification of the error in the response that we wanted. We then adjust all the connection weights between the nodes, and we do so in a way that will reduce this error.

There are different algorithms for doing this. In fact, those algorithms are so important that they themselves have become a little bit of a sub-area in this pursuit to try to find the best algorithms. In all cases, though, the concept is the same. It's like when little Sammy reads the word b-i-g as "beg," and we say, "No, Sammy, not beg, big." The hope is that Sammy then adjusts something within his reading system so that in the future, the proper pronunciation will occur. In neural networks, the thing that is adjusted is the weights, the connections between the nodes. Does that sound familiar? Neuroplasticity. Connection. Of course all words use the same set of weights, so when you change things to enhance the pronunciation of one word, that will affect the pronunciation of other words. In brain terms then, when we adjust the impact that one neuron has on another, that will affect all of the processing contexts in which that pair of neurons play a role.

What that means is a change made to enhance some specific processing simulation has more general implications. As you can imagine, then, getting that algorithm right is a major area. As suggested, it literally has spawned an entire separate research effort that involves people trying to think up and compare different algorithms to see which one produces, first of all, strong performance but also one that seems to map on to the different algorithms that the brain may be using.

The Seidenberg and McClelland model that I have highlighted throughout this talk is a model of reading. Previously I've described reading as a dance of a sort between the procedural memory, the memory we use to speak words, and semantic system, that ties words to the meanings.

But what about other memory systems, especially episodic memory? Can these sorts of models also describe our rich memories for episodes? Probably the most advanced neural network model of human memory is the model proposed by Randy O'Reilly, a professor at the University of Colorado in Boulder. O'Reilly's model of the brain combines what he calls slow learning systems and fast learning systems. The slow learning systems are intended to model association cortex. According to this model, this is where the patterns that underlie durable long-term memories reside or, better said, are re-created. The fast learning system is identified much more directly with the hippocampus. This system is able to very quickly represent new information and, during the process of consolidation, it's able to repeatedly represent that information in a manner that essentially trains the slow-learning cortical systems.

For something to become well integrated into the cortical system, it needs to first be represented in the hippocampus, maybe even across multiple episodes. If I ask you what the capitol city of Florida is, and assuming that you know the answer is Tallahassee, you are retrieving that information from your cortical system, but the information got into your cortical system thanks to repeated encounters with it in your hippocampus.

The system in O'Reilly's model can also work in reverse. If you are recollecting some episodic memory, the relevant information that is stored in the cortical system is loaded into the hippocampal system. There, it can be combined with other information to effectively re-create the initial episode. So the hippocampus is critical for episodic-type memories, and the cortical system is critical for semantic-type memories, but of course episodic memory utilizes information from the semantic system, and things get into the semantic system via episodic memory. It's a true network, and that's why network models hold such promise.

So O'Reilly's model essentially performs the sort of processing that I told you about when I discussed episodic and semantic memory in the mapping memory lecture. This is a realization of the promise of these neural network models. And, in this sense, the model provides a working theory of the processes and representations that give rise to memory phenomena, and it does so in a way that mimics the sort of processes and representations used by the brain. That said, the approach that I have been highlighting in this lecture so far represents an attempt by psychologists to produce a theoretical and computational model. The goal is to produce a model that is sufficiently complex to capture very rich interactions between brain systems, the brain systems that give rise to memory phenomena.

In many ways then this is still a relatively pure academic pursuit. These models are still just theories for the most part, theories that can make predictions we can test and to advance our understanding of memory systems. However, there are some relevant points one can take away from this. For example, O'Reilly's work on fast versus slow learning systems suggests the following. The fast learning system, the one that underlies episodic memory, is relatively prone to error. It's fragile. Sometimes that system simply fails to provide an answer to some query.

For example, maybe we are retracing some route to an old friend's house, and we get to an intersection. As we look both ways, we simply cannot consciously remember going left or right. Our episodic memory has failed us. What do we do? According to O'Reilly's model, we should literally trust our intuition. What sometimes used to be called "woman's intuition" or, as manly men like to say, we should go with our gut.

In O'Reilly's model, the "gut" is the slow learning system. It may have represented our past travels in a way that does not support episodic memory and yet does support a general sense that one direction feels right. When all else fails, we should trust that sense. So if you want just one take-home point to remember from all that's happening in neural network models, you could remember it as this: "Use the Force, Luke."

Learning from Brain Damage and Amnesias
Lecture 16

Damage to specific brain areas related to memory can give rise to very specific functional deficits, deficits that take a real human toll. Studying these patients demonstrates the importance of memory systems to our ability to interact with our world. Studying patients with brain damage has also helped neuropsychologists better understand how the brain executes the various functions related to the different memory systems.

Neuropsychologists are doctors who treat patients who have suffered some form of brain injury. They also study such patients to discover links between the brain and behavior. Patients who have suffered brain damage often show complex behavior patterns; one memory system may be damaged while others are fine.

The famous case of musician and conductor Clive Wearing demonstrates what happens when a person has damage to his frontal lobes and his hippocampus. Clive cannot retrieve any episodes from his life before the damage (a condition called **retrograde amnesia**), and he cannot form any new episodic memories (a condition called **anterograde amnesia**).

Clive hasn't actually lost his episodic memories. From imaging studies, we know that the frontal lobes play an important role in the initiation of action, and retrieving memories is a form of action. We see similar retrieval problems in patients who have undergone frontal lobotomies—the severing of connections between the frontal cortex and the rest of the brain. Less extreme versions of retrograde amnesia are quite common and usually short-lived. A concussion causing swelling of the frontal lobes commonly causes **temporary graded amnesia**, where the person first has no episodic memories, then slowly regains them, starting with those furthest in the past and moving toward the present.

Anterograde amnesia was first linked to hippocampus damage because of an epilepsy patient known as HM. HM volunteered for experimental surgery to remove his hippocampus and amygdale in an attempt to stop his severe and frequent seizures. The surgery worked, but it also caused anterograde amnesia.

Both Clive and HM retained functioning working memories. You can ask them questions, and they will try to answer, although their memory problems may prevent an accurate response. Their semantic memories are also intact. They still know things about the world, and they can show that knowledge either declaratively or nondeclaratively. Both Clive and HM also retained their procedural memories, but the interesting thing is that HM and other patients with anterograde amnesia can learn new procedures.

The interesting thing is that ... patients with anterograde amnesia can learn new procedures.

Another form of memory loss related to brain damage is **agnosia**, meaning "lack of knowledge." Those who suffer from it show a disconnect between their ability to see and hear versus their ability to understand what they are seeing and hearing. So a person with agnosia might see a glove on a table and not understand what it is but can identify it when seeing someone put it on. This is semantic memory—knowledge of the world and the things within it.

Agnosias demonstrate how once memories are created and stored, we use them to interpret what we see, feel, hear, taste, or smell. People with agnosia tend to have damage to cortical areas surrounding the primary cortex of the affected sense. There is an especially interesting form of agnosia called **prosapagnosia**, the inability to recognize human faces. Prosapagnosia occurs when the fusiform gyrus is damaged. We now believe this area is critical for forming holistic perceptions—that is, perceptions based on how collections of features occur together.

Neuropsychological cases can be especially interesting when one finds 2 syndromes that are essentially opposites of one another. Patients who suffer from **Capgras delusions** can recognize objects or people just fine, but the things they recognize do not feel familiar to them. They may report that their spouse has been replaced with a duplicate, for example. Since familiarity arises from implicit learning, this disorder reflects failure of nondeclarative memory in a context where declarative memory is working fine.

Tourette's syndrome is a disorder of procedural memory, ranging from the well-publicized blurting of obscenities to simple tics. Patients with Tourette's are slower to acquire procedural memories. By comparison, patients with HIV/AIDS may show a decreased ability to execute procedural behaviors. Both conditions negatively affect a brain area called the **striatum**. In contrast, patients with obsessive-compulsive disorder have enlarged striata. ∎

Important Terms

agnosia: The failure to comprehend the meaning or function of things otherwise correctly and accurately perceived.

anterograde amnesia: The inability to form new memories after a triggering neurological event.

Capgras delusions: A failure of memory that allows a person to recognize objects or people they have encountered before, but recognition is accompanied by a strong sensation that those objects or people are unfamiliar.

prosopagnosia: The inability to recognize faces, despite being able to recognize other objects without difficulty, caused by damage to the fusiform gyrus.

retrograde amnesia: The loss of memories from before a triggering neurological event.

striatum: A brain region associated with procedural memory.

temporary graded amnesia: The temporary loss of memory of events leading up to the triggering neurological event; the victim's older memories return before the more recent ones, and events immediately before the event may never return (e.g., a concussion patient may never remember being hit on the head).

Baddeley, Kopelman, and Wilson, *The Handbook of Memory Disorders*.

Cermack, *Human Memory and Amnesia*.

Emilien et al., *Memory*.

Questions to Consider

1. The current approach to dealing with extreme aggressive behavior is to tranquilize the patient with drugs. In what ways is this actually a worse solution than, say, a frontal lobotomy?

2. Would you rather have retrograde amnesia or anterograde amnesia? Why?

Exercise

Sometime when you are out, pretend (if only to yourself) that you have no memory of your past at all. How many of your interactions would be different? Pick a time of day—say, 2 pm—and think what it would be like if anything that happened after that time was lost completely. What would you have lost over, say, a 3-hour period?

Learning from Brain Damage and Amnesias
Lecture 16—Transcript

Welcome back. In this lecture we are going to leave the research labs for a while and, instead, we're going to play doctor. In the last few lectures I've told you about links between brain systems and memory, but I've done so in a way that seems rather academic. This seems to be here, that seems to be there, and here is how we might try to simulate it all using neural network models. All that is cool, but in this lecture I hope to put a human face, or actually several human faces, on the relation between brain and mind, all in the context of memory.

I told you, we were going to play doctor, and that's because the field of psychology that we are going to visit is a field called neuropsychology. Neuropsychologists are doctors who treat patients that have suffered from some severe form of brain injury and, in so doing, they get a clearer indication of the link, again, between the brain and behavior.

For many years psychologists have lesioned or, in some other way, damaged the brains of animals in an attempt, again, to understand the relevance of specific brain areas. While those studies can be informative, they always come with a shadow of doubt. We know that human brains are far more complex than the brains of animals, and we don't know if what is true of the rat is also true of the human. How can we be sure? The findings of neuropsychological patients give us one way of doing just that. So let's dive in a little deeper and see what we learn.

Let's begin with the famous anecdote of a Swiss doctor named Edouard Claparede. Claparede worked in a hospital that included patients suffering from various forms of amnesia. One female patient at that hospital could remember events from her youth just fine, but she could no longer lay down any new memories. Each morning Claparede would greet her, and each time she would not remember ever meeting him before.

One morning Claparede had a little pin in his hand, and as he shook her hand to say good morning, he intentionally pricked her with the pin. The next day the patient again did not recognize him, but as he reached out his hand to shake her hand, she pulled her hand back. She did not want to shake his hand although she couldn't say why.

This example shows the complex behavior patterns that can be seen from patients suffering with brain damage. One memory system may be damaged, while others are fine. This patient, for example, could retrieve old episodic memories, but she couldn't form new ones. However, she clearly could form some sort of new memory, one that could aid her in avoiding pain, but did so without any conscious sense of what she was doing.

At this point in the course, you likely do not find this complexity as surprising, at least not as surprising as you might have earlier. You now know that there are a variety of memory systems, and that different systems support us in different ways. So it's not really surprising that damage to the brain might affect some of these systems more than others. So armed with our current knowledge of the brain and how its links to memory, let's see some other patients and put some of these pieces together in the context of real people.

Let's return to a character we met a little earlier, the musician and conductor named Clive Wearing. Clive was a very high functioning artistic man until an infection [caused] by herpes encephalitis produced a very high fever that essentially cooked the neurons in several parts of Clive's brain. The two sites of damage that I want to focus on most are damage to his frontal lobes and damage to his hippocampus.

Let me also highlight two distinct memory problems that Clive lives with. First, he cannot retrieve any events from his life prior to the fever and, second, he cannot form any new episodic memories for events that occurred after his fever. Often patients have just one or the other of these problems. Clive has both. And that is why Clive is essentially living in the moment for every moment of his life.

Clive's two memory problems are separately linked to the damage to his frontal lobes and his hippocampus respectively. So let's take them one at a time. First, let's address Clive's inability to relive episodes of his life that occurred prior to the fever. This form of amnesia is termed retrograde amnesia, retro as in old, like retro clothes or retro music. It's likely the case, by the way, that Clive hasn't really lost those memories, instead he just likely has trouble retrieving them. They're still there. He just can't get at them.

From imaging studies we know that the frontal lobes play an important role in terms of the initiation of action. His frontal lobe damage likely prevents him from initiating retrieval processes. If you never start a retrieval process, you can never ultimately experience a memory, even if the memory is there. It's just like that mayonnaise hiding behind the pickle jar: It may be there, but if you don't look for it, you won't find it.

Can we really conclude all of this simply because brain imaging shows that the frontal lobes are active when people retrieve? Well, there are other results that also support that interpretation. For example, you've likely heard of frontal lobotomies, which is literally the severing of connections between the frontal cortex and the rest of the brain. Why did anybody permit such a procedure to be performed on their loved ones? It sounds pretty extreme.

Well, some people with mental disorders simply become aggressive, to themselves, and to anyone that gets too close to them. In the day before widespread use of tranquilizing drugs, the only thing to do with such patients was to tie them down, 24 hours a day. There were special chairs called restraining chairs for exactly this purpose. So imagine now that this is your family member, and a doctor mentions to you a new procedure that will make the aggression simply disappear. They will no longer have to be restrained. Sounds pretty good I would think.

A frontal lobotomy does exactly that. Like retrieval, aggression must be initiated, and when the frontal lobe is disconnected, it simply is not. It should not surprise you to learn that the patients who underwent these lobotomies have poor memories, and they often prefer to engage in habitual behavior: watching TV, playing card games they know well, or smoking. Those seem to be their favorite past times. But of course they are no longer aggressive. That was a big plus at that time.

Less extreme versions of retrograde amnesia are actually quite common, though they're typically short-lived. In fact, you or a close loved one may even have suffered from it at some point in your own life. Have you ever been hit very hard on the head? Typically when somebody suffers a concussion, there's a swelling of the brain, and that includes a swelling of the frontal lobes.

In those cases, it's quite common that people who suffer from these concussions will initially have little memory of themselves, but then slowly they regain their memories, beginning with those furthest in the past and, eventually, recovering memories up to the last bit of time just prior to the concussion. Some patients never recover the last few hours prior to the accident, but otherwise their memory is fine. Given this progression, this sort of amnesia is sometimes called temporally graded amnesia.

Memory recovery may indeed take some time, and patients can find this time uncomfortable, especially when interacting with those who know them well. Imagine not knowing someone who treats you like a friend or a lover. It will likely be a little odd. But as the patient becomes exposed to retrieval cues, memories are recovered, and often recovered memories then cue the recovery of more memories, making retrograde amnesia a typically short-term problem. It's really only in cases like Clive's, where the damage to the frontal lobes is permanent, that it becomes a much more enduring problem.

So now let's move on to Clive's second memory problem, his inability to lay down new episodic memory traces. This form of memory loss is called anterograde amnesia, where anterior is a fancy word for forward. It is a forward-acting memory problem, one that prevents the formation of new episodic memories.

Clive's anterograde amnesia is most certainly linked to the damage to his hippocampus, which is a structure we've already discussed at several points in this course. We know that the hippocampus is critical as relevant to the transfer of information from working memory to long-term memory, both at the time of encoding and afterwards at the time of consolidation. In fact, we initially learned about the importance of the hippocampus, not from Clive, but from another neuropsychological patient studied decades ago. His name was HM.

HM is a special kind of neuropsychology patient because the damage to his brain was performed surgically, and that allows a much clearer understanding of the damage and the behavioral issues that it causes. Now why would anybody have parts of their brains surgical removed? Well, it's yet another story of the lesser of two evils.

You see, HM initially suffered from a very severe form of epilepsy. It was one that resulted in him having upwards of about ten grand mal seizures a day. So literally, at any moment, HM could experience a seizure that would ultimately result in him dropping to the ground, becoming unconscious, and having his entire body convulsing. Given this, he hated to even leave his home, and he was willing to consider any procedure that might prevent these seizures from happening.

Seizures are caused by what we call negative feedback loops in the brain. A brain area on, say, the left side of the brain sends a signal to a mirrored area on the right, and that signal is bounced back to the left side, the originating spot. The signal then keeps going back and forth, back and forth. As it does so, it strengthens. It becomes stronger. So imagine this electrical signal becoming stronger, and stronger, and stronger, as it goes back and forth. Literally at some point, the brain short circuits. That results in a loss of consciousness. In fact the convulsions that you see are due to the motor areas in the brain that we mentioned that literally control our bodies, and that the electrical activity that is now surging all through the brain is causing random activity in those motor areas, which are then passing this random activity on to the muscles they control, and that results in the kind of spastic muscle movement that we think of when we think of seizures.

Given all this, the process for preventing such seizures is actually straightforward. One needs only to remove the brain areas partaking in this negative feedback loop. Doctors weren't exactly sure which areas were producing HM's seizures, but they suspected the midbrain regions, so they removed the hippocampus and the amygdala from both the left and right sides of HM's brain, again, a very nice clear surgical removal of brain tissue.

The good news is that the seizures stopped, and this was good news indeed, and we need to stress that. HM could now leave his house and experience the world. The bad news is, that just like Clive Wearing, HM could no longer lay down any new episodic memories. If you met him, you could have a perfectly good conversation with him as long as it wasn't about recent events, but the moment you left the room, and the moment he thought about something other than you, you would be completely forgotten. If you walked back into the room, HM would insist that he had no memory of ever meeting you before. This sort of damage, by the way, is well depicted in the movie *Memento*, a movie I highly recommend, especially now that you guys all know so much about memory. I think you'll find it very interesting.

So clearly, though, a functioning hippocampus is critical to the formation of episodic memories, and it's important to highlight that while the formation of episodic memories is impaired, many other memory systems are clearly intact. For example, unlike Clive Wearing, HM has no trouble reliving memories that were encoded prior to his surgery. We assume this is the case because HM's frontal lobes were not affected by the surgery. So while the hippocampus is needed to form new episodic memories, it would be incorrect to view it as the home of episodic memories. Patients with damage to the hippocampus, or even no hippocampus at all, can still experience episodic memories.

By the way, both Clive and HM also clearly have a functioning working memory. As I said, you could have a conversation with either Clive or HM. You could ask them questions, and they would try to answer. Depending on the question, their memory problems may get in the way. For example, if you asked them how high could you reach sitting on a camel, that thing we talked about earlier, I expect HM could probably work his way to an answer, because he could rely on past episodic memories. Clive might have trouble, and that would depend on whether the needed information is episodic or semantic memory. Does he know how tall a camel's back is? If he just sort of knows that, if it's in his semantic memory, then maybe he'll do fine. But if needs to remember a specific instance of standing beside a camel, he just won't be able to do that. HM still will.

Within the confines, though, of the memory problems, both of these gentlemen can think just fine when they are in the moment. Their working memory is intact. As I just implied, their semantic memory system is also intact. With respect to semantic memory, they still know things about the world, and they can show that knowledge either declaratively or nondeclaratively. So for example, if you showed them a toothbrush and asked them what it was, they could tell you. They could also tell you in a sort of nondeclarative way by simply brushing their teeth each morning. Clearly they understand the function of a toothbrush if they can use it properly.

Now let's talk about procedural memory. Procedural memory is perhaps an especially interesting story in the context of these amnesias. First, both Clive and HM clearly retain their procedural memories even after the brain insult. Clive, in fact, can still play the piano, and he can play it very well, and he can sing, and he can conduct. He can also still read and write. I mentioned to you earlier that he writes in his journal constantly. In a more mundane sense, both Clive and HM also care for themselves. So they know all the procedures that you need to know in terms of cleaning and getting dressed for that sort of morning ritual that we all engage in.

But what is perhaps even more interesting is that patients like them, patients suffering from anterograde amnesia, can also learn new procedural memories. Procedural learning seems to still be intact. One procedural learning task that's been studied in some detail is called mirror line tracing. Imagine the outline of a medium sized star within the outline of a slightly larger star. Patients are given a pencil, and they are allowed to see a mirror reflection of the star and of their hand with the pencil. But they can't see their hand directly. So they are seeing everything through a mirror reflection. And they are now asked to draw within the lines, so that they are tracing between the two stars as they do so.

Initially this is a very difficult task because one has to learn to reverse all the directions of your actions given you are seeing a mirror reflection. When healthy participants are given this task, they also find it initially challenging but, with practice, they get better and better. But here is the interesting thing. Amnesiacs also get better and better. And in fact, their improvement is very much similar to the improvement you see in healthy adults. So each day they improve while they insist that they have never performed this task before.

If all this makes you think back to Claparede and the patient that would no longer shake his hand, Bravo. This is exactly what was going on in that example. The patient learned not to reach out her hand after just one experience of being stuck with a pin. She couldn't explain her behavior consciously because she did not recall the episode that shaped it, but shape it, it did.

So the amnesias then represent problems with episodic memory, but are there also other neuropsychological cases that show specific damage to other forms of memory? Yes there are. And the one I want to focus on and spend a bit more time on next is a pattern of damage that goes under the term agnosia. The word "agnosia" means a "lack of knowledge." And those who suffer from it, clearly show a disconnect between their ability to see and hear relative to their ability to understand what it is they are seeing or hearing. In his book, *The Man Who Mistook His Wife for a Hat*, the author Oliver Sacks describes one male patient who suffered from a visual form of agnosia.

Let me give you an example. That patient was shown a glove, kind of like this. I happen to have one right here. It was just held up for the patient, like this. And the patient was asked what it was that he was seeing. The man was not allowed to touch the glove; he could only look at it. And that'll be important, as I'll tell you in a moment. But when he was asked to think aloud about what he thought it was as he looked at it, he would say things like the following. He would say, "Hmmm. Well, there seems to be these five pouches. They're different sizes." Now, obviously, he couldn't touch it. I'm touching it, but he could not touch it. And he would look at this and say, "What could that be?" Well, maybe this could be a purse that one might use to carry coins of different sizes, so you could put bigger coins in the thumb hole, which is bigger than the other ones. Obviously this patient didn't even view it as a thumb hole seeing this as a purse.

When I first read about agnosias I found them completely fascinating. This guy can clearly see the glove. He's describing it. In fact, he can see well enough to read the small print without any trouble. This patient reads all the time. His problem is not a problem with vision; it's a problem of connecting what he is seeing to things he has seen in the past. This is semantic memory, our knowledge of the world and all the things that are within in.

Somehow this man's perceptual system has become disconnected from his semantic memory.

I say it in this way because he has not lost his semantic memory. If we were to tell him it's a glove, he would exclaim, "A glove. Of course." And, also, as I alluded to a little earlier, if you actually let him touch and hold it, he would recognize it as a glove pretty quickly. If you ask him what gloves are used for, he'll tell you: to keep hands warm. He hasn't lost his knowledge of gloves, but he's lost the access to that knowledge via sight.

When I discuss agnosias with my class there's a demonstration I like to use. It's difficult to give somebody a really clear sense of what it's like to suffer from visual agnosia. But it's quite easy to create the sense of what it would be like to have auditory agnosia. As I'm speaking to you now, your auditory brain, those systems in there that are receiving the sounds. But they almost instantly recode those sounds into words that you know and understand. That latter part again represents your semantic memory, and its linking the sounds to their meaning. What would it be like if that system was not able to do what it does? Well, listen to this sound clip. Notice what you hear. <Audio clip plays.>

So you could hear the sounds just fine, right? Your hearing works just as it should. But all you get is the sounds. You can't translate those sounds into meanings. To do that you would have to learn the language; that is, you would need the semantic memory that allows the translation. This is what it's like to suffer from agnosia. You see things. You hear things. But you just cannot understand what it is that you're seeing or hearing.

I want to take this opportunity to return to a common misconception of memory. It's one I mentioned a little earlier, and it's the tendency to think of memory as a final step of processing. For example in my lecture about transferring information from working memory to episodic memory, the basic scenario was that you encountered some new information, you then worked on encoding it, and if you did everything really well, then it would be transferred to long-term storage, making it feel kind of like that's the last stop.

But what the agnosias show us so clearly is that memory is not just an end point. Once memories are created and stored, they literally affect the way we perceive the world. We use our memories to interpret what it is we see, feel, hear, taste, or smell. Every time we recognize something or someone, it is memory that has allowed that recognition. So memory is as much about forming an experience as it is about holding onto the experience for later. All of this is especially true of semantic memory.

By the way, patients with the sort of agnosia I have been highlighting so far tend to have damage to cortical areas that surround the primary cortex of the effected sense. For visual agnosia, for example, I mentioned that vision is primarily processed in the occipital lobe, the place right at the back of the head. Well, the raw visual signals of vision are processed in the middle of that area. It's a subarea called primary visual cortex. If you damage that area you would literally have trouble seeing properly.

Before going on let me highlight what is going on in that primary visual cortex. In 1981 psychologists David Hubel and Torsten Wiesel of Harvard University won the Nobel Prize for demonstrating that neurons in the primary visual cortex act as feature detectors. That is, each neuron fires when some very specific stimulus, some very specific feature, is present in the environment. For example, a single neuron might fire when a line is present at a 60-degree angle at some very specific point in the environment. Other neurons may respond to different orientations, and still others may respond to specific colors or movement. So the primary visual cortex is essentially deconstructing the visual input into raw sensory features, and then these raw features are then reconstructed by the brain by passing these features up to further processing areas that are sensitive to say certain combinations of features. Thus, the visual scene is broken down and then reconstructed as objects located at very specific spatial locations.

This reconstructed visual input is then passed on to the area around the primary cortex, the area termed secondary or association cortex. This is the area that we think is responsible for recognizing what it is we are seeing. Damage to this area leads to a sense-specific agnosias. That's what we've been talking about. To some extent, very basic sensory memories are apparently represented in these brain regions, and each lobe has its own cortex relevant to the kind of stimulation it deals with.

Sometimes these agnosias can even be much more domain specific than just affecting things that, for example, we hear. There is an especially interesting form of agnosia called prosopagnosia. Prosopagnosia refers to a distinct inability to recognize human faces. To kind of make this clear and concrete, let's imagine that my sister suffered from this, and she was lying asleep in a hospital bed. I might then walk into the room and stand quietly in front of her. Not move, just stand there.

If a nurse were then to wake her up and say, "Hey, Look who is here." When she looked at me she might not be sure who I was at all. She would sense the familiarity of my features, which is likely the result of her implicit learning, but she might not explicitly recognize me. She might be thinking things like the following: "Is this someone I know from work? Maybe this is a TV star or a rock star? Or maybe it's my brother?" All of these options would seem possible.

As soon as I spoke or moved, she would recognize me right away. But based only on the visual features of my face that recognition would not occur. So the conscious declarative memory is blocked, but a general sense of familiarity remains. We're going to be talking about this familiarity in detail in subsequent lectures.

Prosopagnosia occurs really when a very specific part of the brain is damaged, an area called the fusiform gyrus. We now are pretty sure this brain area is critical for allowing us to form what are call holistic perceptions, which are perceptions that are based on how collections of features occur together. So let's think about faces for a moment again. We don't recognize somebody's face based on any specific feature, not the shape of their nose or their lips or their eyes. It's not one feature that defines you by your facial appearance. Rather, it's the way the various features of your face combine. That's what makes us all unique, and that's what the fusiform gyrus seems critical for: allowing perception and recognition at this holistic level this combination of features.

Neuropsychological cases can be especially interesting when one finds two syndromes that are essentially opposites of one another. With respect to the agnosias, a fascinating mirrored disorder to prosopagnosia is something called Capgras delusions. Remember, prosopagnosia is familiarity without recognition. People with Capgras delusions suffer from the opposite kind of state of affairs. They can recognize things just fine, but the things they recognize do not feel familiar to them. In fact, they feel decidedly unfamiliar. Patients with Capgras syndrome who live with a spouse may report that while that person they live with looks like their spouse and sounds like their spouse or somebody close to them often report things like the following. They will say that their spouse is them. The sound of their voice is them. I can recognize them as them. But they don't feel right. There's something about them that feels wrong. They don't feel familiar. In fact, they sometimes become so convinced that this person is wrong that they come up with extreme ideas, like maybe this is a robot, or maybe this is an alien that is somehow within their spouse's body.

In fact, in a few dramatic cases, they have even killed their spouse and done things like removed their heads. Why? Because they want to show the wires or the alien anatomy to convince others that they are not crazy. To the extent that familiarity arises from these implicit learning systems we talked about, this disorder reflects a failure of nondeclarative memory in a context where declarative memory—recognition—is working just fine.

Some disorders also target procedural memory. You may have heard of Tourette's syndrome and perhaps when you think of it you think of patients who suddenly and uncontrollably blurt out obscenities. It turns out that only a minority of patients display that behavior. Most just show some sign of what we would call tics, like compulsive eye blinking, throat clearing, coughing, or sniffing, things like that that occur in the background of otherwise normal behavior.

In addition, patients with Tourette's are also slower to acquire procedural memories. Patients with HIV show a decreased ability to execute procedural behavior, and that suggests some deterioration of the brain system is going on there as well. What do these two health issues have in common, Tourette's and AIDs? They both negatively affect a brain area called the striatum, and that's an area that lies just below the hippocampus. Perhaps this brain region controls learning and performance of procedural memory?

There is further evidence to support this possibility, and that evidence comes from patients with obsessive-compulsive disorder, patients who can't help but obsessively engage in specific thoughts or behaviors. For example, an obsessive-compulsive patient might feel the need to repeatedly check to ensure that the oven has been turned off. And they may have to do this ten or more times to be convinced that it was. What makes these patients especially interesting is that they actually have a larger striatum than is normal. If the striatum underlies procedural memory, these patients should have an enhanced ability to learn and to perform procedural memory tasks, and they do.

It turns out the motor movement itself is very complex, especially when performed with the level of precision and grace typical of human performance. Other brain regions also play roles in the initiation and the smooth execution of behavior, including the frontal lobes and the cerebellum. When those areas become damaged, as they are for example in Parkinson's disease, movements can become much less graceful and harder to initiate. But in terms of procedural memory, it really seems that it's the striatum where most of the learning occurs.

As the various conditions show, damage to specific brain areas related to memory can give rise to various specific deficits, and these deficits can have a real human toll. My hope is that by introducing you to some of these patients, I could communicate the relation between the brain and memory in a different and more human way, one that shows just how important these systems are to our abilities to smoothly interact with our world.

All of these conditions I described represent situations where specific memory systems are impaired, but really these situations all pale when compared to the greatest thief of memory. That thief is Alzheimer's disease, and it will be the subject of our next lecture.

The Many Challenges of Alzheimer's Disease
Lecture 17

Alzheimer's disease is the greatest thief of memory we have ever known in terms of how much it steals and how many it steals from—both patients and their caregivers. Much is understood about the progression of the disease, but little is known about its causes or cure. That said, there are many lifestyle interventions that may slow or prevent disease onset, and researchers are developing technologies to improve quality of life for both patient and caregiver.

Alzheimer's disease is predicted to strike 1 in 85 people globally by the year 2050, and for each patient, there will be another 1 to 3 caregivers whose lives may change almost as dramatically as the patient's. Alzheimer's disease is an entirely different process from age-related dementia. We may lose some memory function as we age,

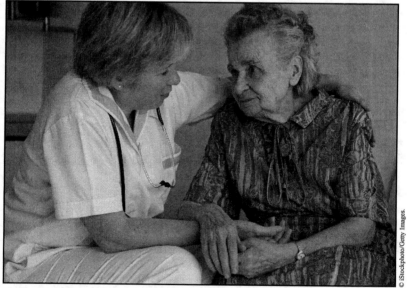

© iStockphoto/Getty Images.

Although there is no cure for Alzheimer's disease, there are many interventions that can improve quality of life for patients and their loved ones.

but nothing nearly as dramatic and progressive as that experienced by an Alzheimer's patient.

The progression of Alzheimer's disease is typically broken down into 3 stages, sometimes preceded by a preliminary stage. The preliminary stage is characterized by mild cognitive impairment, which is worse than average for the person's age and is marked by episodes of complete memory loss. Such symptoms typically, though not definitively, progress to Alzheimer's within 2 to 5 years.

Movement through the 3 main stages of Alzheimer's takes between 7 and 14 years, with only 3 percent of patients living more than 14 years beyond diagnosis. The disease typically strikes later in life, when the patient is 60 or older, although a small percentage of patients show early onset in their 40s or even younger; this version of the disease has a strong genetic link.

The disease targets memory systems, destroying them almost in the order that they were built. At first, episodic memory of the most recently learned information is most likely to be impaired. There will also be instances of almost complete memory loss, a catastrophic loss of personal identity. The sufferer is usually aware the experience is not normal but is embarrassed to tell others about it.

Sometimes during the early stage, patients also become hyperactive. They may have serious insomnia and sometimes just feel the need to get out and walk. This need becomes dangerous when a loss of self-awareness occurs while a patient is walking alone. In many communities, Alzheimer's patients are asked to wear medical alert bracelets for this reason. The patient may also have language problems, both with finding words and language fluency in general. Semantic memory is breaking down. All of this combines to make this disease one that targets social relationships as it targets memory.

In the moderate stage of the disease, patients experience further deteriorations in both semantic and procedural memory. They forget how to brush their teeth, keep clean, get dressed, and so forth. They begin to lose their independence. Language becomes further impaired, wandering becomes even more pronounced, and mood is greatly affected. The patient may also lose disease awareness at this stage, despite all that is happening.

In the advanced stage of Alzheimer's, patients are completely dependent on the care of others. Language is reduced to words or short phrases. Patients exhibit exhaustion and cannot perform even the simplest task without assistance. Sometime during this stage, patients become bedridden. Eventually they will pass away, though typically not from the disease itself.

Available medications can only provide a small reduction in symptoms; they cannot stop or even slow the disease.

Currently, we do not have a good understanding of Alzheimer's disease. We know that patients show abnormal clumps (called **amyloid plaques**) and tangled fibers (called **neurofibrillary tangles**) in their brains, the latter starting in an area called the entorhinal cortex and spreading to the hippocampus. As plaques and tangles spread, they interfere with the functioning of more and more healthy neurons. As neurons lose the ability to communicate, they die.

Available medications can only provide a small reduction in symptoms; they cannot stop or even slow the disease. Lifestyle may play a role in Alzheimer's prevention, as do genetics and early childhood environment. Behaviors with the most potential benefit include a Mediterranean diet, lots of cognitive stimulation (like playing chess and socializing), and medical marijuana. On the flip side, Alzheimer's disease is more prevalent in industrialized areas and among smokers, so avoiding such pollutants may help.

Technology may soon be able to help Alzheimer's patients fill in for some of their lost cognitive abilities. My students and I are currently working on such **cognitive prosthetics**. One example is a GPS-based software system housed in a mobile device like a phone that can detect when the patient is wandering and provide information and assistance to help them get safely home.

An approach like this is more crutch than cure, but it could also aid in the search for a cure when used in combination with drug trials to measure the frequency of wandering episodes among trial subjects. Some people worry that too much reliance on technology may be robbing us of useful cognitive exercise, but in the case of patients suffering from debilitating memory problems, it is hard to see such tools as anything but positive. ■

Important Terms

Alzheimer's disease: A degenerative neurological disorder characterized by memory loss caused by loss of cortical neurons, amyloid plaque formation, and neurofibrillary tangles.

amyloid plaque: Abnormal clumps of beta amyloid protein found in the brains of patients with Alzheimer's disease.

cognitive prosthetics: Technologies that help replace lost cognitive functions.

neurofibrillary tangles: Clumps of tau protein that are found in the brains of patients with Alzheimer's disease.

Suggested Reading

Baddeley, Kopelman, and Wilson, *The Handbook of Memory Disorders.*

Cole and Baecker, *Cognitive Prosthetics for Brain Injury.*

Gruetzner, *Alzheimer's: A Caregiver's Guide and Sourcebook.*

Wayman, *A Loving Approach to Dementia Care.*

Questions to Consider

1. If you saw someone who seemed lost and who you thought might be suffering from Alzheimer's disease, what would be the best way to try to help them?

2. To get a sense of how prevalent Alzheimer's disease is becoming, ask some of your friends if anyone in their family has it. I suspect you will be surprised at how many lives are being directly or indirectly affected.

Exercise

At various points in your day, imagine suddenly forgetting who you are, where you were going, and what you were doing. Imagine how it would feel to lose more and more of your conscious memories, starting from those you most recently acquired backward. So first you forget yesterday, then last week, then last year, then everything from just before the time you met your best friend (at which point that person becomes a stranger), and so forth. At what point in the process do you completely lose the sense of the person you now see in the mirror? When your most recent memory is of a decade ago, does the reflection you see make sense? Imagine remembering nothing from the past 2 decades ... 3 decades ... 4 decades. The actual progression of Alzheimer's is not that orderly, but is it any wonder that Alzheimer's patients become completely and utterly confused and that they lose all sense of who they are and what is happening to them?

The Many Challenges of Alzheimer's Disease
Lecture 17—Transcript

At the end of the last lecture I described Alzheimer's disease as the greatest thief of memory we have ever known. That characterization applies both to how much it steals, and how many it steals from. What's more, those whose memories are stolen are not the only victims.

In fact, the odds are very high that many of you watching this lecture will have either been touched by the disease itself or you know someone who has. In fact, it is estimated that the disease itself will affect 1 in 85 people globally by the year 2050, and for each person directly affected there will be another 1 to 3 caregivers whose lives may also be changed almost as dramatically as the life of the patient herself.

It really is not exaggeration to say that Alzheimer's disease often attacks two people at once, the patient who suffers from it, and typically a very close family member who becomes the primary caregiver. Often it seems that the caregiver experiences a sort of pain and suffering that is in some ways worse than that suffered by the patient.

In this lecture I will be highlighting some of the characteristics of Alzheimer's disease and emphasizing the way it affects the memory of the patient, but also the social bonds between the caregiver and the patient. I have to say in advance, this is not a pleasant story. Alzheimer's disease is progressive and terminal, meaning it only gets worse with time, and it is invariably fatal. As one caregiver states in a documentary on this subject, it is "the long goodbye" as caregivers watch their loved ones slowly receded into themselves and ultimately into death itself.

As horrible as this all sounds, I am also going to try to bring some hopeful and useful information forward. Specifically, I'm going to highlight some of the factors that may help to prevent Alzheimer's disease, factors that you may wish to introduce into your own daily living. In addition, I will use this disease as an example of how technology can be used to provide what some are calling cognitive prosthetics. These are aids that can help patients maintain their dignity and their abilities, and that may even provide tools that can help the search for successful treatments.

Let's first be clear that those who are suffering with Alzheimer's disease are going through an entirely different process than those who simply age. Aging is sometimes referred to as reflecting "normal dementia." As I'll argue in a subsequent lecture, the use of the term "dementia" seems a bit misleading to me. I prefer the expression "cognitive transition" or "cognitive transformation." These terms emphasize a change, a change that's perhaps not entirely unlike the transition from adolescence to early adulthood.

But however one refers to it, the normal characteristics of aging are very different from what happens in a case of Alzheimer's. We may lose some memory function as we age, but nothing nearly as dramatic or as progressive as that experienced by an Alzheimer's patient.

In fact, one of my goals in this lecture, and in this course, is to help you recognize the difference between changes that are normal in the aging brain versus what happens in Alzheimer's. As widespread as Alzheimer's has become, misinformed fear is perhaps even more widespread. Whole neighborhoods can sometimes devolve into gossip and worry over who might or might not be showing signs of "it." Understanding the differences between Alzheimer's and normal aging can relieve some needless anxiety.

So let's look at what actually happens in Alzheimer's. The progression of the disease is typically broken down into three stages, sometimes preceded by a preliminary stage. It's this preliminary stage, which some are hesitant to definitively link to the disease at all. It is a stage characterized by what is termed "mild cognitive impairment."

It's the preliminary stage of mild cognitive impairment that triggers more widespread anxiety. Patients suffering from this sort of impairment do not exhibit symptoms severe or constant enough to be identified as Alzheimer's patients, given the tests that we have to detect the disease. But even though the clinical term is "mild impairment," this refers to memory impairment that is worse than normal for people of the same age. I'll discuss that more in a moment.

Moreover, it is also not clear whether all of those experiencing mild cognitive impairment progress to full blown Alzheimer's disease at all. So, this preliminary stage doesn't show actual symptoms of Alzheimer's and it's not clear it leads to Alzheimer's. Furthermore, although it's likely that those with who did have Alzheimer's disease did previously experience a period of mild cognitive impairment, that's seems not always to be the case. So even someone suffering from mild cognitive impairment may not progress to Alzheimer's disease.

Mild cognitive impairment does typically progress to Alzheimer's, and does so after a period of perhaps two to five years. From there, the disease progresses to early stage Alzheimer's, then moderate, and then to advanced stage Alzheimer's. Movement through these various stages can take between 7 and 14 years, with only 3 percent of patients living more than 14 years beyond diagnosis. This progression through the three stages is the period of the "long goodbye.".

I should also mention that while this disease typically strikes later in life, when the patient is 60 years or older, a small percentage of patients suffer from what's called early onset Alzheimer's disease. This version of the disease has a very strong genetic link.

Patients in their 40s or younger may already begin experiencing the symptoms, and it is not uncommon that more than 60 percent of the deaths in a family may be due to Alzheimer's when the family has a specific gene that's linked to early onset Alzheimer's. But regardless of the age of onset, the general progression of symptoms is the same, so let's visit those symptoms now.

Generally speaking, the disease targets memory systems, and it destroys them almost in the order that they were built up earlier in life. Early on it is the episodic memory of most recently learned information that is most likely to be impaired. Note that this sort of memory loss is also typical of normal dementia. That's one of the reasons it can be difficult to detect the difference from very early on.

However, even during the preliminary stage, that stage characterized as mild cognitive impairment, there will be times when the patient will suffer periods of almost complete memory loss. They literally forget who they are, where they live and, if they happen to be in an unfamiliar location, they may also forget where they are and where they were going.

In essence, it is like they suddenly suffer a catastrophic loss of all of their personal information. And note, this is just the preliminary stage, and there has already been a catastrophic loss of personal information. The practical point is this: You are not showing early signs of Alzheimer's disease when you are having the normal experience of forgetting.

The person suffering a catastrophic loss of personal identity is aware that what they are experiencing is not normal. Unfortunately, they very often react to that experience with an inward sense of embarrassment. They feel like they should know these things, and that they must be stupid not to know them. So a patient may enter a room, for example, where family members are, and they may begin saying something. But then they might suddenly, completely forget who they are and what they were saying. But rather than just admitting this to the people in front of them, people that they suddenly might not even recognize as their family anymore, they try to cover this up, cover up what they are experiencing. Perhaps they try to make some sort of joke or head for a bathroom.

Eventually their memory returns, and they kind of forget about the experience. And if they do remember, their understandable but misplaced shame can prevent them from admitting their symptoms, and that really leaves it up to the family members to detect. What's worse, if a family member does detect something odd, and even if they are proactive enough to book a screening for Alzheimer's, if the patient is not suffering such a bout during the test, the Alzheimer's may not even be detected.

I've been trying to give you tips now and then throughout this course so my tip here is to be aware of these signs of Alzheimer's and to make sure that older people you interact with are also aware of them. These bouts are not subtle. Losing your sense of identity is rather dramatic. If, say, your mother knows about this, and then she acts in a manner that you worry about, you think perhaps she has suffered one of these bouts. Well, perhaps knowing about them will give you an opportunity to figure things out early.

Now that said, even this can be tricky. When it happens, when the patient is in the midst of a bout like that, they're confused, they're embarrassed, they're defensive, and they may not respond to queries saying, "You know, you're right. I don't know who I am right now, and I don't know who you are." Don't expect a calm intellectual discussion. But I do think it's OK to ask a question or two if only to assess if the response is more defensive than you would expect. Once the person is feeling better, maybe then you can talk about it, and then you can try to get a better sense of what may or may not be going on.

These bouts continue into the early stages of diagnosed Alzheimer's and, in both of these stages, mild cognitive impairment and the early stages of Alzheimer's, this symptom, these bouts of memory loss, can become especially dangerous when they occur in the combination with another common symptom. That is, sometimes during these early stages, patients also become very hyperactive. They may have really serious problems sleeping, and they may sometimes just feel they have to get out and walk.

Of course, at a very general level exercise is great, however it becomes dangerous when a loss of self-awareness occurs while a patient is walking. Remember, patients feel stupid and embarrassed when these bouts occur. So let's imagine a patient walking down a road only to suddenly lose all their personal information. They don't know which way to go, and they don't want to ask anyone for help because they feel stupid. So they walk and they walk and they walk without any sense of where they are going or what they are hoping to find.

In fact, in many communities patients are asked to wear bracelets that include information that this person does indeed suffer from Alzheimer's disease, bracelets that also tend to include a phone number and some sort of identifying information. When the number is called, the person answering consults what is usually called a "wandering database," and that database identifies the patient, and it provides information on the caregivers who are then called to pick up their family member. Either that or a police officer comes and brings the patient home.

I'd like you to imagine this though from the perspective of the patient for a moment. You are walking, suddenly you forget everything, and you feel like an idiot. You keep walking and walking, probably doubling back and taking different streets, until eventually someone notices that you are acting lost and confronts you about it, likely offering assistance, so they confront you in a positive way, but still, they confront you.

You must admit to this stranger that you don't know who you are or where you're going. Hopefully they notice your bracelet, and they bring you to an unfamiliar home, and ultimately the police or some family member you may not even recognize in the moment, brings you home. When you arrive at home you see many worried faces, and it is obvious that you have caused all sorts of distress by being such an idiot. At least, that's how it may feel to you. What emotional state this likely produced? What will be the consequences of all this?

Well, if it happens repeatedly, and it will, then sooner or later your caregiver will insist on controlling your movements. Doors will be locked, you will essentially be jailed, and the next time you suffer a bout of memory loss you will find yourself locked in some strange place. If you make a fuss then some person you may or may not recognize will not let you out. You're confused, you're angry, and you may even say something very nasty.

From the caregivers' perspective this is also a horrible situation. In trying to do their very best for a loved one, they are forced to control them and that often results in frustration and anger being direct at them. This is an extremely bitter reward for perhaps the highest demonstration of love and caring.

During this early stage, patients will also often forget recently learned information, even when not suffering one of these bouts of complete memory loss. So a caregiver might ask them to do something when they are at work, and the patient might forget that. And when it's not done, the patient might say something like, "You never told me to do that. You never asked me to do that." You can see how this can lead to frustration and friction within that caregiver/patient relationship.

The patient is also frustrated during this period by language problems. They will have problems finding specific words for things they want to say. Now we all have that problem sometimes, so-called "word-finding errors." But it's worse with Alzheimer's patients. They experience this much more commonly, and they also have language fluency problems in general. Their semantic memory is breaking down. All of this combines to make the disease one that targets social relationships also as much as it targets memory. In fact, that's one thing to take from: that's the realization of how important memory is in terms of supporting strong social relationships. When memory fails in such a catastrophic way, it can take down even our closest social relationships along with it.

Eventually the symptoms become worse as the patient moves into the so-called moderate stage of the disease. From a memory perspective, this is where we begin to see further deteriorations in both semantic and procedural memory. Patients forget how to brush their teeth or good hygiene habits more generally. They may forget how to get dressed, how to take a shower, and how to do many of the things they used to do routinely and do on their own. Even their habits are lost and without reliable habits, they also lose their independence.

So at this point they need a lot of assistance just to function. At this point, some caregivers will move the patient to a nursing home. That alone is a very expensive and also very heart-rending decision. To the patient, it may seem that they are being abandoned. Because of this some caregivers will try not to make this move. Those caregivers will have to become nurses themselves. They have to take control. So either way if you make the move, and sometimes the patient is feeling angry and abandoned, but if you become the nurse, you are now nurse to a patient who is place, is still angry, frustrated, confused, and seemingly ungrateful.

During this moderate stage the language problems become further increased. And wandering can become even more pronounced, and mood is also greatly affected. A patient may cry or become aggressive out of the blue, and the decreased language abilities make it even harder for the caregiver to connect with that person they love and remember. It can seem this person is transforming before their eyes, and they are losing touch with the person they once knew. This complicates things considerably.

In the advanced stage of Alzheimer's, patients are completely dependent on the care of others. Language is reduced to words or very short phrases. Patients typically exhibit exhaustion and will not be able to perform even the simplest task without assistance. Sometime during this stage patients typically become bedridden. Eventually they will pass away, though typically not from the disease itself. Usually they will die of pneumonia or adrenal failure or the loss of some other critical system.

As I warned, this is a grim and potentially depressing progression. Personally, I find it absolutely horrible that we could have a rich warm relationship with someone we love dearly, and then have it end this way. Our typical notion of a caregiver-patient relationship we think of the patient as understanding the sacrifice of the caregiver and responding with love and deep thanks.

In the case of Alzheimer's disease, the lack of disease awareness and the general confusion, frustration, and embarrassment that patients feel can make them react negatively to someone they no longer even recognize as a loving family member, and instead they come to see this as someone who is controlling them or confining them. This can break the hearts of those who are showing their love in the strongest way they can.

So what can be done about this? Well, many people are trying hard to understand the disease better and how to treat it. However, the punch line is this: We currently just don't have a good understanding of the disease. We do know that patients with Alzheimer's disease show abnormalities in their brains. They have more abnormal clumps (called amyloid plaques) and they have more tangled fibers (called neurofibrillary tangles). The plaques start in several locations, while the tangles start deep in the brain, in an area called the entorhinal cortex. Later they spread to the hippocampus. As plaques and tangles spread, they interfere with the functioning of more and more healthy neurons. As neurons lose this ability to communicate with each other, they die.

This is one reason why agents that reduce plaques and tangles do not reduce symptoms: The brain cells are already dead. The best we can do right now is offer some treatments that provide small benefits in the severity of the symptoms. There is no cure; nor do we even seem able to slow the disease progression to any significant extent. So we have a long way to go in terms of understanding and treating the disease.

Given that no cure is available, I want to spend the remainder of the lecture highlighting two other ways we can react to Alzheimer's disease. The first is the possible role of lifestyle in terms of prevention. As you'll see, there may be some things we can do that may reduce the likelihood of getting Alzheimer's disease, though the evidence is not nearly as firm as we might like. In fact, given that genetics and one's early environment also appear to contribute to the disease, the possible benefits of lifestyle change may vary from person to person.

The second concerns ideas for how to respond once the disease has been diagnosed. One idea is something that I myself have been working on, the notion of using technology as a cognitive prosthetic. This is something that might both enhance the life of the patients and caregivers while also offering a new tool that might help us to gather information and perhaps even assess treatments.

Let's start with prevention. First, it's important to stress that it is extremely difficult to perform really tight scientific experiments that firmly link any behavior to higher or lower rates of disease. Instead we are often looking at correlations. For example, we know there is a lower incidence of Alzheimer's disease in Mediterranean regions and, it seems, for those who eat Mediterranean diets. This has led some to suggest that we should be eating a diet rich in fruits, vegetables, olive oil, and of course red wine, and if we do so that may help prevent Alzheimer's disease.

When I say we need to be careful with such claims, it's for the following reason. The people who tend to eat such diets tend to be people of Mediterranean decent, and it may simply be the case that there is some aspect of their genetics that is different, and as a result of that shared heritage, they have that shared genetics, and that's what's actually giving them some insulation to the disease. It may not have to do with the food they eat. Or maybe it does. It's really hard to know for sure.

But with this caveat in place here are some other similar factors. People who engage in activities that involve cognitive stimulation seem less likely to get Alzheimer's disease. This could include activities like playing chess, card games, or crossword puzzles, playing a musical instrument, or even those who commonly engage in social interactions.

The notion is not that these activities prevent Alzheimer's directly, but that they forestall conditions of cognitive decline that may be more hospitable to Alzheimer's. According to this idea, for example, those London taxi drivers we were talking about, the ones with an enlarged hippocampus, are creating a less hospitable environment for Alzheimer's to take off. By engaging in a lot of intellectual activity, you're kind of doing the same thing.

Interestingly, medical marijuana seems to delay the onset of Alzheimer's disease, apparently because the active ingredient in marijuana, THC, prevents the formation of the brain deposits associated with the disease. Alzheimer's disease is also more prevalent in industrialized areas leading some to speculate that exposure to metals, especially aluminum, may be a contributing factor. Smoking also increases the risk of Alzheimer's disease.

So, if you believe in these sorts of findings, then the prescription is obvious. Move to the country, eat lots of fruits and vegetables, drink wine, smoke only marijuana, and take up a musical instrument. In these respects at least, someone like Willie Nelson is not a candidate for Alzheimer's disease!

But what if you or a loved one has Alzheimer's disease, then what? You should be aware that medications already exist to slow the progress of the disease itself, especially during early and moderate Alzheimer's. The specific drugs will change, but one of the reasons to identify the disease early is to seek treatments that have been found to slow its progress for months or years. There are also a variety of treatments to address behavioral consequences of the disease, things like depression and loss of regular sleep.

As for the future of managing this horrible disease, I also want to talk about how technology might help. Just as a prosthetic limb can replace a missing leg and thereby allow someone to walk rather than use a wheelchair, perhaps technology can fill in for at least some missing cognitive abilities. This is a notion sometimes called cognitive prosthetics, and my students and I are currently working on just such an approach to Alzheimer's disease. I want to discuss this, not because such a solution currently exists, because it is yet another example of how science might address this disease, but also because it puts a different light on more general issues of technology and memory as well.

Here's one possible scenario. Patients in the preliminary stage Alzheimer's disease, that is, those in the mild cognitive impairment stage, might be given a mobile computing device that has been equipped with the appropriate software. This device would be capable of receiving global positioning system signals. In addition, the caregiver and the patient would work together, and they would specify certain locations that the patient may frequently wish to visit. The GPS coordinates of those locations would be indicated to the software, each of which is given a very specific and easy label like "the park," or "my brother's house," or "the grocery store," or "home," etc.

Other personal information would also be entered into the device, including the caregivers contact numbers, numbers of the police, and personal information about the patient like their name, age, and where they live. Finally, a number of messages are recorded by the caregiver. And I'll describe the role of those messages in a moment. Now anytime the patient wishes to go for a walk they are allowed to do so, but on the condition that they first indicate the route they plan to take, and they do so by punching it in on the device. They also must take the device with them. The device itself stays dormant, but even while dormant it tracks the GPS coordinates of the patient and constantly monitors them to detect if the patient has become lost. How would it know that the patient is lost?

Well, built-in algorithms might do two things. First they would compare the route the patient is following with the route they said they were going to follow. Second, it would look out for things like double backs, slowdowns and speed ups, or other wandering type behavior suggestive of someone who is not simply walking in a determined purposeful way.

All of this information would be combined to form an assessment of whether or not the patient seems to be acting lost. If the patient acts lost, then the phone rings, and it literally keeps ringing until the patient touches the screen or responds in some other way, something that's designed to be easy for them, something that works. At that point a pre-recorded message from the caregiver could offer advice, which perhaps could include contacting the caregiver himself.

So the idea here is that in this way the patient might actually be able to find their own way home. There might be no need to confess an embarrassing lack of memory, less need to worry caregivers, and less aimless wandering into potential harm. This also means that the caregiver would not need to jail the patient. For example, the device might monitor progress as it gave directions, and if the patient was not following them properly, the device could call the caregiver directly and notify them of the precise location of their family member.

Now, obviously, an approach like this is more of a crutch than cure. But it could also aid in the search for a cure. That is, by keeping track of how often a patient gets lost while they're walking, we would have a clear objective measure of disease progression, one that is measured unobtrusively and in the context of normal life. If some biometric monitoring were added, the data gathered could be even more informative. So let me give you a sense of that.

Let's say that there's some drug that could be potentially beneficial. We could now directly test this possibility by comparing how often a group on the drug became lost compared to a group not on the drug. Thus it is the crutch that can inform a cure, and it could do so while enhancing the lives and relationships of all caught in this horrible situation. Many of us already use our technologies in this way. Anyone who uses some form of electronic calendar is essentially allowing it to remember important meetings and important so that they don't need to. Similarly cell phones remember phone numbers that we previously might have actually held in our own memory.

Some people worry that too much reliance on technology may be robbing us of what otherwise might have been useful cognitive exercise. In this very lecture I stress that cognitive exercise is important in the prevention of Alzheimer's. Perhaps that is true, and perhaps we should consider that. But in the case of patients suffering from a debilitating memory problem, it is hard to see any tool as anything but positive.

Although technology of the future may become a cognitive prosthetic, so too can a caregiver. Alzheimer's disease is, at its core, a horrible disease that is very hard to deal with. But I can offer one small idea. Yes, the patient may sometimes have to be jailed, unpleasant though that can be. But to the extent a caregiver is able to walk with the patient, that can have many benefits, especially if the walk can be shaped to give the patient some freedom, and not feel like the caregiver is just supervising.

In fact, you might even want to plan special walks together, especially during the stages of mild cognitive impairment and early to moderate Alzheimer's. When the patient is lucid, these can be great times for the caregiver to be with the one they love, and when there are bouts of confusion the caregivers will be there to assist. Alzheimer's is a horrible disease, in part, because it destroys everything familiar. In our next lecture we will turn to the subject of familiarity itself.

That Powerful Glow of Warm Familiarity
Lecture 18

Past experiences affect us in ways we often underestimate. Through simple repetition, items come to be perceived fluently, and that fluent perception can make us think we are acting rationally when we are not. This happens most when we are making decisions based on little research or deep thought. Repetition can also form prototypes that are themselves processed fluently, even if we have never experienced the literal prototype.

W e now turn from theoretical and empirical information about how memory works to think about the many ways memory influences our behavior every day, starting with the influence of familiarity, or **perceptual fluency**, the resonance of a current situation with our past experience.

When we experience something over and over, we become better—more fluent—at recognizing it. The semantic information we have about objects in the world is represented in the association cortex. In short, it allows us to know what it is we are seeing, hearing, and so forth. More accurately, the more experience we have with some object, the more quickly we are able to recognize it from its features.

The processes of perception themselves can be thought of in terms of procedural memory. Repeated experience viewing some particular stimulus enhances the fluency with which the stimulus is processed. But in this case, we subjectively experience this fluency as a positive emotional reaction.

We sometimes attribute perceptual fluency to past experience, but not always, and even when we do, we don't always get the specific past experience right. Thus, feelings of familiarity are open to interpretation, and the interpretations we make can allow us to be fooled, or even to fool ourselves.

Experiments involving the **mere exposure effect** demonstrate dramatic effects related to simple exposure to a stimulus. When words are presented to subjects via **rapid serial visual presentation**, the subjects felt like they saw the words but could not remember them. Yet recognition tests show that participants can make accurate guesses about what words they were shown.

What's interesting is, if you instead ask the test subject to categorize words in terms of how much they like them, they tend to like more of the presented words. The feeling of familiarity is undifferentiated; participants interpret or attribute the positive feeling in terms of whatever task is at hand. This is why politicians plaster their names on every available surface just before an election and advertisers throw their brand's name on everything: to increase your fluency and thus your associations with the name.

The success of perceptual fluency depends to a large extent on humans being relatively naive to its powerful effects. It has the most influence in contexts where we have little solid information to rely on. The scary thing is, these contexts are very common, and modern research supports the old saying, "If you say something often enough, it becomes true."

If conditions are right, the brain can be tricked into fluently processing things it has never actually seen.

If conditions are right, the brain can be tricked into fluently processing things it has never actually seen. Implicit memory, our tendency to extract the structure and regularities from stimuli, encodes structures even when they were never explicitly presented. So, for example, the constant presentation of female models who are medically 15 to 20 percent below a healthy weight for their height and age reinforces an idea that thin women are beautiful, even though it may be contrary to good health.

Prototypes like these are really just another type of script or schema, and as such they can be extremely useful in helping us negotiate our way through the world—if the stereotypes are valid. However, while we use the prototypes to guide our decisions, we do so in a manner that is often blind to accuracy of the experiences that gave rise to them. ■

Important Terms

mere exposure effect: The surprisingly strong memory effect of brief exposure to a stimulus, even when no effort was made to remember the stimulus.

perceptual fluency: Familiarity; the resonance between present and past experience.

rapid serial visual presentation: A technique used in memory experiments wherein a set of words is flashed before a subject so quickly that the subject feels he or she hasn't seen most of them.

Suggested Reading

Dill, *How Fantasy Becomes Reality*.

Fennis and Stroebe, *The Psychology of Advertising*.

Graf and Masson, *Implicit Memory*.

Questions to Consider

1. Now that you know about the effects of familiarity, do you think you will make your decisions any differently the next time you vote or go shopping?

2. Have you ever met someone from your home country while traveling abroad and felt that you really liked them? Why might this be the case? Do you think you would have liked them as much if you had met them just down the street from where you live?

The next time you are watching television, notice how many commercials really say very little about the true merits of the product they are selling, instead only mentioning the name of the product and trying to associate it with things you already like. Does the prevalence of such commercials suggest that advertisers regard the influence of familiarity as more powerful than any rational claims they could make about why you should buy their product?

That Powerful Glow of Warm Familiarity
Lecture 18—Transcript

Early in this course I introduced you to your memory systems, and the experimental data relevant to them. We then discussed the links between these systems and the brain, and we did that from a number of different perspectives.

With all this groundwork under our belt, the remainder of the lectures will focus on how memory influences us in our daily lives. We're going to talk about contexts that range from ballot boxes (the issue we will discuss quite about in this lecture) to courtrooms, and beyond. Basically, we will take all of the theoretical and empirical knowledge we have been building up, and use it to think about influences of memory as they play out each and every day.

In this lecture we're going to focus on a concept I have already mentioned a few times, an influence that is often called "familiarity." To begin illustrating this concept, think back to your last local election. Do you remember what happened as the election got closer and closer? That's right: Big signs and little signs, containing only names and political affiliations, began to pop up all over the place, like dandelions in the summer. Why do politicians and politician wannabes do this to us? If we thought about it all consciously, shouldn't these be the last people we vote for given their willingness to clutter up our public spaces with seemingly endless repetitions of the same signs?

Of course, the unfortunate truth is that they do this because it works; it does indeed increase the chance we will vote for them. It's the same reason why advertisers insist on getting the name of their product in front of our eyes as often as they can and, if possible, associating their product with other stimuli that produce positive reactions in us.

The world is trying to influence us, and they are using low-level memory processes to do it. The worst part of it is this: Even if you know it's happening, you still fall prey to its power. It's the power of perceptual fluency or what many of us call familiarity.

In the earliest days of psychological research Edward Titchener referred to the "glow of warmth" that one feels when they are in the presence of the familiar. This could be a familiar context like home, the familiar sound of a mother's voice to a newborn baby, a familiar friend, or maybe even a familiar name on a ballot box. How does this familiarity come to exist, and how do we interpret it as humans?

Familiarity is obviously the result of previous experience. It is not so much though the re-experiencing of some past event as it is some form of resonance with that past experience. How are we to think of this in terms of memory systems?

Well, in terms of a specific stimulus feeling more or less familiar, this feeling of familiarity is assumed to arise from something called perceptual fluency. The notion is that when we experience something over and over we become better, that is, more fluent, at recognizing it, and this is what is meant by perceptual fluency.

Remember when I told you about the agnosias, visual agnosia for example? I told you that for most of us the semantic information we have about objects in the world is represented by our association cortex. By contrast, when we see something we originally represent what we are seeing in primary visual cortex, that then passed on to the association cortex and that object is recognized.

Association cortex allows us to know what it is we are seeing, and for those suffering with visual agnosia, this second step sometimes does not occur. By this depiction, the recognition of some object seems to either happen or not. But that is actually an oversimplification. In actuality the process linking visual features to our semantic knowledge of objects is really much more graded.

For those of us with intact association cortices, the more accurate way to think of things is that the more experience we have had with some object, the more quickly we are able to recognize it from its features.

The notion then is that processes of perception themselves can be thought of in terms of procedural memory. Repeated experience viewing some particular stimulus enhances the fluency with which that stimulus is processed, just like repeated experience riding a bike, for example, enhances the fluency of bike riding. The only new aspect of this is the assumption that we can subjectively feel this fluency. Fluent perception is one way in which a stimulus can come to feel familiar to us.

For example, experiments have been performed in which words are presented very briefly and then covered up by strings of random letters. Participants are merely asked to report the word they saw, something called a perceptual identification task. These experiments show that the more common a word is, the more likely that it will be perceived when it is presented, especially when it's presented for very short durations, as I described.

So this fluency of processing can be felt, and when we feel it we often attribute it to past experience, which makes sense because that's what usually produces it. But we don't always attribute it in that way. And even when we do attribute it to past experience, we don't always get the specific past experience right. So feelings of familiarity are open to interpretation, and the interpretations we make can allow us to be fooled or even to fool ourselves.

Some of the most interesting experiments on potential misattributions of familiarity were done in the context of something called the mere exposure effect; that is, dramatic effects related to the mere exposure of a stimulus. In those experiments stimuli are presented to participants, one after the other, in very quick succession, at the same screen location. This is a method called RSVP, or rapid serial visual presentation, and it feels like the moment you see one word it is replaced by another, then another. Boom, boom, boom, boom. All located at the same screen location. So you literally feel bombarded by this stream of words. If the words formed a sentence, you could read the sentence. But in most experiments the words are randomly selected items and, in that case, you feel like all you can do is watch.

In the initial studies, a series of words would first be presented in this way, random words, one after another. Then, either immediately or after a little bit of a delay, some other task is given. If you simply ask people to recall as many words as possible, they will recall almost none. They felt like the words were seen, but the pace of presentation was so quick that no words could be encoded enough to allow subsequent memory.

If you instead present a recognition test, then one can find evidence of memory. Remember, in a recognition test complete items are presented at the time of the test. Typically half of the items would have been part of that RSVP stream and half would not have been part of it (the latter are what we call new items). Participants have to decide whether they think each item at test was on the list, that is, it was an "old" item, or it was not on the list, a new item.

When memory is tested in this way, you do see evidence of memory for the items. Specifically, people say old more to items that were presented than they do to items that were not. So clearly they have a sense of whether or not an item was presented. However, when you ask the participants, they feel like they were just guessing. If you probe them enough they would likely say something like, "I couldn't remember any of the items as occurring, but some felt a little more familiar, so I just guesses that those items were old."

In this case then, participants are explicitly using familiarity to infer previous presentation. Said another way, they attributed the familiarity of the item to its occurring in the earlier RSVP list. Here is what makes all this interesting and relevant to life in the real world. If you change the question that you ask, then familiarity has its influence in different ways.

For example, assume we use a recognition-like experiment, but instead of asking participants whether items were in that RSVP stream or not, we instead ask them to categorize items in terms of how much they like them. So they are basically going to say "I like this item" or "I dislike that time," like, dislike. What you see is that participants will say they like more of the words that had been presented in the RSVP stream. Their mere exposure during the RSVP stream makes them subsequently more likable.

What's going on here? Well, memory researchers would say that by presenting the items, even briefly in that RSVP stream, that presentation is enough to strengthen slightly their pattern in memory. When those items reappear later at test, this strengthening of their memory pattern results in them being perceived a little more fluently than they otherwise would be. You can literally recognize the item more quickly, and you can feel this fluency, the feeling is one of familiarity.

Here's the kicker though. This feeling of familiarity, or warmth in Tichener's words, is what we call undifferentiated. We are not sure of its source, we just feel that feeling. That feeling will then be interpreted or attributed in terms of whatever task we have at hand. If we are asking if an item had been presented earlier in the experiment, as in a typical recognition experiment, then we assume that the fluent items were in the experiment earlier. If we are asked which items we like, then we like the items that we experience as fluent better.

If this sounds a little farfetched, consider a really interesting follow-up study. Again, a set of items are presented in an RSVP stream, and then they are re-presented at test, intermixed with new, non-presented items. In this study, a number of different tasks were presented to different groups of participants. All of the tasks were what we call shams. (I'll explain that in a moment.)

For example, in one context participants were told that while it would be very hard for them to consciously notice this difference, some of the test items would be presented a little longer than others. Their task was to indicate whether or not they think an item was presented longer or not-so-long duration. Now we call it a sham because, in reality, all items are presented for the exact same length of time. But participants were more likely to say that a previously presented item was presented longer. Similarly, if you asked them which ones were presented a little brighter, when really there's not any difference in the brightness at all, they will choose the previously presented items as the ones they think were brighter.

But the really interesting twist is the following. If participants were instead asked which items had been presented for a shorter duration or in a slightly dimmer color they again categorized the previously presented items as either shorter or dimmer. So the question itself doesn't seem to matter. This is one of those points that bears repeating. The specific question you have in your mind doesn't seem to matter. Instead, it seems that whatever the participant is looking for, be it an old stimulus, a likable stimulus, a long or short duration, or a bright or dim font, the relatively fluently processed item gets chosen.

So perceptual fluency is attributed in a very powerful and context-specific way. It essentially makes something fluent stand out from the crowd, allowing it to become the target of whatever the person might be looking for. So now put yourself in the voter's booth, looking at a voting card that features a sea of potential candidates. What's your task? Your task is to choose the person you think would do the best job at whatever they are running for. If you're like many of us, you didn't have the time or the interest to research every candidate for every position. So how do you make your decision?

Well, what the candidates hope is that their name will stand out, and that you will be drawn to them as your selection. How can they help that along? Well, by previously exposing you to their name over and over and over. They don't even care if you think much about their name, they just want that name to be a pattern you know, a pattern that has been primed, and hence a name that feels warmly fluent, a fluency you may indeed attribute to them being the right person for the job.

Of course it is important to again emphasize that this all works out for them because of the specifics of the question that is in your mind, which is, "Which of these people do I think is best for the job?" Had the question instead been something like, "Which of these people do you think is most likely to be involved in a scandal?", your eyes and mind, again, might have been drawn to the most fluently processed name.

Another important aspect of this phenomenon is that it depends to a large extent on human beings being relatively naive to this powerful effect of perceptual fluency. Sure when we look at the names on the ballot we might remember seeing some election signs bearing those names, and maybe even understand that this may make that name more familiar, or stand out, but we don't think we are making our choices on this basis. We feel like our decisions reflect some higher level of thinking that is not influenced by the mere repeated viewing of a name.

Well, the research suggests that our decisions are indeed affected by simply experiencing things, and advertisers make heavy use of this phenomenon when trying to get us to buy certain products. Let's say you are in a store trying to decide which laptop to buy. Maybe you did a lot of research, and maybe you have analytically decided on the best one to buy. Or maybe you didn't, and you're just looking at them, trying to find one that looks good, whatever that means. If you see a brand name that is fluent, that feels warmly familiar, that one might pass the "looks good" test. We might attribute the fluency to quality of the product. You might have even noticed that in both of these examples, I have suggested that maybe you had done some research on say who to vote for or which laptop to purchase, or maybe not. Perceptual fluency has its largest effects in contexts where we really have little real information to rely on.

The scary thing is there are a lot of those contexts. We very often make choices based on very little research. Instead we might say that we just went with the choice that felt right. Well, that feeling we are relying on is fluency, and given that fluency can be manipulated, it doesn't always provide us with the right choice. It's because of this sort of research that people say things like, "If you say something often enough it becomes true." It's another thing that politicians clearly believe in. Literally, if you hear something over and over again, it will become a fluently processed, familiar message. Should you be in a position of deciding if that message is true, a familiar message will be more likely to feel true. All I can really add to this is the following: I am doing a fantastic job giving these lectures. I am doing a really fantastic job giving these lectures. I am—well, you get the picture.

This notion of attributing familiarity in an undifferentiated manner also explains a phenomenon that some call unconscious plagiarism. Let's say that you are a writer, and you are currently writing a novel. As a writer you have likely read a lot of books yourself. So now you're looking for that perfect thing for your male character to say to a woman who he is angry with. And you mull it over and over in your mind, and it suddenly it comes to you: "Frankly, Violet, I don't give a damn." The more you think about the line, the more it feels just right.

Of course, that's actually a rather famous line from *Gone with the Wind*, although the heroine of that was Scarlett O'Hara, of course, not Violet. But, in fact, this line is so famous you probably would remember it from that book. But had I chosen something a little less famous, something you may have read but you read it without really making note of it. Then when you later come up with the same line yourself, it could feel familiar, and you could attribute that familiarity to your brilliance.

Many writers of books and songs, when faced with the similarity of their work to previous work, have made just this claim. Yes, they know that other book or song. Yes, they agree that what they created is pretty darn similar. But, no, they did not realize they were plagiarizing from it. This sort of plagiarism isn't reserved for writers either. Sometimes we unconsciously plagiarize other people's ideas. Again, we heard an idea voiced by another at some point but maybe we didn't think about it too deeply at the time. Later we are thinking about the same issue, and that very idea comes to mind, quite fluently. It feels like a good idea. It feels warm. Once again, we assume that's because we are brilliant. When in doubt, assume you're brilliant.

Of course, the unfortunate reality of these situations is that, as highlighted earlier, most humans don't understand how powerful the effects of perceptual fluency can be, and how open they themselves are to misattribution. So if you find yourself in a courtroom trying to argue that yes, apparently you plagiarized something, but that there was no intent to plagiarize and, therefore, there should be no punishment, it's unlikely you'll get far. Most jurors would simply see the similarity across the original writing, the original song or idea, and whatever it was you provided, and would find the evidence overwhelmingly strong. Surely you had to know. In fact, courts have ruled that your intent doesn't even matter. If you plagiarized, you plagiarized. Whether it was a conscious plagiarism or unconscious is irrelevant.

So the brain is biased to process fluently anything that it has seen before. But, interestingly, if the conditions are right, it can also be tricked into fluently processing things that it has never actually seen. To get a sense of how this can happen, consider the following experiment. We first create some random pattern of dots, say 10 dots arranged in some relatively random way. We're going to refer to this pattern as our prototype pattern. We then create 10 new patterns. We start with the prototype in each case, but then we slightly move one dot or several dots a little one way or a little another way. And we do that in a different way for each of the 10 patterns.

Each of those 10 that we create from the prototype is called an exemplar of the prototype. They each represent instances, or exemplars, of that class defined by the prototype. So all the new patterns have as many dots in the same position as there are in the prototype pattern, but all the new patterns are different slightly from the prototype.

We then select randomly 5 of our new patterns, and we present them to people to study. Following that, we have a test in which all 10 patterns are shown, and we also show the prototype. Participants are asked whether each pattern they see was or was not one of the 5 that they studied. Generally they have a very hard time telling the difference between presented and non-presented patterns, but they do all show one consistent tendency. When the prototype is shown it is almost always called old. Even though that particular pattern was never shown itself, it seems to be the most familiar of them all. Why?

Remember implicit memory? That tendency we have to extract the structure, the regularities, from the stimuli we see? Well, when we do that the structure becomes encoded even when it was never explicitly presented. Each stimulus we showed had a lot of overlap with the prototype. So parts of the prototype pattern were learned every time a new stimulus was presented. What's more, the manner in which those patterns did not match the prototype was random. As a result, over the course of presentation, all parts of the prototype pattern were seen. So even though it was never presented as an intact whole pattern, the consistency with which its parts were shown lead its pattern to also be reinforced, reinforced enough to produce all the same sorts of tendencies as we see in the mere exposure effect.

So the prototype fits the implied structure of the experience even better than the exemplars that were created do. This complete alignment with the implied structure allows it to be processed fluently, which again makes it feel familiar. Slightly different source this time but same end result: familiarity.

The conditions I just outlined may seem a little contrived, but they are not really too far removed from situations we all experience daily. For example, let's consider our concept of female beauty. Many of the female actresses that ultimately portray beautiful women got their start in modeling, and female models themselves are often projected as images of beauty. Is it fair to say that most of these models have something in common, like the new patterns we made from some prototype pattern?

Well, the average model weighs perhaps 25 percent less than the average female and may maintain a percentage of body fat that 15 to 20 percent below what is considered to be healthy given the model's height and age. This is what they have in common. Most project variants of a body that is likely to be too thin to be healthy. In fact, modeling agencies have been reported to actively pursue models known to be anorexic. We see these women, each beautiful in their own right, and we form a prototype of beauty, that pattern of features that we find the most "warm."

Is this innocent enough? I mean, the Greeks had mythology to entertain them, and the gods and goddesses in their pantheon were absolutely beautiful or abnormally strong or fast or intelligent. We find extremes entertaining. So maybe this is just another such case of the same thing. Maybe the media is our Mount Olympus.

Of course the problem is that the abnormality of the prototype becomes lost. The women we see are not seen as abnormally thin and beautiful in that way, rather they come to define beauty and thus the thinness they represent becomes viewed as how one should look. Young girls are seeing these images, and they're attempting to become them because when they do they, others see them as beautiful. And that's concerning. Again, the general idea is that when we see exemplars of some prototype, we come to form a representation of the prototype, even though it, itself, may never have been presented.

And that representation can guide the decisions we make about the general class of items from which the exemplars have been drawn, beautiful women for example. This isn't necessarily a bad thing. It isn't if the exemplars we see are truly representative of the category to which they belong. In that case, the prototype ends up being a sort of average, and it makes sense that this average would feel familiar or "right" in terms of representing the stereotypical exemplar of the category. So using that prototype as a basis for our decisions might seem appropriate.

If any of this sounds (dare I say) familiar, well prototypes are really just another word for scripts or schemas. That is, we could talk about some restaurant as being a stereotypical fast-food restaurant, meaning everything you do in that place follows the standard or prototypical fast-food experience. As I have highlighted before, such these stereotypes or scripts can be extremely useful in helping us to negotiate our way through the world— when the stereotypes are valid. So if the exemplar experiences that give rise to the stereotype are real and accurate depictions of fast-food restaurants, then we end up with an accurate schema. However, the problem is that, once again, while we use the prototypes to guide our decisions, we do so in a manner that is often blind to the accurateness of the experiences that gave rise to them, and sometimes these experiences are not representative.

For example, those who write scripts for movies are sometimes accused of consistently portraying women or people of various minority groups in non-representative ways. When I was a young boy, it was during the Cold War, and the "bad guys" in many of the movies that I watched were Russians. I doubt that I ever saw a Russian portrayed in any sort of positive way. Thus my stereotype of the prototypical Russian was pretty negative, which could clearly affect the way that I might interact with Russians. Luckily I have met many very friendly Russians since, but this example does show you the power that prototypes can have.

So the main point of this lecture is that past experiences have a power to affect us in ways that we often underestimate. Through simple repetition, or through similarity to something we have seen repeatedly, items come to be perceived fluently, and that fluent perception can be misattributed in ways that make us think we are acting rationally when we are not. This happens most when we are making decisions based on very little research or deep thought. If you don't like the idea of being influenced by familiarity, it's a good idea to research your decisions.

In addition, experiences of exemplars from some category can also form prototypes that are themselves processed fluently even if never actually experienced. These prototypes can guide the way we interact with subsequent exemplars from that category, all without us truly appreciating the power that those previous experiences have had on our current behavior.

So the next time you are tempted to make some generalized comment about some group or some concept, it is worth taking the time to ask whether you think you've really interacted with a representative sample of that group or concept. If not, accept the possibility that your perspective may be biased and, again, seek out more information that might help you form a more representative viewpoint.

The situations I have discussed in this lecture are real world situations involving perceptions of familiarity, and the attributions that can arise from that. But in the next lecture, we are going to leave the real world—at least the physical world—and we're going to enter the metaphysical, as we consider attributions of familiarity in the context of that creepy feeling we all love to experience. That's right. It's finally time to talk about déjà vu.

Déjà Vu and the Illusion of Memory
Lecture 19

Many people are inclined to attribute déjà vu to a metaphysical cause—a premonition, a message from God, and so on. But there are several sound this-worldly theories to explain the phenomenon. Most are related to our brains making mistakes in perceptual fluency, interpreting the unfamiliar as the familiar, either through priming, episodic memory degradation, or a parahippocampus glitch.

The experience of **déjà vu**—a French phrase meaning "already seen"—is a common but unsettling one. This sudden, overwhelming feeling of familiarity in a situation that we rationally know is brand new can seem almost mystical in the moment, but most scientific theories describe déjà vu as an illusion of memory.

Two common explanations of déjà vu are not memory based. The first suggests that déjà vu arises from random electrical stimulation in the temporal lobes, not unlike the stimulation epileptics experience right before a seizure. Another theory is that sensory information from each of our eyes or ears reaches our brains at a slightly different rate; when the message arrives from the slower eye, it feels familiar because we really have already seen it. The theory that déjà vu arises from a misattribution of perceptual fluency is a better fit for the evidence. Humans are very uncomfortable when something feels familiar and they don't know why, so they feel compelled to attribute the familiarity to something.

Virtually all of the memory experiments that inform our understanding of déjà vu utilize the recognition memory test. Researchers are especially interested in the false alarms that occur on a recognition task. Some false alarms are caused by words with **semantic overlap**; for example, subjects who were shown the word "rose" might register a false sense of familiarity with "tulip." If the text contains a mix of words that are in everyday use with more obscure words, they are more likely to falsely register any common words as familiar.

False alarms on a recognition test are interesting, but they are not really déjà vu. Déjà vu also includes that sense of oddness, the subjective creepy feeling. This is very hard, if not impossible, to re-create in a laboratory, so most theories of déjà vu will be just that—theories.

Another possible explanation for déjà vu is **priming**. Our memories are always preparing us for what we are about to experience; for example, you might start a conversation expecting a certain language to be spoken. This allows us to react more quickly and efficiently in any situation. Stimuli can prime us even when we are not aware of them. In déjà vu, priming may happen via a subconscious glance.

> **Our memories are always preparing us for what we are about to experience. ... Stimuli can prime us even when we are not aware of them.**

If you see just enough of a scene to begin processing it, glance away for a moment, and then return to the original scene, your memory may already be primed for what it is seeing, even if you weren't aware of that first glance. You are left with an intense feeling of familiarity that you cannot attribute to anything.

Neuropsychological theories of déjà vu focus on a brain region just below the hippocampus called the **parahippocampus**. Imaging studies show that this region is active when stimuli feel familiar, irrespective of whether those stimuli are consciously recognized or not. So in brain terms, déjà vu may be a situation in which the parahippocampus is active but no conscious memory is retrieved because there is no memory to be retrieved.

Alternatively, the hologram theory of memory argues that memories, like holograms, are re-created out of bits of themselves; the smaller the bit, the more blurred the ultimate memory. In déjà vu, some small aspect of our current experience may be enough to retrieve a very blurry version of some past experience. If this ghost of a memory is strong enough, it may trigger brain regions that respond to familiarity without retrieving an episodic memory. A similar theory suggests that our indirect experiences— say, through books or movies—might be enough to trigger a strong sense of familiarity that cannot be easily attributed to anything. Both of these are really alternate forms of the priming-attribution theory.

What do all these theories of déjà vu tell us about memory? For one thing, they tell us that declarative and nondeclarative forms of memory can become dissociated and that we can feel it when they do. The reverse can happen, too. If you take any word and repeat it over and over and over, eventually that word will not feel familiar anymore. Experiences like this are called **jamais vu**, which translates to "never seen." The Capgras delusion is an extreme form of this. ∎

Important Terms

déjà vu: A disquietingly strong sense that a new event has already been experienced; from the French term meaning "already seen."

jamais vu: A disquietingly strong sense that a familiar event has never been experienced before; from the French term meaning "never seen."

priming: A process of being prepared for a stimulus by some previous experience.

parahippocampus: A brain region involved in sensations of familiarity.

semantic overlap: In a recognition test, a word that evokes a sense of familiarity because it has a meaning similar to or belongs in a category with a word presented earlier (e.g., red and crimson; rose and tulip).

Suggested Reading

Graf and Masson, *Implicit Memory*.

Koonce, *The Deja Vu Experience*.

1. Why do humans seem to need to explain every experience in some way? Which explanation of déjà vu do you find most convincing from your own experience or what you have heard about déjà vu from others?

2. So called date-rape drugs cause the body to release the hormones usually released by physical attraction. Someone unaware of being drugged might misattribute their response to the drug as true feelings of attraction for someone who happens to be nearby. How is this like the déjà vu theories described in this lecture?

Exercise

Can you think of someone who you will likely run into in the near future? If so, think about that future meeting now, and practice something you will say to that person—anything, even something simple like "Good morning. Very nice to see you today." Imagine yourself meeting that person and saying that as many times as possible. Then, when you do meet, go right up and say those words just as you have been practicing. What does it feel like when you say the words? How is this situation like the one that theoretically produces déjà vu, and how is it different?

Déjà Vu and the Illusion of Memory
Lecture 19—Transcript

I remember the first time my wife and I visited Amsterdam together, which is when I experienced a distinct episode of déjà vu. We approached a bridge over a canal on one of those typical streets of Amsterdam. Like most streets it featured a canal and 4-to-5–story stone buildings on either side and a pair of roads flanking each side of the canal. I remember looking to my left, and as I watched a group of bicycles approaching me, and that clearly European vehicle backing onto the street, and even the birds flying over the way they did, it all felt eerily familiar. Just like I was watching something I had seen before. But I'd never been here before with my wife; I was sure of it. Yet everything felt so familiar, leaving me with this unsettled feeling and the desire to make sense of it all. Could I have dreamed this event before? Was it some sort of prophecy almost? Did I experience it in some past or some parallel life? Is some force trying to tell me that this experience is in some manner important, no matter how benign it may seem? These are the feelings that we associate with déjà vu, seeing again.

As humans we really do enjoy the abnormalities of life. The vast majority of things that we encounter in our lives are explainable, often in relatively mundane ways. But every now and then we come across something that seems unexplainable, something that seems to defy all we know to be true of the world, and those things really capture our thoughts and imaginations. We want to understand them. Is the experience of déjà vu one of those things? On its surface, it feels like an intense reliving in the flesh of an experience that we can't consciously recall ever having. It is almost like we are the actors in the re-creation of an episodic memory, and yet we cannot form the true episodic memory of that event as occurring in the past.

Are there scientific explanations of déjà vu? Well there certainly are theories, and most of them describe déjà vu as an illusion of memory. Sometimes illusions have a very important place in science. So for example: Perhaps you've been to a science museum and you've experienced some so-called optical illusions, things that trick the eye into seeing something that really isn't there at all. As researchers discovered these illusions they tried to understand them because often in understanding the illusions they gained a better understanding of the system that was prone to them, in that case the visual system. Well, is déjà vu an illusion of memory? If so, can we learn more about memory by trying to understand how déjà vu comes about? Many believe so, and in this lecture we'll explore some of the theories that have been forwarded so far, and we'll see what those theories tell us about memory.

Before diving in too deeply into these memory-based theories though, let me highlight two explanations of déjà vu that are not memory based really. The first suggests that déjà vu arises from random electrical stimulation of the temporal lobes. This argument is based on reports from people who suffer from epileptic seizures. It turns out that they often report a déjà vu–like experience just prior to each seizure. From monitoring their brains we know that just prior to the seizures there are small amounts of random electrical activity in their temporal lobes, and that's the area where most epileptic seizures originate. So, maybe we all experience that kind of random activity once in a while, and maybe that's what causes the déjà vu experience in us all. It's not a very exciting explanation, and many people argue that the sort of experience that epileptics have is distinctly different from typical déjà vu experiences. Still, it is possible that the cause of déjà vu is as simple as occasional random activation of some brain areas that lead to a feeling of strangeness and an illusion of previously experiencing the current event.

Now, another relatively simple explanation of déjà vu is that it reflects the very small time difference with which visual information sometimes reaches one of our eyes relative to the other. The claim is that sometimes one eye gets information just a little before the other. The first eye gets processing started, essentially greasing the path for when that exact same information follows just milliseconds later through the other eye. This slight temporal displacement of processing makes the processing feel familiar despite all other information suggesting this is a novel experience.

I want to make two points about this theory of déjà vu. First, in terms of the specifics, it does not fare well as a general theory of déjà vu. Déjà vu is not always a visual experience, and it also occurs for people with only one eye. So again, it's likely incorrect. But the second point is this. The idea that déjà vu may reflect some misattribution of perceptual fluency may have some merit, even if the specifics of the theory do not. We talked about misattribution of familiarity in the previous lecture; we know it does occur in the situations that I described. So it may provide a good way of thinking about déjà vu. As you'll see several of the current theories fit with this notion, including the way I will highlight.

Well, I guess if we're trying to be somewhat inclusive in our consideration of déjà vu, we should also consider the most common theory people have. Clearly déjà vu reflects us dreaming about the experience in detail before it happens, or perhaps even living that experience already in some past or parallel life. OK. Clearly this is not a scientific theory, but I mention it primarily to emphasize the following. When we have intense feelings that something has that warm glow of familiarity we often feel the need to attribute that glow to something, and we are willing to stretch credibility pretty far sometimes to find a source. In the memory theories I will now turn to, this aspect of déjà vu is explained by assuming two things. Humans are very uncomfortable when something feels familiar, and they don't know why, so they feel compelled to attribute the familiarity to something. If they miss the true cause of the feelings of familiarity, then they are quite willing to accept even bizarre metaphysical possibilities.

With respect to this latter point, I think an analogy to magic is useful. Even when we are sure that magicians are really illusionists, and we know that they perform the tricks they do by somehow diverting our attention at critical times, we can still feel the metaphysical aspects of magic. That is, if we miss the sleight of hand, then we are left with an event that we have no explanation for, and somehow that gives us this creepy feeling. It's metaphysics at work—it's magic! But if we see the sleight of hand, then the feeling of magic does not happen. We just appreciate the trick. Déjà vu is not a sleight of hand, but it may be a sleight of mind, with familiarity being caused by something the mind simply missed. That is the sort of illusion we're looking for.

Virtually all of the memory experiments that inform our understanding of déjà vu utilize the recognition test. In previous experiments that we've done together we usually used the free recall test. I would just read you a list of items, then perhaps wait for a bit, and then simply ask you to recall what you can remember. That recall test is very much a test of your declarative memory systems, and there isn't much role for perceptual fluency, and thus familiarity, to play in that sort of task. However, as I emphasized in the previous lecture, perceptual fluency plays its largest role when there are options to choose between, like the names on a voting list. So, to create this sort of context we use the recognition test.

And, as you know, in a standard recognition test, items are first presented on a study list. These items are presented and then referred to as "old" items. After the study, there may be a pause, or not, and then the test is presented. The test items consist of the old items shuffled up and intermixed with an equal number of "new" items, items that were not on the study list. For each item on the test list the participant must make an old/new decision that is, do you think the current item was or was not on the study list? When people perform this kind of test they typically report calling items old for one of two reasons Either they explicitly remember seeing the item on the list, or they don't, but that item felt familiar so they assume it was on the list. So, familiarity plays a role in this task, and that's why it's appealing for studying déjà vu, or any potential illusion of familiarity using recognition.

In fact, when studying illusions of familiarity, researchers are especially interested in what are called the false alarms on a recognition task. Now, false alarms are said to occur when participants incorrectly categorize new items as old. That is, they think these new items were on the list, even though they were not. Given that new items were not presented on the study list, it would be impossible for these old responses to reflect the person remembering the items occurrence, so instead it must reflect the item just feeling familiar. So, if familiarity is your focus of interest, then false alarms on a recognition test provide the best instrument for measuring it.

So now let's jump into an experiment to make this all a little bit more concrete. Let's say you present a study list that maybe has many items but includes items like the following: "rose," "tractor," "pistol," "platter," and "currency." Now, when we present the test, we again have all sorts of items but among the new items are "tulip," "plow," "gun," "plate," and "money." The critical point is that some of these new items are very closely related to the study items in terms of the meanings they convey and that's a variable we call semantic overlap. So, given our discussion in the previous lecture, it may not be surprising to learn that participants will often false alarm to those semantically related items. That is, a relation between the items can allow fluency to bridge from one item to another item it's related to, for example, from "rose," which was presented, to "tulip," which was not. Thus, the overlap in semantics allows this new related item to be processed more fluently, and this fluency translates into a feeling of familiarity. That increased familiarity makes participants want to call those related new items old. The participants themselves do not realize that the feeling of familiarity comes from the similarity to the studied items, and, instead, they assume it is due to those items specifically being on the study list that's why they call them old. So this is already a very basic illusion of memory.

This again points to the general point that fluency of processing can be caused by one source and attributed to another. The real source of the feeling of familiarity is missed, and another is blamed. Let me give you one more less exotic example of that. Let's imagine another recognition experiment. This time our experiment includes some new items that are words that are common in the English language and some that are not. So an uncommon word would be a word like "chassis," for example; a common word might be "table." Even though these are both new items, participants will false alarm more to the common words, more to "table" than to "chassis." Again, in psychological terms, because common words have been processed so often, outside the experiment of course, but they've been processed so often that their patterns of activation have been repeatedly reinforced, and thus, they can be perceived very fluently. They are like a well-developed procedural memory. This fluent perception, caused by them being experienced commonly in life, makes them feel familiar. However, when the participants feel this familiarity they do not attribute it to the commonness of the word. Within the experimental context, they falsely attribute the fluency of that word to presentation of the item in the study list and therefore they call that item old.

The point here is not that different from the point I emphasized in the previous lecture. We can feel familiarity, but we often aren't very good at knowing its true source, and we're prone to misattribute it. This is one part of the story we need to explain déjà vu now let's move to the second part, and it's with respect to something called priming.

Some of the situations that we've discussed in these lectures have involved priming, but I haven't really highlighted it until now. So, to make the concept of priming explicit let's talk about a couple of other experiments. Across a number of trials let's say I show you letter strings, and some of those letter strings are correctly spelled English words like "table." Others are what we call non-words like "thair." Your task is to decide, as quickly and accurately as you can, for each item presented, is it a word or is it a non-word, and I record your speed and your accuracy. Now let's say I show you a bunch of words and non-words, but the critical ones are the words. Let's pick on four words: let's say "doctor," "notes," "class," and "scalpel." Those are four of the words that are within this larger experiment. Note that two of these words are related to medicine, "doctor" and "scalpel," and two are related to learning contexts, "notes" and "class." Now imagine I do this exact same experiment, but I test some people within a hospital, and I test other people within a university. What you would see is that decisions to these medically related words are faster when tested within a hospital so they can respond to the doctor, and any medically related word at all, faster in a hospital than they could respond to those university related words. But, if you do the test in the university the opposite is true. So that suggests there is something about the context in which you're tested that literally prepares you to perceive certain items. When you're in a hospital, you're ready to perceive hospital items; when you're in a university setting you're ready to perceive university items.

So the associations that you've formed in the past, perhaps between places and concepts, but also between pairs of concepts, are preparing you in advance for things that might occur in that context. Remember when I was discussing agnosia, and I told you that memory is critical for understanding what it is that you are currently seeing or hearing. Well really, the truth is that memory is actually preparing you in advance for what you may be about to see or hear. When we walk into any situation we walk in primed for what may happen, and this is really great because it allows us to react more quickly and more efficiently when these expectations, even the very low-level ones, are correct.

What makes priming potentially relevant to déjà vu is that stimuli can prime us even when we are not aware of them occurring at all. Many studies, in fact, have documented so-called subliminal priming effects. For example, let's again say that we are presenting words and non-words, and we're asking participants to categorize them as quickly as possible. But this time, just before each word or non-word we very quickly present a prime, and that prime is either semantically related to the critical item, or it's not. So, for example, if the critical item was "nurse," we might just before it present either "doctor," which is related, or "printer," which is not. We present these words very quickly, so quickly that participants say they only see a flicker. So it's like there's a flicker and then "nurse" comes, and they decide. Despite not seeing that initial word, the prime, decisions to "nurse" are faster when it is preceded by a related item, like "doctor." That's subliminal prime.

So now let's return to Amsterdam, figuratively speaking of course, and let me specify what we're going to call the priming-misattribution theory of déjà vu. There I was at that street corner. Maybe, just maybe, the following happened. I glanced down the street to the left but, just as I did so, something to the right grabbed my attention; maybe it was a loud noise, maybe it was a paddleboat tipping over in the canal. Whatever it was, I glanced over very quickly, but whatever it was caught my attention so quickly that I didn't even remember glancing to the left. I just remember being pulled over here. However, that glance, brief as it was, may have been enough to begin processing of the scene, enough so that when I looked left again my perceptual system had a head start; it was primed. So now, as I look at that scene I am able to process it more fluently than I think I should be able to given that I've never seen it before. I can only conclude that I have seen this scene before, which of course is correct at some level. I saw it just milliseconds ago. I just wasn't aware that I'd seen it. So, since I do not realize it's the glance to my left, the true source of my fluent perception, I don't notice. I cannot correctly attribute the familiarity to its real source. This is my mind missing the sleight of memory, which in this case was that quick first glance. As a result I am left with an intense feeling of familiarity that I cannot attribute to anything, not anything that makes sense. This is not a comfortable feeling, just as it is not comfortable to see a magician do something you cannot understand. When we have intense feelings that something has that warm glow of familiarity we often feel the need to attribute that glow to something, and we are willing to stretch credibility pretty far sometimes to find a source.

Whoa, did you feel that? Did you just experience some sort of déjà vu? Honestly, I have no idea if you did or not, but I just tried to create it using the principles of priming-attribution theory to give you an experience of how it might work. Specifically, I asked the producers to splice in that last sentence in the exact form it was in when I said it earlier in this lecture. Therefore, it was an exact copy of my words and how I said them, repeated. My hope is that, given that earlier presentation, this sentence was nicely primed, and thus, its relatively fluent processing gave you a sense of familiarity, but one that you couldn't immediately figure out. Perhaps this led to a creepy feeling of a sort as you struggled to figure out why that sentence felt so familiar, a feeling not totally unlike déjà vu.

If we did actually cause even some of you to experience déjà vu, then that might be a procedure that could be used to produce, and therefore study, this phenomenon more directly. False alarms are interesting, but they are not really déjà vu. Déjà vu needs to include that sense of oddness, that subjective creepy feeling that makes the soundtrack from the twilight zone play in our heads. That is a very hard, if not impossible, to create in a laboratory, and that's why most theories of déjà vu will be just that, theories.

I have focused so much on the priming-attribution theory because it's the one that I think makes the most sense from all we know about memory. However, there are also other theories, some of which are similar in some ways but different in others. While it may be hard to experimentally show that one is superior to another, they are each worth visiting if only to see what they may tell us about memory and the interaction between memory systems and the way those interactions can lead to illusions of previous experience. So let's consider some of the other memory-based theories as well.

The first one I want to discuss isn't so much a theory of déjà vu per se, nor is it really even a competitor to the notion I've just described. But it does allow us to connect some of this to the brain, including some of the regions we've been discussing. I told you about work suggesting that the hippocampus is critical to conscious memory. Well, other imaging studies have suggested that a brain region just below the hippocampus, an area called the parahippocampus, is active when stimuli feel familiar, irrespective of whether those stimuli are consciously recognized or not. So in brain terms it seems that déjà vu reflects situations in which the parahippocampus is active, but no conscious memory is retrieved, because there is no memory to be retrieved. So, something activates the parahippocampus; perhaps it's just the sort of random activation that was previously discussed in the context of epilepsy, or perhaps it's the sort of perceptual head start I highlighted in the perceptual priming theory.

What other experiences could cause a sense of spooky familiarity? Based on a hologram theory of memory, a Dutch researcher named Hermon Sno argues that memories, like holograms, are re-created out of bits of themselves, the smaller the bit, the more blurry the ultimate memory. He claims that some small aspect of our current experience may be enough to retrieve a very blurry version of some past experience. For example, perhaps you go on a ride with a friend in his 1964 Plymouth. As you ride you begin to experience intense déjà vu. Although you have no conscious memory of it, perhaps your grandfather owned just this kind of car and you rode in it when you were very young. Thus, the look, the smell and the feel of the car may bring that memory back, but in such a degraded form that it is really more like the ghost of a memory. Perhaps this ghost is strong enough to trigger brain regions that respond to familiarity, like the parahippocampus, but not strong enough to give rise to an episodic memory.

Another somewhat similar theory highlights the potential role of memories that we have indirectly experienced through, say, books or movies. For example, imagine that as a child you watched a movie in which some character drove up to a famous landmark, maybe the CN tower in Toronto, and then much later in your life you yourself are visiting Toronto for the first time, and you drive up to that landmark. That might be enough to trigger a strong sense of familiarity that cannot be easily attributed. After all, you have never been to Toronto. Unless you remember that movie distinctly, you again have familiarity that you know cannot be derived from personal past experience. This is your first time in Toronto. Perhaps the most interesting aspect of this theory is its suggestion that some of our memories may not be directly personal memories but, rather, may be memories indirectly derived from other characters that we have been associated with. In that sense, their memories become ours, and yet they're still distinct.

One thing to notice about both of these latter theories I've described to you, the hologram theory and the indirect experience theory, is that they're really both alternate forms of that priming-attribution theory. Instead of arguing that a quick glance might have caused the priming, they argue that a vague memory, or an indirect memory from a book or movie, might cause the fluent perception. Like the priming-attribution theory they assume we are unaware of the true source of the priming, and hence we resort to these metaphysical explanations.

In the case of my Amsterdam story, for example, well, my last name is Joordens, which perhaps is a clue to you that I'm Dutch. Maybe on some past trip to Amsterdam with my parents when I was very young, maybe I saw scenes much like the one that caused déjà vu for me later when I was with my wife, that sort of ghostly memory that I cannot recall. Or maybe in home movies that Dad used to show us there were scenes that I experienced indirectly, scenes that included scenes like the one I saw with my wife. That may have produced the déjà vu experience. So yes, the source of the priming is different, but the basic explanation of the memory illusion is the same.

So maybe despite the difficulty of showing déjà vu in lab we are nonetheless converging on a theory that explains the illusion, and what we can then ask, well, what do these converging theories tell us about memory? Well, one thing that it tells us quite clearly is that declarative and non-declarative forms of memory can become dissociated, decoupled, and that we feel it when they do. That is, usually when we experience some event it increases the likelihood both that it will be fluently perceived and that we will remember it episodically. So things we remember usually feel familiar, and that's great. But occasionally things can feel familiar without us remembering the events that caused the increase of familiarity. Now actually, the reverse can happen as well.

If you take any word and you repeat it over and over and over, eventually that word will not feel like the familiar word you know anymore. You will know it's a word, and you will know it's a word you know. You will have a memory of it as a word. But through repetition it somehow loses its sense of familiarity, which sounds odd, but it's true. Give it a try. Take any word. Let's say "truck." Say it a hundred times. Just listen to me say it a few times: "truck," "truck," "truck," "truck," "truck," "truck," "truck," "truck," "truck." You say that over and over again, it becomes a sound. It doesn't become a word. Its "wordness" slips away. This sort of experience is called *jamais vu*, which translates to never seen. It's the odd feeling of seeing a stimulus that you know you've had previous experience with but that stimulus does not seem familiar, almost like you've never really encountered it before. So it's really the opposite of déjà vu. Remember the Capgras delusion that I told you about? It's like this. So yes, recognition and familiarity can become detached. And when they do, they give rise to desire in us to understand and explain the odd feelings that that creates. Déjà vu and jamais vu are perhaps extreme versions of this. But there is also a much more common version.

So imagine the following. You step on a bus, you see that face in the back and know that you know that person, but you don't know where you know them from—familiarity without any conscious memory. Once again, this is an uncomfortable feeling. And I want to stress this. It's one that seems to demand some form of resolution. And we've all been there. We initially ignore the person in case we don't really know them or in case we end up in a situation where we have to talk to them and we can't remember why we don't know them at all. So instead we cast these furtive glances their way as we try to figure out where we know them from, and our minds are working hard to do just that. So this is the next thing we have learned from this discussion. When our memories do become dissociated that event kicks of a cognitive investigation. Where do I know that person from? Why does this scene seem so familiar? Just like a good detective, our memory systems do not like loose ends.

Recovered Memories or False Memories?
Lecture 20

Human memory is not like a camera; it does not store and replay perfect copies of events. We all forget or misremember details of our past, but astonishingly, we can even "remember" events that never occurred at all. These so-called false memories are more than a quirk of human psychology; they can have powerful effects on our interpersonal relationships, as well as profound ramifications within the legal and judicial system.

Our episodic memories, just like our sense of familiarity, can sometimes go awry for some of the same broad reasons. Memories so fundamentally false are fascinating, raising all sorts of questions about the basis of conscious memory.

In the 1980s and 1990s, more and more prosecutors began submitting witnesses' **recovered memories** as evidence in major cases, but not without stirring controversy. Even as these uses became more frequent, debate flared over whether recovered memories are accurate or whether they are creations of the therapeutic process.

The idea of repressed and recovered memories is as old as psychology itself. Sigmund Freud believed that mental health issues are best viewed as symptoms of some deep internal conflict. As such, a therapist should not attempt to treat the symptoms but to uncover the conflict and help the patient acknowledge and deal with it. This theory is based on 2 assumptions: first, that the patient does not know what the conflict could be, and second, that active cognitive processes exist to keep these conflicts buried.

Given these assumptions, psychoanalysts believe that the only way to uncover the conflict is to use indirect methods that gently probe the mind and allow the painful memories to expose themselves, methods like inkblot tests and free association. If therapy goes well, the patient reaches **catharsis**, a realization of the internal conflict that makes all the patient's troubles make sense. The memories obtained from this process tend to feel clear and accurate, and the patient is certain they are real.

Unfortunately, these assumptions are not based on scientific findings, and doubts about them have only increased over time. The first doubts were raised by psychologist James Deese in the late 1950s; his research suggested that people could have episodic memories for things that never occurred. In the 1980s and 1990s, psychologists Roddy Roediger and Kathleen McDermott returned to Deese's findings and devised a method for creating false memories that bears striking similarities to aspects of clinical psychotherapy.

After undergoing Roediger and McDermott's false memory experiment, some people are more confident of their false memories than they are of their real memories. Roediger and McDermott's experiments also suggest that even a well-meaning therapist can make assumptions about what the patient is suppressing and inadvertently lead the patient to create a memory that fulfills those expectations—a form of priming.

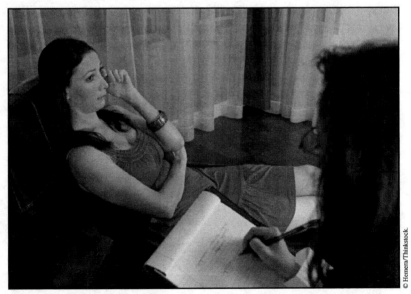

Repressed memory is one of the central principles of psychoanalytic theory, and recovering or releasing them is the main goal of talk therapy.

That said, just because you can create false memories in a lab doesn't prove that all memories recovered in a psychoanalytic setting are false. Dismissing all recovered memories risks re-victimizing the patient and compounding his or her mental health issues. It is a problem with no easy solution; the justice system has compromised by continuing to allow recovered memories as testimony but requiring them to be backed up by other forms of evidence.

Separating real from imagined events means distinguishing between mental experiences prompted by external events versus mental experiences prompted by internal events—things we think or imagine. What is quite fascinating, given how memory seems to work, is how well most of us do distinguish real from imagined most of the time. Episodic memory can go drastically astray because we exist in highly complex environments that require us to switch attention rapidly among various stimuli that our memory must piece together. But our memory systems hate loose ends, and it is in tying those ends up that our memories sometimes fail us. ■

Important Terms

catharsis: In psychoanalytic theory, the release of blocked psychic energy, typically by way of free association and sustained talk.

recovered memory: A memory, usually a traumatic one, thought unrecoverable that is retrieved with the aid of hypnosis or psychoanalytic techniques.

Suggested Reading

Bjorklund, *False-Memory Creation in Children and Adults.*

Brainerd and Reyna, *The Science of False Memory.*

Davies and Dalgleish, *Recovered Memories.*

Sandler, Fonagy, and Baddeley, *Recovered Memories of Abuse.*

1. Have you ever suddenly remembered something that you feel had been forgotten for years? If so, does this mean that memories can be repressed, or is there some other explanation?

2. Have you ever been in the situation where you had to ask someone if you had already told them some bit of information or not? Or maybe you wondered whether something really happened or whether you merely dreamed about it happening? How are these situations similar or different from the false memory situation described in the lecture?

Exercise

Here is a list of words related to sleep: bed, tired, sheet, blanket, night, exhausted, snooze, pillow, refresh, doze. Read those to a friend one day and ask them to try to remember them. Then test them the next day and include the word "sleep" in the test. Do they claim to remember "sleep" being in the original list? How confident are they in their memory?

Recovered Memories or False Memories?
Lecture 20—Transcript

I ended the last lecture by saying that our memory systems do not like loose ends, and I highlighted some illusions of memory that can follow from that.

Well, what is true of familiarity, as supported by non-declarative memory, can also be true of episodic memory. Of course, we all forget or misremember details of past events, but the claim here is much stronger: the claim is that you can actually remember past events that never occurred at all. Memories so fundamentally false are truly fascinating, and they raise all sorts of questions about the true basis of conscious memories. We'll begin our exploration of this topic in the context of a famous debate that occurred in the 1990s. One that pits Freudian psychodynamic therapy against laboratory studies of false memory. The main context for this debate, the courtroom. But the academic and public debate in the media was even more intense.

So let's talk about the story that initiated this all. In 1990 George Franklin was convicted of murdering a girl named Susan Nason, a murder that was committed 21 years earlier. The sole basis of his prosecution was testimony from his daughter, Eileen, testimony based on a memory that she had had after undergoing therapy. Theoretically, the memory had been repressed but recovered by the therapeutic process.

This conviction, and others based on similar testimony, raised many questions about the accuracy of memory in general and of recovered memories in particular. The Franklin case opened a decade in which many more cases based on repressed memories began to be heard throughout the decade. Until that time, cases not involving murder were bound by the statute of limitations for prosecuting someone for a crime. After the Franklin case, some states in the U.S. changed their statute of limitation for some crimes to acknowledge that memories in fact can be repressed and then subsequently recovered, thereby allowing a critical witness to come forward with memories of a crime when a longer period of time had passed.

A large part of what made these cases controversial was debate over when or whether recovered memories are ever accurate, or whether they are just creations of the therapeutic process itself. That debate itself tells us a great deal about memory as it occurs in real-life situations and puts questions about the veracity of human memories squarely at center stage.

But before we get to all that, we have some participants here in the studio as well. They are here because I want to do another memory test with both you and them. When we get to the memory test itself, I want to ask you a question or two about what people remember, so having these guys here will allow me to do that more directly.

Of course I'd like you to participate in the memory test as well. Unexpected memory challenges give you a much better workout than familiar challenges like crossword puzzles, so why not give it a try. I'll explain what I am up to a little later in the lecture when we get to the test itself. For now though, I just want to read you a list of words, and I want you to try your best to remember them. Again, no writing anything down. Just listen to the words as I read them, and try your best to remember. OK. Ready? Here it goes:

"Molehill," "horn," "peak," "melody," "plain," "band," "top," "radio," "summit," "sing," "climb," "piano," "valley," "sound," "hill," "note." Fantastic, thanks. Now let's get back to the interesting issue of recovered memories.

As a first step, I need to explain some aspects of Freudian psychoanalysis since the details are highly relevant to the debate. It's important to be clear that there are actually various approaches that a therapist might use when they're trying to help a client who is suffering from some mental health issues. Freudian psychoanalysis is just one of these approaches, but it's the one that's almost invariably linked to the notions of recovered memories. So for the rest of this lecture that will be the approach I'll be focusing on.

Freud himself believed that when people have mental health issues, the issues they are having are best viewed as symptoms, symptoms of some deeper psychological issues. So, much like a virus, the way it causes say the symptoms of a flu, the psychological trauma causes the behavioral problems. As such, a therapist should attempt to treat that virus and not the symptoms and to do that they need to uncover the psychological conflict, because it is only by acknowledging and dealing with that conflict that one can ultimately become free of the symptoms.

However, the assumptions underlying psychotherapy predict that uncovering these deep-seated psychological traumas will be quite difficult. That's true for two reasons. First, it is assumed that the worse psychological conflicts are buried well below our consciousness. Thus the patient does not even know about them at all. Second, it's further assumed that there are active cognitive processes that attempt to keep those memories buried. They are not available to consciousness because they are being repressed from consciousness by exactly that sort of mechanism, a mechanism that is apparently attempting to spare the individual from some deeply troubling memory.

If the therapist were to try to directly probe the mind to try to uncover this conflict, he will be met with resistance. These defense mechanisms will literally get in the way of such a direct attempt. Given these assumptions, psychoanalysts believe that the only way to uncover the conflict is to use indirect methods, methods that gently probe the mind and try to allow the painful memories to essentially expose themselves.

You've likely heard of things like the inkblot tests. They might try to show a patient perhaps a somewhat ominous looking inkblot, and perhaps the patient when they look at it, the first thing they say is "uncle." Maybe they show the same inkblot another time and the patient says "fear." Slowly the psychiatrist, and perhaps the patient as well, begins to see patterns in the responses, patterns assumed to reflect aspects of that internal conflict.

These patterns might also be mined using other free-association tests and, so for example, in the classic free-association test, a psychoanalyst might intentionally include a word like "uncle," to which perhaps the patient says something like "overpowering." The analyst might also ask the patient to do something like draw pictures. So they might say, "Draw a picture of Thanksgiving dinner." Of particular interest might be the way in which the uncle is portrayed in this picture. Does he look scary?

If therapy goes well, the patient might ultimately reach a point called catharsis. Catharsis is the realization of this internal conflict, a sudden understanding of what it is that's been giving rise to all the problems all along. This is the point when the recovered memories might appear. The patient might suddenly remember the uncle, let's say, sexually abusing them, or they might remember their father killing their friend. The memories obtained from this process tend to feel clear and accurate, and the patient is certain they are real. Finally the patient feels like everything makes sense.

Reaching catharsis is typically not considered enough for the patient to achieve true healing. Many patients are advised that they must take the next step, and that means achieving justice. In the case of recovered memories, that often means bringing the culprit to court, charging them, and ultimately sending them to jail for their crime. Only then will the patient be able to move forward with their lives.

Now everything I just told you rests on the assumptions of psychotherapy. These ideas have entered popular culture, but unfortunately these assumptions are not based on scientific findings; instead, they are based primarily on the theories of one man: Sigmund Freud. Doubts about these assumptions have only increased over time, and many other therapies exist that are based on entirely different assumptions.

But that said, in the 1980s and 1990s it seemed that many patients were recovering memories in just this way, and with that change of statute of limitations, more and more court cases were based solely on recovered memories. These cases were tricky because they are often one person's word against another, and again they rely on the assumptions of Freudian psychotherapy being accurate. But often the patients were so sure, so confident that like Mr. Franklin many were prosecuted and found guilty. Jurors tend to be swayed by confident eye-witnesses, even when they are reporting on an episodic memory that they couldn't even retrieve for 20 years.

Are recovered memories to be trusted? Sometimes, maybe? Never? Always? Well, a psychologist named Deese published a study in the late 1950s, and that study suggested that people could actually have episodic memories for things that never actually occurred. That might sound ridiculous, right? How could you have a memory for something that never occurred? When Deese's paper first came out, that seems to have been the reaction of many in the scientific community as well. Deese's work was largely ignored.

However, as all these cases based on testimony of recovered memory began stirring the public in the '80s and '90s, two psychologists named Roddy Roediger and Kathleen McDermott remembered the Deese findings and brought them back to light. They devised a specific methodology for creating false memories, and the really startling thing is that that methodology they came up with bears a striking resemblance and a lot of similarities to some of these aspects of clinical psychotherapy that I've been telling you about.

Before I give you the details of their methodology, I think it's time to test your memory for the items that I read you a few minutes ago. What we're going to do is a recognition test, but it's a recognition test with a twist. I'm going to read out some items to you and for each item I want you to think about the item first, and, if you want you can write them down, and then think about three things about the item: the item itself, whether you think the item was in the list, and how confident you feel that the item was on the list, let's say on a 5-point scale. What we're going to do in the studio here, is when I read these items, I'm going to ask the people in the studio to raise their hand if they think an item is old, that is if it was on the list, and to raise a number of fingers on that hand that reflects how confident you are that that item is on the list.

The first item I'm going to ask you about is the word "table." So think about it for a moment, and then I'll just ask everybody to consider the word, whether you think it's old, how confident you are. OK. Anybody here, go ahead, raise your hands if anybody thinks it's old. OK. And how confident? Five? Three? One person, 3 confident. OK. That's cool. All right, that was not on the list by the way. But it's a good point for me to mention, actually, that when you do recognition tests that happens all the time. People remember items not being on the list; it's called a false alarm. That's OK. No big deal.

So now let's go to another one. How about "melody"? Yeah, go ahead and raise your hands. So we have about 5 hands, and everybody's at about 4 or 5 confidence. "Melody" was on the list. So now how about "snooze"? OK. Nobody thinks "snooze" is on the list. "Snooze" was not on the list. How about "music"? Nope. OK. So we had 3 people and we got 3s and 2s and 3s. OK. Cool. And finally, how about "mountain"? That's the last one I'll ask you about. Think about it. Anybody? OK. Some 5s, 3s, and 4s. Cool. Thank you very much. It turns out neither "music" nor "mountain" were on the list. But these were the classic items we would test in these situations. In both of those cases, we did find some people who thought they were on the list, and in the latter case, in the case of "mountain," we found people who were saying 4s and 5s.

It is in fact a common finding that many people remember at least one of those two absent items as being on the list and that they feel pretty confident about them. Some people actually though are more confident for the items that were not on the list than they are for items that were on the list. And in case you had difficulty experiencing this yourself, let's listen again to the part of the lecture where I'm reading the list so that you can hear the list and you can be assured that I am telling the truth, those two items were not on the list. As you listen, I also want you to notice the structure of the list. Beginning with the first word, I am actually alternating two related lists, two related lists. The first list is a list of words related to the word "mountain." So you'll hear things like "molehill" and "peak" and "plane" and "top." The second list is a list of words related to the word "music." So you'll hear words like "horn," "melody," "band," and "radio." OK. So here's the replay. Ready? Here goes: "molehill," "horn," "peak," "melody," "plane," "band," "top," "radio," "summit," "sing," "climb," "piano," "valley," "sound," "hill," "note."

I would also like to point out that I have often done this same experiment in my university classes. And in those cases, quite a few people do have these false memories and, when they do, they are sometimes very confident that their memory is accurate. The most recent class in which I did this experiment used the same words you just experienced, and about 30 of a 100 or so students demonstrated the illusion of memory we're discussing here by raising their hands when I asked how many of them heard the word "mountain."

How about "mountain"? How many would be able to say, "Yes, 'mountain' was in there"? How many people say, "No. It wasn't"? OK. Mountain's a cool one. "Mountain" was never read, was never shown.

This demonstration that you can create false memories in the lab is relevant to the false memory debate in two ways. First, it clearly shows that people can remember events that didn't happen, for example, hearing the words "music" and "mountain." That in and of itself is not all that surprising, but what is really surprising is that when they do remember these words, they can sometimes be very confident their memory is accurate, just as confident as they were when they remembering words that actually were on the list. That is a true episodic memory. That alone makes it hard to just accept the testimony about a recovered memory as accurate, even when the witness is highly confident.

But there is a second aspect of creating false memories that's even more worrisome. Remember when I said that this process for recovering memories involves getting at the inner trauma in a very indirect way, hinting around it, but never actually saying it directly. The therapist may think that the patient was, let's say sexually abused by an uncle, but the therapist will never say that directly. Instead, situations are created that encourage the client to think of things along the lines of what the therapist is thinking, and at some point the client may remember that target event, even if it never occurred.

In many ways this is very similar to the laboratory way of creating false memories. Think of that again. We don't ever present "music" or "mountain" in the list, but we present a bunch of words that are related to "music" and a bunch of words that are related to "mountain." We essentially hint all around the critical word without ever mentioning it. Then when we tap memory, we find that we have created a memory for that concept we hinted around, perhaps in the way a therapist might help create a memory by hinting around what they hypothesize to be the event causing the inner conflict. Again, if this feels a little like our discussion of prototypes two lectures ago, at its heart it is a very similar illusion of memory, it's just played out in a legal context. The sort of context that can have innocent people end up in jail for decades. Sometimes illusions can have very palpable consequences.

Well, I have described this as a debate, but I likely should have called it a heated debate, and you likely have a better understanding why. After all, rapes and murders really do take place. So imagine listening to the story I just told you from the perspective of a Freudian psychoanalyst. You thought you might be able to help bring criminals to justice and also to give closure for your client. But in essence, you have just been accused of helping to implant false memories that are ultimately used to put innocent people behind bars for horrific crimes that they didn't actually commit.

Clearly some analysts would be, and some were, very upset by such a depiction. What's more, many of them rightfully pointed out that just because you can create false memories in a lab, and just because the procedure used to do it bears some surface similarity to the therapeutic techniques, that certainly doesn't prove that all memories recovered in the psychoanalytic setting are false memories.

Maybe some are false memories. In fact, some have been conclusively shown to be false after the fact. But still, perhaps some are not. Perhaps some are accurate recovered memories. In this case we could end up actually re-victimizing somebody and thereby compound their mental health issues. Let's think about this a little bit. They finally feel like they understand the root cause of their trauma, they reach that state of catharsis, they move forward to get justice, and now we refuse to believe them. We tell them that no matter how clear it may seem to them, their cathartic memory is surely false and they are deluding themselves and making false accusations against innocent people. Wow.

So this really is a fascinating and a multifaceted issue and one that has no easy solution, at least for those who believe in the assumptions of psychoanalysis. To most others though, the assumptions of psychoanalysis lack scientific support, while the evidence is too strong that memories appearing for the first time in a psychoanalytic context may be inaccurate.

The justice system has responded to this more general perception, and now in order to convict there is a need for someone to show some other form of evidence, something in addition to the recovered memory, something that can give at least some sort of further credence to the accuracy of what's being described. Given what we learned about memory during the first decade of the 21st century, it has become extremely unlikely that anyone would be prosecuted on the basis of a recovered memory alone.

These scientific results have also resulted in the overturning of many of the initial prosecutions that were based on recovered memories. Remember the case of George Franklin, the one I mentioned at the beginning of this lecture? George's conviction was overturned in 1995, and no further charges or accusations were ever leveled. In fact, no further evidence could be found to support the memory of his daughter, and what evidence that was still available seemed to refute it. George spent five years of his life in jail for what seemed to have been a false memory created during therapy.

So what does this debate about false memory tell us about the accuracy of our memory systems more generally? Well, if we consider both the experimental technique that's used to create a false memory, and the clinical context in which recovered memories are said to occur, in both cases it is not completely accurate to say that the stimulus was in fact never presented.

It's true that it was never presented in the environment, so I never read the words "music" or "mountain" aloud. But when you hear all those words related to "mountain," it's completely possible that the concept of "mountain" that was so primed by all of those related words did come to mind. So while "mountain" was never explicitly presented at study, it may have occurred in your mind.

This depiction highlights one of the real challenges that our memory systems face when trying to account for things that really happened. When doing so we have to separate the real experiences from the imagined experiences. Of course, all experiences are really experienced in our mind, even those that initially were stimulated by the outside world. The process that allows us to perceive the world around us, they do their thing by essentially bringing information from the outside world into our minds.

So what we really have are mental experiences prompted by external events versus mental experiences prompted by internal events, things that we thought about or imagines. Now of course schizophrenics have a horrible time discriminating real from imagined and can even happily have conversations with people who really aren't there.

What is quite fascinating, given what we're learning about memory, is that why don't most of us do that? Why is it the case that most of us seem to be able to distinguish real from imagined? It's not like we don't hear voices in our heads. We sometimes say that about schizophrenics, they hear voices in their heads. Well, I hear voices in my head all the time. I imagine talking to people; they talk back. So sometimes that voice that I'm hearing isn't even my own voice, it's someone else's voice. And yet, nonetheless, I somehow take ownership of all of that and see it as something that I've generated. And that's what separates us from schizophrenics, not the presence of voices but the attributions we make about them.

Maybe when priming is consistent enough, as it is in the false memory experiment or in the psychoanalytic context, then the imagined events become so well represented that they can begin to feel more and more like events prompted by external experiences.

Studies of the effects of hypnosis support this notion. Hypnosis allows us to imagine things with enhanced clarity. Because of this apparent clarity, hypnosis is sometimes used to help a witness remember some critical details of, say, a crime scene that they witnessed. Through hypnosis, the person can imagine going back in time and retracing events, and it all feels quite real.

What that means is that the cues that we can use to prompt memory are stronger, and that can indeed prompt and promote the recovery of memories. But there's a real problem as well. Hypnotized people are highly suggestible and if pushed slightly they will provide confident answers even when they give inaccurate information.

For example, if you ask somebody who witnessed a bank robbery, "What color were the robber's shoes?" The witness will likely give you an answer; if you push hard enough they will say "red." Maybe that answer is due to enhanced memory. Maybe they were suddenly able to recollect that, or maybe they were just going along with your suggestion, and they provided an answer through a process that we sometimes call confabulation, the filling in of memory gaps by fabricated information, just to provide the answer. The problem with hypnotized people once they've been hypnotized is they believe these things. They believe it's true, and so they're not sure what's real or imagined, and after they've been hypnotized, we can't tell the difference either.

It's because of this that often in criminal investigations, police will really resist the temptation to hypnotize a witness. Once hypnotized it's very difficult to trust the memory that that witness has. Again, we can't separate the confabulations from the real memory. So as a result, this person automatically loses some credibility in a relatively automatic way and that makes it hard, the court system knows this, so it makes it hard to trust anything they say. And because of all this police will usually only hypnotize people as a last resort, when they feel like they have nothing to go on in a case and they hope that the testimony from the hypnotized subject might bring some new leads that ultimately might give them some more concrete way to solve the case even potentially without that witness's testimony.

This adds more suspicion to the memories recovered in the psychoanalytic context because often hypnosis, or other forms of guided imagery, are among the techniques used to indirectly probe the unconscious mind. Have you ever seen those people on TV who first experienced some odd event, and they couldn't make sense of it, and then they went somewhere and they got hypnotized, and then under hypnosis they suddenly remembered it all. It was aliens. They were kidnapped. The aliens kidnapped and probed them. They're very confident in these memories. They go on TV shows and tell you all about it. Once the event is experienced with such rich imagery, once you go through that memory under hypnosis, it becomes very hard to discriminate imagined events from events that really occurred.

It's important that I make clear, though, that everything I've been saying about the fallibility of memory in court cases, it should not be taken to imply that our memory for events is not a sufficient basis for investigation. On the contrary, memory can produce valuable leads that can be confirmed or denied using other evidence. Rape victims may be able to identify their assailants, witnesses may be able to identify a murderer, and so on. It may even be possible for someone to forget a traumatic event entirely, but then later remember it spontaneously. But then all the cautions would apply, just as what we've already discussed. And that's my main point in this lecture: more than we can realize, episodic memory can go drastically astray. Unfortunately, being convinced that we've remembered accurately is no guarantee that we have remembered accurately.

After all, we all interact in highly complex environments. Often we're switching attention between various stimuli that we experience. Memory works to kind of piece together these experiences that were part of some specific event without mixing things up. But our memory hates loose ends, and sometimes memory fails quite dramatically. I'll conclude with an example where no hypnosis or psychoanalytic prompting were involved.

Consider the following case. A woman was home alone watching television when an assailant broke into her apartment and raped her. When the police arrived the victim said that she had a very clear memory of the rapist's face, so a sketch artist was brought in and immediately a sketch was drawn up. Sketch in hand, the police were able to quickly identify the accused perpetrator. His name was Donald Thompson; he was a professor at a nearby university.

However, the police quickly realized that he could not have committed the rape, he had an airtight alibi. He was on live TV at the time. Ironically he was on an educational show talking about distortions of memory. The victim of the crime had indeed seen his face just before or perhaps even during the crime because she was watching him on TV when the assailant broke in.

Somehow the two events, the TV show and the rape, had become fused in her mind. She remembered the face, but the source of the face was distorted in her memory. Somehow it became the face of the rapist. As this example shows, while memories often serve us well, even drastic distortions are possible.

All of this highlights the fallibility of episodic memory. Let's go back to something I said much earlier in the course when I described episodic memory as analogous to the bookshelves in a library or the hard drive on a computer. Clearly we need to revise that. After all, as we've seen, those analogies are too clean for the kinds of cases we've just been discussing. Human memory does not store perfect copies of experience that are then replayed in a manner that provides a perfect copy of that event. Video cameras do that, human memory does not. So how does it work then?

Well, in our next lecture, we'll revisit how we really remember the events of our lives. It's actually more like—well, wait and see. Let's be constructive on this topic, and let's see what sorts of analogies you can come up with.

Mind the Gaps! Memory as Reconstruction
Lecture 21

> The analogy of retrieving memories from our brains the way one retrieves a book from a shelf is actually a false one; in reality, every time we remember an event, we are reconstructing it from specifics stored in our episodic memory and general knowledge of the world stored in our semantic memory. In most contexts, this system is elegantly efficient, but it is also prone to minor errors that may have not-so-minor consequences.

In the late 19th century, Russian neuropsychiatrist Sergey Korsakov discovered that many of his patients who were alcoholics or malnourished had severe trouble laying down new episodic memories. He also noted that these patients had a tendency to confabulate, yet they weren't intending to deceive anyone. These observations were some of our first clues to the nature of memory retrieval.

A few decades later, Cambridge University psychologist Sir Frederic Bartlett tested people's ability to recall details by reciting an American Indian folktale to English men and women and asking them to repeat what they had heard. The test subjects were likely to remember aspects of the story that were culturally familiar but tended to forget or alter unfamiliar details; for example, they tended to Christianize the story's spiritual and supernatural aspects.

Bartlett's conclusion was that we do not retrieve memories as complete episodes but reconstruct them by piecing together newly stored bits with things we already know. In other words, our semantic memories fill in gaps within our episodic memories. On close examination, this system makes a lot of sense; because most of the details of any experience are mundane, they can be left to semantic memory, while the episodic memory takes care of unusual or unique details. The problem is that people have trouble knowing the difference between the facts and the filler.

So we know memories are often inaccurate, and that these inaccuracies are due to the reconstructive nature of memory. We also know that these inaccuracies may be accompanied by high levels of confidence. Most of the time, these errors are trivial, but in a legal context, errors in memory can have huge consequences.

Every year, more than 70,000 Americans are charged with crimes solely on the basis of eyewitness testimony—that is, on the basis of episodic memory—and studies show that eyewitness testimony is the single most convincing form of evidence for the average jury, even when that testimony has been discredited. This is worrisome because a number of studies demonstrate how inaccurate eyewitnesses often are. Also, jurors are heavily swayed by a witness's appearance of confidence, and we know how confident people can be about their false memories.

The American justice system does what it can to find jurors with unaltered memories and weak biases and then to control the details of the case those

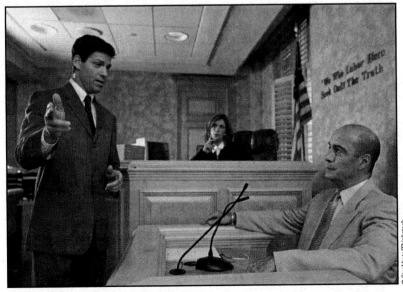

Juries put more faith in eyewitness testimony—another human's episodic memory—than any other form of evidence.

jurors are exposed to. This begins with voir dire, an Old French term that means "to speak the truth." Lawyers get to interview prospective jurors, and with highly publicized cases, a judge may go so far as to order jury sequestration before or during the trial.

Lawyers also sometimes try to use memory re-creation to their advantage through carefully choosing the way they word their questions. Most of us know this as "leading the witness"—namely, asking a question in a way that suggests a certain answer.

It's important to emphasize that these sorts of errors don't just happen in the courtroom; they happen to each of us on a daily basis. In the vast majority of cases, the important aspects of our episodic memories are correct— "important" meaning the aspects we thought were important at the time of encoding. Semantic memory pieces those aspects together to provide a seamless replaying of the event.

So why did Dr. Korsakov's malnourished patients confabulate for no apparent reason? Because their condition caused thiamine deficiency, which damaged the hippocampus, they simply had less accurate memories to go on. They tried to make sense of the bits they had; they just weren't very good at it. ■

Suggested Reading

Best and Intons-Peterson, *Memory Distortions and Their Prevention.*

Memon, Vrij, and Bull, *Psychology and Law.*

Schacter, *The Seven Sins of Memory.*

Questions to Consider

1. The more you understand how things work in various contexts, the better you are able to fill in the gaps between remembered details, and the more vivid your memory will be. What does this say about the link between the accuracy of memory and how vivid, and therefore real, it might seem?

2. The next time you and someone else have very different memories of some event, pay attention to the specific bits you disagree about. Are these bits things you likely felt were really important at the time of encoding?

Exercise

Find the folktale Sir Frederic Bartlett told to his subjects, "The War of the Ghosts," online. Read it once, then in about a week try to rewrite it. Compare your recounting to the original. Even knowing all you now know about memory, do you still make interesting errors of omission and regularization?

Mind the Gaps! Memory as Reconstruction
Lecture 21—Transcript

We follow the progression in this course that mimics in some ways how the study of a memory itself has evolved. Tricks to improve memory, understand the different systems of memory, figure out the underlying biology, and bring everything to bear to what we're learning back into our everyday life. And in recent lectures, we've also been chipping away at a major oversimplification. It's a simplification that can be very misleading, as we've begun to see as we consider how memory hates these loose ends.

The pair of images I gave you much earlier about long-term memory, the notion of files being retrieved from a hard drive or books from a library, that clearly needs to be revised. In actuality, our long-term memories are not really like either, and we don't retrieve them from memory in that way either. We in fact re-create our memories anew each and every time. And this is especially true for episodic memories, and they are our most personal connection to our past. It's very important to me that you leave this lecture series with an accurate sense of how episodic memories work. In so doing, you'll also gain a more nuanced picture of how these memories have also created your ongoing sense of who you are.

To frame this discussion I want to briefly tell you about another neuropsychological syndrome, one that also involves anterograde amnesia. Here's the story. A Russian neuropsychiatrist named Sergei Korsakov noted that many patients he encountered shared the same two symptoms. First, they had severe trouble laying down new episodic memories. Why? Well, one thing that Korsakov noted about these patients is that the vast majority of them were alcoholics, and those who weren't alcoholics had suffered from some form of malnutrition. And while it turns out that one can indeed survive on alcohol, that is, there's enough calories to sustain life, it doesn't have many nutrients, and thiamine especially is critical for a healthy hippocampus. Without thiamine, the hippocampus slowly dies, resulting in progressively more severe anterograde amnesia.

The second symptom that Korsakov noted is also going to be important to this lecture. He noticed that the patients suffering from this progressively worsening anterograde amnesia also showed a tendency for confabulation, saying things that just were not true. They weren't lying per se, and what I mean by that is they weren't really intending to deceive anyone. So why were they confabulating then? Understanding the answer to this question will also provide a deeper understanding of episodic memory just as this lecture is meant to do. So we're going to return to these patients at the end of the lecture to explain their behavior in light of this new understanding.

To move towards an understanding of confabulation, let's use our working memories to transport ourselves to Cambridge University in England early 1900s, and once there we will to meet a professor named Frederic Bartlett, now Sir Frederic Bartlett. Like many British professors of the time, he would travel from his flat to the university on a bicycle, and he would meet many of the same people each day, and he would stop and chat with them all a little.

At some point, Bartlett decided that he would use this daily routine as a context for a memory study—no, not in the sense of the method of loci, in a different sense. Specifically, he found a somewhat oddly written American Indian legend, and it's called *The War of the Ghosts*. At least it was oddly written by British standards. It used language in different ways, it referred to spiritual notions that few Brits knew, and generally it told the tale in a manner that seemed to leave out some details. If you're interested, I'm sure you can find this online.

Bartlett decided one day to read *The War of the Ghosts* to each person he met, asking them to try to remember it. Then after various intervals had passed he would ask these people to recount the tale back to him, and he recorded and analyzed what they said.

Virtually nobody was able to recount the story correctly, everyone made errors. Some of these errors would be what we could call omission errors, that is, parts of the legend were actually missing. These errors could perhaps be attributable to forgetting, but Bartlett noticed that all parts of the legend were not equally forgotten. The parts that made the least sense, or that fit least with the stories that were commonly told in Britain, those were the parts most likely to be forgotten. That alone was potentially interesting, but these were not the only errors made.

Another very common error was what Bartlett termed regularization errors. Essentially, when people recounted the legend they did so in a way that fit more closely with the sorts of stories people were accustomed to, and they also were made to fit with the beliefs that the people had. So, for example, Christian references ended up replacing the references to native spirituality, the legend itself was generally made more flowing, and sometimes parts were added to bridge these perceived gaps that were present in the original legend.

Also, the legend ends in way that seems abrupt and confusing to many British people, and they would tend to alter the ending to make it more, well, more like a conclusion.

Based on these data and other experiments, Bartlett published a book in 1932 that made a strong claim about memory. He claimed that we do not retrieve memories and we certainly do not retrieve them as complete wholes, but rather we reconstruct memories by piecing together certain bits that we had newly stored and bringing these together with things we already know.

For example, if I asked you to recall your last visit to some nice sunny beach location, Bartlett would claim that the memory you would recount to me would first have to be constructed, not retrieved as a whole. The construction would begin with the retrieval of certain specific facts that you had stored, perhaps where you went, perhaps some memory of fellow travelers you met there, perhaps even some event that occurred on the beach, that sort of thing.

You would then take these bits of retrieved memories and then you would glue them together into a story and make that movie of the mind that we see. Of course you aren't going to remember every little detail of the trip, so to piece together the story you use your semantic memory to fill in the gaps, your general knowledge of geography and beaches and resorts and how all those things work. The problem is we sometimes have trouble knowing the differences between the bits we actually remembered, and the bits we filled in to complete the story. We have to mind those gaps, and sometimes that can be trouble. The facts and the filler are hard to discriminate. The entire memory can seem like one seamless and accurate recounting.

When you think of the sort of memory system described by this account it actually makes a lot of sense. Using semantic memory in this way allows us to not have to episodically remember every single event that occurred in some past experience. Really that sounds pretty inefficient when you think of it, because most of the details of any experience are just mundane common aspects of the way the world works. Why store all that information over and over with each new experience? Why not just store the relevant bits of some experience then use our knowledge of the world to paint in all of those less relevant details?

For this to be effective, though, for it to provide a seamless feeling of replaying that past event, it would also make sense to not make the distinction between retrieved and overlaid memory clear. We'd like them all to blend together to provide one nice movie in our minds. This seems like a pretty good outcome, even if we do sometimes feel overly confident that the details we filled in were really part of the real episode.

By the way, you've likely repeatedly experienced a much more everyday version of how the accuracy of your memory can differ from your confidence in it. I remember one occasion when my wife and I had been invited to a colleague's house for dinner. Sometime thereafter she made a remark to a friend about the odd shade of green on the outside of the house we visited. I found the comment strange because I distinctly remembered the house being painted brown. I said as much, and the two of us began nicely debating the issue, each of us though sure that our memories were correct.

But of course, despite the fact that we were both absolutely confident in our memories, one of us had to be completely wrong. One of us was both confident and inaccurate. Who? Well, I can't really remember, and that's not really the point anyway. The point's this: You have likely experienced a similar situation sometime when you and somebody else were both sure about different versions of the same memory.

So we know that memories are often inaccurate and that these inaccuracies are often due to the reconstructive nature of memory. We also know that these inaccuracies are sometimes accompanied by high levels of confidence. What are the consequences of all this?

Well, the consequences are minor. We seem to remember the important aspects of shared memory, and if we quibble over details now and then that's really no big deal. Or is it? Let's return again to the courtroom. Why the courtroom again? Well, as our previous lecture on false memories so clearly illustrated, the consequences of inaccurate memories are amplified when one's freedom may be on the line. Thus it is perhaps not surprising that many experimental studies of inaccurate memories are conducted within a legal context. These are the studies that tell us the most about how episodic memories are formed, and the distortions that may be part of that process. So if we must follow them into the courtroom, so be it.

Let's actually begin with some sobering statistics. According to the textbook I use when I teach Psychology and the Law, over 70,000 Americans a year are charged with crimes solely on the basis of eyewitness testimony, and of course eyewitness testimony is episodic memory. These are not necessarily weak cases.

For example, in one experiment Elizabeth Loftus, a leader in the study of memory in the legal context, provided participants with a description of a hypothetical case in which a grocery store owner was robbed and murdered and the suspect was arrested. Three groups of participants were asked to pretend they were jurors in the case.

One group was provided with circumstantial evidence that the suspect was guilty; he had money in his apartment, he had traces of ammonia on his shoe that matched that of a common floor cleaner that was used in the store. Eighteen percent of this group voted for conviction based on this circumstantial evidence. A second group was given the same evidence, but they were also told that a witness had seen the suspect shoot the grocery clerk. Seventy-two percent of this group voted for conviction, so clearly the eyewitness account had a strong effect. But here's the really interesting part.

There was also a third group. The third group was told the same thing as the second, but this time the defendant's lawyer discredited the witness by showing that the witness's vision was extremely poor, 20/400 to be precise. Thus the witness couldn't have seen the suspect clearly at all. Sixty-eight percent of the third group voted for conviction.

So only 4 percent of the jurors seemed to see this discrediting of the witness as important. Even with his horrible eyesight, his testimony still had a powerful effect. Why? Some psychologists believe that eye-witness testimony is itself highly memorable to jurors and that's why it has such a big impact on their deliberations and on their decisions, and it doesn't really matter whether the testimony is discredited or not.

This is worrisome because a number of psychological studies have detailed how inaccurate eye-witness testimonies often are. For example in one study customers were asked to engage in an unusual but otherwise safe interaction with a store employee. For example, a customer might enter a shoe store and insist that he wanted the clerk to sell him some milk. When the employee refused on the grounds that they just don't sell milk, the customer pushed the point further, then left frustrated.

Later the employees were shown line-ups consisting of the bizarre customers along with other faces. While 42 percent made a correct identification, 22 percent could not recall well enough to make a choice; more scary though, 36 percent choose someone else—an innocent person.

Thus one can indeed accurately remember a perpetrator, but they can also get it wrong at startlingly high rates. This wouldn't be a major issue if jurors could tell the difference between accurate and inaccurate memories. One could imagine that maybe some feature of the recounting might tip them off. However, there is good reason to doubt that even this is true.

For example, in another study witnesses viewed a perpetrator in the act of a robbery. For some witnesses the perpetrator had on a hat that covered most of his hair; for others, the hat was a little higher, showing quite a bit of his hair. For a third group there was no hat at all, so all of the perpetrator's head was visible. These groups identified the correct individual at rates of 33, 40, and 74 percent, respectively, so they showed clear differences in the accuracy of their memories.

However, when mock jurors were completely informed of what the witness had seen, they convicted at rates of 62, 66, and 74 percent, respectively. Said another way, even under conditions where the witnesses were choosing the correct perpetrator only a third of the time, choosing an innocent person the other two-thirds, jurors still found whoever they chose to be guilty 62 percent of the time.

Part of the explanation of this has to do with the confidence with which witnesses testify. There are two issues here really. First, jurors are heavily swayed by confidence. If a witness says, "I am absolutely certain that that is the man I saw," jurors are more likely to convict them than if a witness says, "I'm pretty sure that was the man."

Troublingly though, the second issue is that confidence is often only weakly correlated with the actual accuracy of a memory. In fact, most of the research examining the relation between memory confidence and memory accuracy suggests that most of us are as confident in our inaccurate memories as we are in our accurate memories. People deprived of adequate sleep, for example, have been found to be more confident in their memories and to become even more confident about memories that turn out to be inaccurate. Our memory systems hate loose ends.

This all comes back to Bartlett's notion of memory reconstruction. Our reconstructions are part retrieved fact and part filled in fiction, but we ourselves have a lot of trouble telling the difference. Consider the following study. In 1992 a cargo El Al Boeing 747 crashed into a tall apartment building in Amsterdam. This disaster was covered extensively in the media, including many images of the aftermath of the crash, but given that there was no video of the crash itself, only the aftermath was shown.

Despite this, when psychologists questioned students about their memory of the event, 66 percent claimed to remember seeing the airplane crash into the building. In addition, they also offered further details. Some remembered the plane hitting vertically, others remembered it hitting horizontally, and some claimed seeing it already on fire before crashing into the building.

There's no doubt that when we hear about such an event, our mental re-creation of the event includes details we may not have actually witnessed, details like those just described. But this all becomes tricky when, upon repeated remembering of the event, these details become indistinguishable from the details we actually saw.

This sensitivity of memory to additional details can be especially problematic when one becomes exposed to the information after experiencing the event, before recounting it. In the Dutch study described before, the student might well have read accounts from witnesses at the scene, some of whom may have described their memories, memories which may have included details that were not included in the news reports.

So, a little like that rape victim described in the last lecture, the students may actually experience problems with what we call source memory. They did indeed hear some things, and they saw some things, but those things became merged and that's what they saw in the movie in their minds. When the psychologists only asks them about what they actually saw, they have trouble separating those seen-only events from the larger movie, and they remember actually experiencing events that only the witnesses on the ground actually experienced.

Now of course the justice system does what it can to try to find jurors with relatively pure memories and weak biases and then to control the details of the case those jurors are exposed to. This first part of the trial is sometimes called *voir dire*, and it's a term from Old French which translates as "to speak the truth." During this phase lawyers question prospective jurors in hopes of uncovering any biases that they might bring to the case that could color the way they remember the trial details, and also they want to ascertain whether potential jurors have already been exposed to biasing details about the case from media sources or things like that.

The hope is to find jurors who currently know very little about the case and who seem to have no preconceptions that would bias the way they consider evidence. After all other controls are in place, with respect to what evidence is even considered admissible, and the goal is to have jurors make their decision based on a balanced consideration of the evidence that they were exposed to in the courtroom. Thus we really want to make sure that they aren't already bringing other evidence in with them, evidence that they may have read or they may have heard about already.

In very high profile cases, the justice system, their attempts to kind of keep this juror memory pure, can also continue throughout the duration of the case. That is, jurors might be sequestered, kept apart from their jobs, from their friends, from family, and of course from the media. This sometimes means that jurors end up living in a controlled bubble within a hotel room, allowed to speak only with other jurors or with other members of the justice system. They may be allowed to speak with family members as well, but on strict condition that they not talk about any of the details of the case.

But is that sufficient? Does that mean we've started out with pure jurors, we've insulated them from all their biases and details that might come from media or friends? If we do that, have we handled everything we need to handle? That all works as long as the information they hear in court is presented in an unbiased manner. But is that true? Can we accept that that is in fact occurring? Well, lawyers know a little bit about memory re-creation as well, and given the chance, they will use that knowledge to their advantage. Consider the following experiment also performed by Loftus and colleagues.

Participants first saw a short slideshow in which a red car went through a stop sign before running into a white car. Sometime later the participants were questioned about what they had remembered. However, the way they were questioned was varied across groups.

The first group was asked, "How fast was the red car going when it contacted the white car?" For the remaining groups the term "contacted" was changed, and it was changed to either "hit," "bumped," "collided," or "smashed." So the fifth group, for example, was asked, "How fast was the red car going when it smashed into the white car?"

The speed estimates mirrored the verb that was used, with estimates of 31, 34, 38, 39, and 41 miles per hour respectively across the five groups. Simply by changing the wording of the question the participants seemed to remember the red car going up to ten miles an hour more.

But was this really how they remembered it or were they just kind of trying to match the context presented by the questioner? That's actually a hard question to answer definitively, but the experimenters tried. They called the participants back a week after they had viewed the slideshow, and they asked them to remember the event again in their minds and then asked them if there was any broken glass on the ground after the accident.

Note that all participants were asked the same question this time. The correct answer was no, there was no broken glass. But those exposed to the more extreme verbs earlier were also more likely to remember broken glass being present, in fact, 32 percent of the participants in the "smashed" condition remembered seeing broken glass despite the fact that it wasn't there. Once again, a false memory, perhaps caused by the suggestion of broken glass and supported by the use of the word "smashed."

If you watch court shows at all you've probably heard some lawyer exclaim at some point, "Objection! She's leading the witness, your Honor!" The term "leading the witness" refers explicitly to the situation in which a lawyer has asked a question in a way that suggests a certain answer.

This is the extreme form of what we've just been discussing. Often they do the same thing in much more subtle ways. Now as Loftus's work shows, one can definitely lead a witness, and thereby they can indeed affect the way they remember events in much more subtle ways, so for instance, by selecting the words one uses carefully when asking questions. Good lawyers know this, and they use it. It's one of the things that makes them good lawyers.

So I've been talking a lot about memory in the context of the courtroom. This really is an interesting context because, as mentioned earlier, nowhere else is memory usually under such scrutiny because nowhere else are the consequences of incorrect memories so severe. It seems that we hear almost every week about someone who was falsely imprisoned, often for decades, only to be released when new DNA procedures conclusively show that some witness's memory was inaccurate. So to some extent, the legal context has indeed become the primary laboratory for investigating errors of memory.

However, it's important to emphasize that all the sorts of errors that we've been discussing occur for each of us in our daily lives on a regular basis. I often find myself in situations where my memory of some event conflicts with someone else's memory of the very same event. Knowing all I do about memory, I cannot help but now say things like the following: "Well, I may very well be wrong about this, but all I can really say is this is how I remember things occurring."

Occasionally I may try to highlight some detail that I recalled, some detail that I'm pretty sure is correct, a detail that perhaps corroborates my recounting relative to that of somebody else, and I hope that when they think about this detail they will also recall it and in so doing will realize my reconstruction is more accurate than theirs. But often I must simply agree to disagree. I remember things the way I do, and I'm hesitant to believe deeply that any memory I have is actually a completely accurate rendition of the actual event I witnessed.

I am very far from being the only memory researcher whose education has resulted in an appreciation of the dangers of believing all the details of my episodic memory. I have mentioned Elizabeth Loftus and her work a couple of times in this lecture. In fact, she is *the* expert on the sort of memory distortions we've been discussing. In light of that, consider the following story.

One day, the 44-year-old Loftus was horrified to hear from her uncle that at the age of 14 she had been the one to discover her mother's body floating in a pool. Until then, she had no memory of discovering her mother; she didn't even precisely know how her mother had died. But after hearing this from her uncle, she began to remember some horrifying details. For example, in her words, "My mother, dressed in her nightgown, was floating face down. I started to scream. I remembered the police cars, the lights flashing. For three days my memory expanded and swelled. But then early one morning my brother called to tell me, my uncle had made a mistake."

That's right, Loftus had not discovered the body, her aunt did. This was all a false episodic memory, and even the leading scholar in the field of eyewitness testimony (who had published important books on the subject before this incident)—well, not even she was immune to the effects of memory distortion.

As incredible as some of these distortions are, though, it is important to put all of this in context. These distortions arise from a memory system that efficiently provides us records of past events, and in the vast majority of cases, the important aspects of those events are correct. Usually it is just the details of an event that are prone to distortion and confabulation.

The false memory of Elizabeth Loftus is obviously much more extreme, and it does show how dramatic memory distortions can be, especially under the influence of powerful new stimulus together with circumstances that make it more suggestible.

But like the creation of memories in the psychoanalytic setting, the way that Loftus reconfigured her memories at the prompting of her uncle is really the exception that shows the rule. Usually our episodic memories reflect a combination of accurate memory for aspects we thought were important at the time of encoding, then semantic memory pieces the aspects we thought were important together to provide a seamless replaying of the event.

So what does this all tell us about the Korsakov patients that were suffering from bad nutrition and confabulation? Well, their anterograde amnesia was not as dense as the cases of Clive Wearing and H.M. that I described earlier. They could still encode some parts of what was happening and remember those parts subsequently, so they didn't have a complete loss of memory going forward. But they had much smaller pieces than you or I had, and so they had much bigger gaps to fill in. That's what was causing their confabulation—their attempt to fill in these large gaps.

So just like us, they really were trying to make sense of what they had, and they were piecing it together using assumptions about what must have happened; that was an attempt to link the events. They just weren't very good at it. The gaps they had to fill were too large. Thus, their confabulations were obvious. We all do the same thing as Korsakov's alcoholics, just to a less noticeable extent—when it is noticeable at all. So now it all makes sense.

Well, this leads us all very nicely to our next lecture. The implication of all we've discussed today is that at encoding we must somehow decide which details of an event to encode and which to not worry about so much. What factors do we base that decision on? Well, we've mostly focused so far on how the stimulus fits with other memories that we may already have.

But other factors are also relevant to this, including the relevance of some aspects of the experience to our lives and the emotions that some events produce. So, our subject for next time is how do we choose what to remember?

How We Choose What's Important to Remember
Lecture 22

Now that we know our episodic memory only encodes part of every experience, we must ask how and why those parts are chosen while others are allowed to fade away. When we allow our brains to do the choosing (which is most of the time), they encode elements that are most similar to our previous experiences and elements that immediately affect our survival. However, we can, with some effort, choose what we encode as well.

Effective deliberate memory encoding takes effort. We have so many experiences in the course of any given day that we simply cannot engage in this sort of effort for each one. Therefore, the brain uses 2 main criteria to decide what is important: personal relevance and survival relevance.

Things that are personally relevant to us are easy to associate with other things in our life and in our existing memories, and therefore they are easier to organize. We also think more about the relevant, which increases the chance such things will enter our episodic memories. The problem with this is that what is relevant now might not be relevant later.

There are other cases when relevance is thrust upon us. Perhaps the most extreme example is the **weapon focus effect**. When someone is the victim of or witness to a crime, that person can often describe the weapon better than he or she can describe the perpetrator. At that moment in time, the weapon literally means the difference between life and death, so the person has a hard time looking at or thinking about anything else. There's a straightforward evolutionary explanation for the weapon focus effect: We likely descend from those who best attended to factors in their environment linked to survival.

In situations of extreme stress, it is easy to tell if an organism—humans included—has recognized some stimulus as relevant to their survival. We all have 2 modes of central nervous system operation: the **parasympathetic** mode and the **sympathetic mode**. We can only be in one of these modes at any given time.

- The parasympathetic mode, which we are in when we are relaxed and calm, is concerned with the long-term survival of the body. When it is in control, heart rate slows, muscles relax, and basic housekeeping functions like digestion kick into gear.

- When a crisis occurs—say, you hear a loud explosion—the sympathetic mode takes over. Heart rate increases, respiration increases, adrenalin pulses through the body, attention snaps to the situation at hand. You are ready to fight or flee.

The part of the brain that flips the switch between the modes is the **amygdala**, an almond-shaped region of the midbrain whose primary job is to sense threat in the environment. Evidence from fMRI studies show that when the amygdala senses danger, it also activates the hippocampus, which results in deeper encoding of everything that is happening. This interaction is the basis for the **emotional binding hypothesis**, the notion that the amygdala's job is not just to get us through the present crisis but to ensure we encode the experience to improve our chances of survival in the future.

The amygdala's job is not just to get us through the present crisis but to ensure we encode the experience to improve our chances of survival in the future.

Even if you've never been in a major crisis yourself, you likely have a vivid memory of crises you experienced through the news. Many Americans say they remember the tiniest details of where they were and what they were doing when they heard the news of the terrorist attacks of September 11, 2001. Such detailed mental snapshots are called **flashbulb memories**.

Are flashbulb memories really as accurate as they seem? The experimental data is mixed. Studies suggest that for people who felt more personally attached to the event (say, people who had friends or family scheduled to fly that September 11), flashbulb memories retain greater accuracy over longer periods, so personal relevance may be a factor. Then again, those with a personal connection to the event are also more likely to tell many people their story in the hours and days right after the event, so perhaps the stronger encoding comes from repetition. Note also that such cumulative retellings get attached to and may distort our original memories, so even those flashbulb memories may lose accuracy over time.

Aside from these automatic processes of encoding, you can to some extent take control of which details enter your episodic memory by using the basic mnemonic techniques discussed early in this course: association, dual encoding, and repetition. If you want to remember the positive events of your life, then cherish them as they occur by organizing them and sharing them with others. ■

Important Terms

amygdala: An almond-shaped region of the brain involved in the processing of emotions, particularly fear.

emotional binding hypothesis: The notion that memories with powerful emotional content are more strongly encoded than those without.

flashbulb memory: A brief and highly detailed memory usually associated with a traumatic experience; often found in patients with post-traumatic stress disorder.

parasympathetic mode: The state of the nervous system during periods of calm, associated with "rest and digest" functions.

sympathetic mode: The state of the nervous system during crisis situations, associated with the "fight or flight" response.

weapon focus effect: The tendency of a witness to or victim of a crime to be able to recall details of a weapon (i.e., the immediate perceived threat) more clearly than he or she can recall the perpetrator.

Mason, Kohn, and Clark, *The Memory Workbook.*

Nelson and Gilbert, *Harvard Medical School Guide to Achieving Optimal Memory.*

Uttl, Ohta, and Siegenthaler. *Memory and Emotion.*

Questions to Consider

1. The amygdala triggers the body's stress response when it is active. Without an amygdala, we would never feel fear or worry. Why don't we all just have our amygdalas removed?

2. I mentioned that people who were in horrific crashes and ended up concussed often have trouble remembering the terrifying events just prior to their accident, and yet people who witness terrifying events without being subsequently concussed remember the events very clearly. What does this suggest about the importance of consolidation to the effects of emotion on memory?

Exercise

The next time you embark on some sort of adventure, test the rule that 3 things will go wrong and count them off as they do. Does this somehow make them less annoying and less worthy of dwelling on and remembering? Then think about what you might do to remember more vividly the highlights from your adventure.

How We Choose What's Important to Remember
Lecture 22—Transcript

Last time we developed a picture of memory, episodic memory specifically, that makes a lot of sense yet that also differs from how we typically feel about our memory. That is, memory feels like you are replaying some previous event exactly as it happened, but really, what you're seeing is only partly true retrieval of that event. A lot of that internal movie is filler and the context that's provided by semantic memory.

This explains both why human memory is so powerfully efficient while at the same time also explaining why we get minor details wrong all the time. It's two sides of the same incredible story.

But sometimes we care about those minor details, at least after the fact. That's what happens in court cases, and that's what happens with lots of ordinary details throughout daily life. The picture of memory we developed last time makes it urgent to figure out how our memory systems decide which parts of an actual experience to encode.

If we remember some features directly, while we just fill in the rest, it becomes critical to understand which parts of the things we experience end up being stored in our memories and which are just glued, cooked together using pieces from other memories that we already have.

So there are two things we would really like to know. First, do we usually have any control over which aspects of an experience are stored as memories, or does our brain just make these decisions for us, with maybe little or no help from working memory? Second, during an experience, how can we tell what parts of that experience we might want to be accurately retrieved when we retrieve the memory later? Those are the questions we will try to address in the current lecture.

Let's begin with the question of how much control you have over what details you might later remember with accuracy. The answer seems to be this: You can have some control, indeed more than most of us normally exert. Most of us, though, often seem content to just let our brain handle things. Why?

Well, as demonstrated in that early lecture on mnemonic strategies, effective encoding is effortful, but by now you should know the mantra well. If there is some detail that you wish to never forget, or misremember, then encode that detail in a way that optimizes the use of organization, association, and when possible dual coding. If you do that you will be maximizing the chance that that specific detail will be one of the facts that your subsequent episodic memory of the event will get right.

Of course, the problem is that we have so many experiences in the course of any given day. We simply cannot engage in this sort of effortful encoding for every one, or even for very many. Usually we are too busy just living, which means that, yes, for the most part, we let encoding happen itself without much intentional interference from our working memory. So if we are just leaving things up to the brain, how does the brain decide what is important?

The first factor I want to highlight is something called personal relevance. In some studies participants are first shown a set of pictures, and they are asked simply to rate how relevant each picture is to their lives. So if it were me, for example, I might rate a picture of a guitar as quite relevant but a picture of a flute as less relevant. After all the pictures had been rated there was a bit of a break, and then memory for the pictures was tested. Now note, participants were not warned of this memory test, they assumed that the purpose of the first phase was just to get those ratings of relevance. But when memory is tested, the more relevant pictures are remembered better.

This likely reflects a more natural, less effortful version of those same mnemonic principles. Things that are relevant to us are easy to associate to other things in our life and therefore easier to naturally organize. I see a guitar, I automatically think of one of my guitars, especially perhaps one that it might resemble. Or perhaps I even imagine playing that guitar, giving me both a more complex image than the one that was present and maybe even some proprioceptive form of representation, a dual-code, what it feels like to play that guitar.

So as we go through life, some of the things we experience seem relevant, the vast majority do not. We think more about the relevant ones and that increases the chance they will become future facts in our episodic memory.

Of course, the problem with this is that what is relevant later might not seem relevant now. Relevance of information can change over time. But what can we do? We can only know our future selves so well.

There are some other cases when relevance though is literally thrust upon us and sometimes in very dramatic ways. Perhaps the most extreme example of this is something called the "weapon focus effect." Police are often frustrated when they are interviewing witnesses of some crime with the hope of trying to get a better sense of the perpetrator and specifically, obviously, of what that perpetrator may have looked like. If the perpetrator was brandishing a weapon then it is very common that the witnesses don't provide many details about the perpetrator himself, but they can tell the police a whole lot about that weapon he was wielding.

At that moment in time, that weapon could literally mean the difference between the witness's life or death, and apparently they have a very hard time looking at or thinking about anything else. Their attention focuses in on the one thing that really matters and encoding of all other details is minimal at best.

In fact, the weapon focus effect allows us to highlight a more basic principle that the brain uses when deciding which experiences to encode deeply. Generally speaking, if some detail of current experience is relevant to your future survival, then it should be encoded. To justify this we can just resort to a pretty straightforward evolutionary argument. Imagine that some of our ancestors took particular note of things linked to future survival and others did not. Which group is most likely to have the greatest subsequent reproductive success? Obviously those who noted the relevance of such items. So yes, we have likely evolved from those who attended to factors in their environment that were linked to survival, and attention to some factor now increases memory for it later.

In fact, in extreme situations at least, it is actually very easy to tell if some organism, humans included, have recognized some stimulus as relevant to their future survival. You see, we all actually have two modes of operation, and they're governed by something called our central nervous system. These modes are called the parasympathetic and the sympathetic modes, respectively, and they are kind of like two sides of a coin. One can only be in one of these modes at any given time.

When all is peaceful and we are relaxing, then the parasympathetic mode takes over. The parasympathetic mode is worried about long-term survival of our bodies. And so, when it's in control our heart rate slows, our muscles relax, and basic housekeeping functions like those involved in digestion kick into gear. So we digest the foods we eat, we extract the nutrients, we ship those nutrients out to body tissues that need them, we prepare the waste for disposal, that sort of thing.

However, imagine you are laying back on your couch when suddenly an explosion occurs and blows in the front window of your house—boom! What happens then? Well, almost instantly your heart rate increases, your breath increases, adrenalin pulses through your body, your muscles are ready for action, your mind sharpens.

Oh, by the way, your digestive processes also slow to an almost stop. That's why your mouth can feel dry in those situations. There's no need to worry about long-term survival right now, you are in the midst of threat, and it's your short-term survival that matters. You are now in what some call fight-or-flight mode, and that's what it feels like when your sympathetic nervous system switch has been flipped, and it's very dramatic.

By the way, when all of this happens, things are also happening in your brain. In fact, if there is a part of you that actually flipped that switch, that part is you is your amygdala. It's an almond-sized area in your midbrain whose primary job is to sense threat in your environment. When it does, it triggers the sympathetic nervous system into action. When people suffer from so-called panic attacks, it is often an overactive amygdala that is typically to blame. These people can suddenly feel like they are under threat, but they can't even say why because, in fact, there was no stimulus that triggered the threat, it was internal, and that can be even more scary.

Anyway, when the amygdala triggers the sympathetic nervous system, it also does something else, though; it also activates the hippocampus, which results in deeper encoding of everything that's happening. It is almost as if the amygdala is saying, "Hey! Danger is present. Record everything that happens, because we may need to know about this later so that we can avoid being in the situation again." By the way, if you're a Spiderman fan, the amygdala is pretty much akin to his so-called "spider sense," that feeling he would have anytime danger is present.

This close interaction between the amygdala and the hippocampus is the basis for a theoretical notion called the emotional-binding hypothesis. The hypothesis suggests that events that have a direct link to our future survival stimulate the amygdala, which then activates the hippocampus, and the result of this is a binding together of as many details of the event as possible. Remember we've talked before about the hippocampus performing binding functions. So the claim is that this circuit, this brain circuit, is indeed working to remember as much as possible about the details of the event and to form associations among those details that bind it all together.

At some level one could ask, "Why is it so important to do all this binding? I mean the body is essentially under attack, right? Shouldn't we be worried about surviving right now?" Of course the notion is that the vast majority of threats we encounter in life are not fatal. By definition only one can be fatal, cats aside of course. So usually we live another day, and if we have formed strong associations between all the details of the event related to the threat, then maybe, in the future, sensing the presence of one of those details could allow us to prepare for the threat in advance. That's a true spider sense.

Remember my dogs learning that when I opened a certain cupboard a treat might be coming soon? Well, maybe we will learn that when a snake with that specific color pattern is present, a nasty bite is coming real soon unless we detect it earlier next time, in which case forming the association might literally allow us to avoid the bite.

Evidence from MRI studies appears to confirm the basic tenets of this emotion binding hypothesis. That is, when emotional stimuli are presented the amygdala definitely becomes activate, and it definitely activates the hippocampus. So we know that system does indeed react to threat. But is it really binding together all sorts of contextually relevant information as the emotional binding hypothesis suggests?

Please take a moment and think about the morning of September 11, 2001. What do you remember? Of course you remember the horrific events of the day, made even more horrific by the fact that a group of humans had actually wanted them to happen and had actually made them happen. So we all have those terrible images etched into our minds; planes crashing into buildings, waves of dust clouds, smoke billowing across the New York skyline, dazed-looking news reporters trying to understand what had just happened.

But do you also remember where you were, and who you were with, and what TV you were watching? Some people even claim to remember what they were wearing or other such details, almost like those details had been burned into our memory. The term "flashbulb memory" was first coined by Brown and Kilik in 1977 to describe such detailed memories.

While 9/11 provides the most dramatic case of a flashbulb memory for many of us today, similar sorts of dramatically detailed memories have been reported for a range of world events, these include things like the assassination of JFK, the death of Princess Diana, the explosion of the space shuttle *Challenger*, and various other tragic events of that sort.

In fact, the emotional binding hypothesis was primarily proposed to account for these kinds of flashbulb memories. Why can we remember the details of those events so well? Well, perhaps because the hippocampus has bound all of those details together into a very rich episodic memory, one that is far more fact than filler, and somehow just the sheer amount of those details that we remember convinces us of this. Flashbulb memories feel like very accurate, very detailed memories.

Are they really as accurate as they seem? Flashbulb memories themselves can be somewhat difficult to study scientifically, but some try. When some highly emotional event of that sort happens, there's a group of researchers that scramble to test memories right after the event and then at various intervals after that. The goal is to examine how stable and accurate these flashbulb memories truly are.

Unfortunately, the data from such studies have been mixed and complicated. For example, studies of the *Challenger* space shuttle explosion have suggested that although people reported clear and vivid flashbulb memories 6 months after the disaster, the details of the memories they reported had actually changed a fair amount. These findings challenged the notion that flashbulb memories are actually accurate. Perhaps reliving any emotional event stimulates the amygdala, perhaps only slightly. But that may be enough to make any memory we have feel more vivid, more powerful, regardless of the actual accuracy.

However, follow-up studies have also examined some personal characteristics in more detail, and these studies suggest that for people who felt more personally attached to the event, their flashbulb memories did retain accuracy even over long periods. So relevance comes in here, too.

For example, one study examined memories for the 1989 earthquake that occurred in California during the World Series. Many of us witnessed that earthquake unfolding as we tuned in to the baseball game on television, and given the reaction of the announcers we realized the emotional significance of the event that we were witnessing. Many TV watchers reported flashbulb-like memories.

Of course, for those people who were actually in California, the earthquake was much more relevant, much more personally relevant. When memory was examined months after the event, the flashbulb memories of TV watchers were found to be quite unstable, but the memories of Californians were much more stable. So perhaps one has to literally feel that sort of personal danger for the flashbulb system to really do its thing?

Unfortunately, even here there are complicating factors that also get in the way of a really clear understanding. For example, the study of the California earthquake just examined how often people talked about their flashbulb memories with others. Perhaps not surprisingly, the study found that those directly involved in the event talked to many people about it during the time right after the event. So they told and retold and retold their story in the hours just after the event occurred. It's likely not a stretch to say that little else was probably discussed in California during that time. Virtually all conversations were about that earthquake.

Those who watched TV, they also swapped flashbulb memory stories, but not nearly to the same degree. It is entirely possible then that the durable memory trace is due, at least in part, to a rehearsal process of the reliving the events over and over when they were still fresh. This should remind you of our earlier discussions of working memory as the gatekeeper to long-term memory. The more often we rehearse some bit of information, the more likely that it will be accurately transferred to episodic memory. So maybe the emotionality of the event simply promotes discussion rather than enhancing memory more directly.

This is a good point to think about, the cumulative effect of retellings, and how that can kind of affect memory in general, including flashbulb memories. Each time we retell some memory we first retrieve it, and what we get, of course, is a mix of these accurately stored details along with inferences, the facts and the filler. As we exchange this story with someone else, our discussion brings up more information, including, for example, information that the other person's version has that ours may not have. Of course, we then store a memory of this discussion in memory, and the newer memory is not entirely separate from the original one.

So the original memory was now exposed to new information that is highly related to it, information that is so similar it could be very easy to include some of the new details in our new reliving of the event. Perhaps something the other person said made a lot of sense, so we incorporate it into our version of events, and then we now store this new altered version of the memory.

If we do this over and over, we are both strengthening some of the core parts of our memory through rehearsal, but we are also allowing the memory to morph somewhat thanks to this exposure to new related information. To some extent this is a little like that telephone game we used to play as kids, where some bit of information is heard and then repeated, and while new bits are added as the information goes down the line, and eventually we end up with a very different story. It may not be so different in case of flashbulb memories, but the same notion could be acting.

This example points to the difficulties in studying memory in real-life contexts. There are so many variables, and there are only so many that a researcher can control. It would be fantastic to find some group of participants right after some emotional event and then to ask them not to talk about the event to anybody, thereby allowing you to see how much of a role talking plays in terms of shaping the eventual memory. However, researchers would have to swoop in as fast as first responders, and even if they did, even if the traumatized people agreed not to talk about the event to anyone else, those people would still have time think about the event over and over.

So it is really difficult to rely on real-world studies of flashbulb memory as either support for, or refutation of, the emotional binding hypothesis. What we would like to do is test this in the lab instead. But of course, it's considered unethical to make some participant feel some form of large or direct threat. So we really can't simulate some event of the magnitude of say 9/11. We must, instead, turn down the threat level to a point where it is not as psychologically shocking.

I suggest this may be an opportunity, because maybe this emotional binding hypothesis is a more general theory. Perhaps this circuit always operates to some extent, not just when the threat level is very high. Sure, it would likely work at a level appropriate to the threat, but we may even see it operating at much lower threat levels. If so, that would make a clearer link to the events of everyday life.

So with this in mind, let me describe an experiment by someone named Donald MacKay. MacKay's study relied heavily on so-called taboo words. Some of these words are the kinds of words that would give a movie an *R* rating. Some, for example, were racially or sexually charged words. Generally speaking, these are the sorts of words one would never say around their religious leader or their grandmother, the sort that might get your mouth washed out with soap if you spoke them.

In MacKay's study these kinds of words were intermixed with neutral words and then were presented to participants in various colors. So on a given trial, one of these words would appear, either a neutral or a taboo word, and it would be presented in some color of ink. The participants were simply asked to categorize the ink color of each item by pressing an appropriate key on a keyboard as quickly as they possibly could.

Two findings from this study are of interest. First, participants were slower to indicate the color of taboo words than they were to indicate the color of neutral words. According to MacKay, this is because the taboo words initiated an emotional binding process, and that took some time. Of course, these words were no direct threat to the participants, but seeing those sorts of charged words in the context of a psychology experiment is definitely odd, and the claim is that this oddness was sufficient to trigger the amygdala. And there seems to be evidence that this is true in the form of their second major finding. After indicating the color of all those words, both neutral and taboo, participants were given a recognition test for the items.

The recognition test asked two questions for each item that was presented. Was this item one of the items you saw in the earlier color categorization part of the experiment? If so, what color was it presented in? The data showed that participants did indeed remember the taboo items better than the neutral items, so some sort of memory enhancement was happening there. Perhaps even more important, they could also remember the color of the taboo items better than they could remember the color of the neutral items. This is exactly what the emotional binding hypothesis predicts—that various aspects of the stimulus, what it was and what color it was presented in, seem to be bound together. The memory may not be a flashbulb memory in the sense of our memories of 9/11, but it does seem to have more details in the context in the way that is similar to a flashbulb memory. However, it also may be operating to a lesser extent all the time, and it is likely a major player in terms of deciding which stimuli we encode deeply enough so that they will subsequently form the facts of our episodic memories. Well, in considering then how the brain decides which events to encode deeply, we've ended up in some pretty dark lands, and I'm a little worried that I could leave you with the wrong impression. So let me highlight a couple of points.

First, in this lecture I have highlighted both relevance and a general notion of threat as factors that affect what information we naturally encode more deeply. Yes, the threat examples are more dramatic, but when we look back at our memories they're not full of all these dangerous incidents. Why? Simply because encountering things that are relevant is very common, encountering threats is relatively rare. If one of these factors is more dominant, it is relevance.

What's more, the studies that have been done on relevance likely underestimate its, well, its relevance by a lot. I mentioned the study where participants were presented with sort of generic pictures, and they were asked to categorize them as relevant to their lives or not. Well really, how relevant can a generic picture be? A little, sure, but the things we encounter regularly in our lives are much more specifically relevant to us, to our lives. It's hard to do psychology studies that are sensitive to the details of a particular participant's life. But in skipping over the personal details, we inevitability underestimate how important relevance is.

And again, relevance and threat are the factors that I am highlighting with respect to things your brain uses when it decides what to encode. This is only part of the story, of course, the unintentional encoding part. Yes, we are often busy just living our lives, but at the same time we do often run into situations where we explicitly decide we want to attend to some fact or experience, and this is the important other side of the story.

So one thing I'd like to really emphasize is that you can play a very central role in determining what sorts of episodic memories the future version of yourself will reconstruct, and what details are prominent in that reconstruction. You have learned the basic techniques of deep and powerful encoding. If you want your future memories to be based on the positive events of your life, then cherish those positive events as they occur. By cherish I mean, organize them and share them.

We seem to have a natural tendency to take pictures or videos of great events in our lives, think of weddings or the birth of a child, for example. So we take the time and effort to create externalized memories, ones that we sometimes only seldom revisit. My suggestion is to do the same with your internalized memories. Think about them when you can, and talk to your friends about them. If there is a good lesson to take from that discussion of flashbulb memories, it is that events we choose to discuss with one another will have an impact on our subsequent memories. So, if something really great happens to you, or someone close to you, talk about it.

If you want to take it a step further, then, right after some personal event maybe even organize it carefully in your memory and form dual codes using mnemonic strategies. Doing that sort of thing will increase the chance that in the future those memories will come to mind and again color your life in a positive way. At the same time, do the opposite for your negative experiences. Obviously, learn what you must from them, but don't dwell on them, especially the seemingly random negative events in your life. As they say, the only path to success leads through failure. Look at negative experiences that way, as opportunities to learn and to move closer to success.

Whenever my wife and I are about to engage in some new adventure, I have a rule for myself. It's obviously an imprecise rule, but it's one that I use to kind of downplay negative events. It goes like this. At the beginning of the adventure, just assume that at least 3 things will go wrong. Expect it, and when it happens don't get angry. Just count them off. So if you get to your vacation but your bags don't, oh well, there's one negative thing down already. Don't let your amygdala get in a knot over it. Just let it go. And that's the larger point. What you encode as important is something that you do have some control over, and you have even more control when you begin taking that control in advance.

Aging, Memory, and Cognitive Transition
Lecture 23

Our semantic and procedural memory systems continue to function quite effectively into normal old age. While early researchers turned up dramatic effects of aging on episodic memory, a lot of those studies were confounded by time-of-day effects; it turns out that the changes are small and are better thought of as a transition than a decline. Some aspects of memory, including creativity and big-picture thinking, actually improve with age.

As we age, many of us feel our memories are less accurate than they once were, and we often look for ways to minimize memory deterioration. But as you are now aware, memory is not a single thing. When it comes to the question of memory declining with age, we must realize that any one question about memory—even just long-term memory—is actually 3 questions.

For the most part, procedural and semantic memory show little decline with age. Problems with procedures usually have little to do with memory and more to do with the physical effects of aging—arthritis, vision or hearing loss, and the like. And for the most part, we don't complain that we're losing our semantic memory; we can still recite the multiplication tables we learned as children. The classic complaint is a decline in episodic memory, in terms of both recall and encoding.

One interesting feature of this episodic memory loss is a tendency among older people to tell the same story to the same person over and over, forgetting that they've told it before. It has been suggested that this is actually an evolutionary advantage, ensuring that each generation remembers and passes on important information to the next.

When does an individual's episodic memory begin to decline, and how dramatic is the impairment? The earliest major studies on this, performed in the late 1980s, suggested that memory decline began as early as the age of 50 and was rapid and dramatic. But in the early 1990s, psychologist

Lynn Hasher noticed something about these studies. One of her areas of expertise was **circadian rhythms**, the natural hormone and neurochemical cycles of the human body, which affect both physical and cognitive behavior. Knowing that our circadian rhythms shift as we age—in adolescence, we are more likely to be night owls, and as we age, we become morning people— she noted that most of these tests were performed in the afternoon and evening, when the graduate students conducting the tests and the young subjects were at their mental peak but the older subjects were becoming tired.

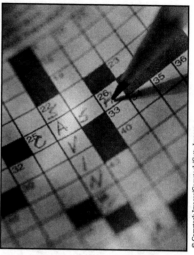

Crossword puzzles are good for sharpening certain memory skills, but better still are complex hobbies that engage more than one memory system at a time.

Hasher conducted similar studies, but she ran them both early and late in the day. She discovered that, when you control for the time variable, the performance gap between old and young subjects shrank considerably, although it did not disappear. What's more, the data indicated that the time of day had a far stronger effect on memory in both groups than did age. Hasher and her colleagues' further studies also revealed that younger people were better at focusing their attention, while older people were more easily distracted by extraneous detail. Interestingly, you see this same contrast between so-called normal people and creative people—writers, composers, painters, and so on.

From this evidence, Hasher suggested that the way our brains change as we age is not a form of cognitive decline; rather, it is cognitive transition. In most cases, the way we interact with the world changes as we age. We do not need to attend to as many things at once. As a result, we literally change the way we interact with the world, and we spend less time thinking about details and more time thinking about the big picture. Accurate episodic memory, of course, is all about the details, so episodic memory does show a slight decline. However, creativity shows an improvement, as demonstrated by how many people take up creative hobbies during retirement. So the way our minds change during normal aging is not so much a loss as a trade-off.

That said, it is possible to sharpen our episodic memory as we age. Many researchers have recommended brain exercise like crossword puzzles, Sudoku, and so on, but more complex and general hobbies can be even more beneficial—hobbies like dancing, painting, or writing, which require constantly learning new things and repeatedly recalling what you have learned. ■

Important Term

circadian rhythms: The daily ebb and flow cycles of hormones and neurotransmitters.

Suggested Reading

Craik and Salthouse, *The Handbook of Aging and Cognition.*

Kausler, *Learning and Memory in Normal Aging.*

Langone, *Growing Older.*

Questions to Consider

1. If you could choose a life where you were very worried about details all the time but as a result were really good at remembering details, is that the sort of life you would choose?

2. We say that you can't teach an old dog new tricks, and yet procedural and implicit memory seem not to decline with age. As you've gotten older, have you tried learning "tricks" unrelated to your existing skills? Which seem easiest, and which seem more challenging?

Exercise

As you go about your day, think about the various tasks you perform. Which ones exercise which forms of memory? Is there any form of memory that you are not exercising much within your current behaviors? Given that semantic, procedural, and implicit memory are so important to effective functioning in the present, episodic memory is often the one form of memory that gets the least exercise. Could you think of some new behavior that you might like that would fill the gaps in your current memory workout? If it could become some new hobby or activity that you truly enjoy, you would be keeping your mind young in a way that would be easy to continue.

Aging, Memory, and Cognitive Transition
Lecture 23—Transcript

Do you feel your memory isn't as accurate as it once was? Maybe it seems that you can seldom remember the details of some event, the people you met, their names, the order with which things happened, or the little parts of some experience. Or maybe your kids keep complaining that you are telling them the same things over and over again.

If none of this is yet happening to you, maybe you have seen this behavior in others. Perhaps older relatives that are telling you the same stories over and over again, and you're worried that one day this will be you. Are changes in memory just part of the normal aging process? If so, how dramatic are they? Is there anything you can do to minimize deterioration in memory if it does occur?

In the late 1980s, many of the so-called baby boomers were approaching 50 years old, and they were beginning to worry about their memory decline with age. Given their numbers, baby boomers represent a big voting block and, as a result, wise politicians are often attuned to their concerns, and would like to act in ways that reflect this sensitivity. So it is no coincidence that the story of what we know about aging effects on memory begins in the 80s when funding for research on the effects of aging became available.

The story I am going to tell you is one with a number of twists. These twists and turns are interesting because they reveal a lot about the scientific process. I look forward to telling you this story because, as I do so, I'll have the opportunity to emphasize why even scientific results need to be viewed with caution.

As well intentioned as scientists generally are, they can sometimes miss important variables, or they can get locked into seeing things a certain way and, in so doing, they sometimes miss a bigger picture that tells a more accurate overall story. Ah, but I'm getting ahead of myself. Let's start in the 80s and move forward.

First though, it is important to again stress that memory is not a single thing. As you know very well now, we humans possess a number of memory systems including procedural memory, semantic memory, and episodic memory. So when it comes to the question of whether memory declines with age, it's important to realize that any one question about memory is actually three questions, and that's if we focus on just long-term memory.

So let's start with some good news. Many of the initial studies of aging effects on memory included episodic memory, semantic memory, and procedural memory tasks. For the most part, semantic and procedural memory seem to show very little decline. In fact, it seems that as we age we simply continue to gain new knowledge about the world and new motor skills, and there seems to be no apparent "cognitive" degeneration with respect to the knowledge and skills we've had all along. I say "cognitive" degeneration because the actual performance on procedural memories may decline due to things like arthritis, muscle atrophy, or other conditions that make it harder to move in certain ways, but this is really a decline in motor abilities not in the cognitive processes that support them.

Similarly, if one's sight or hearing is not good, they may seem to not be as good at some skill like driving for instance, but again, this isn't a reflection of procedural memory per se. It's a reflection of the input to procedural memory. So, again, some good news. No need to worry about your semantic or procedural memory systems. They seem to age pretty well, especially if you take good care of your body and listen to your eye and ear doctors.

But of course, it isn't semantic or procedural memory that older people or those that interact with them complain about. It is episodic memory. The classic complaints are things like not being able to remember the name of a person we just met. Now clearly that's episodic memory. And it's an episodic problem, perhaps a problem with the encoding step.

And again, nearly everyone notices the tendency of an older person to tell the same joke or story repeatedly to the same person. This again is an episodic memory issue. The only reason most of us do not tell the same people the same stories repeatedly is because we remember that we already told them. That is, we recall a previous episode of telling that story to that person. If a story or joke comes to mind, and I don't recall telling it to this person, why not tell it, especially, for example, if it's a really good joke?

Let's talk about that specific tendency for a moment, because I once gave a talk about aging and the effects of aging on memory, and someone said something very interesting to me, something that really resonated, at least for me. They said that maybe this tendency of older people to retell stories was actually a good thing, a tendency that occurs naturally and serves a very important role at a more general level. That is, most of the stories older people retell are stories about the past, stories full of our ancestors, our aunts, our uncles, our grandparents, and cousins, what life was like when they were young.

In a very real sense, this is the oral history of our families the episodes of our family members who went before us. And unless written down, these episodes could be lost with the passing of the older person who is now telling the stories to us. It is, in a sense, a cross-generational memory system.

Sure they tell us the same stories over and over as you know very well now. But as you also know repetition is an effective method for passing along a memory. Perhaps that's exactly what's going on. It's a passing of memories from one generation to the next in a manner perfected over years of evolution.

I told you that story resonated with me. Well, I heard this perspective less than a year after the passing of my father. (I love ya, Dad.) As it turned out, I had just been bringing my mother to visit her brothers and sisters, a kind of reconnection for a woman I love deeply who suddenly felt very alone. As we drove from one relative to another, Mom would relate stories about all of them as kids. I knew these stories. I had heard them many times. I still hear them many times. But this time, with the grief of losing my father still heavy in my heart as it still is, and in the context of literally spending time with each as we arrived at their place, the stories gained a new significance, a new dimension of reality and importance.

So what the questioner at my talk spoke of, those repetitions as serving an important role in telling families their oral history, really hit home for me. So, one take home message from all this is the following: If someone complains that you keep telling them the same stories, or if you ever want to complain to an older relative for the same reason, remember the role this behavior might serve.

All that aside, the tendency to repeat a story to the same person still does suggest a decline in episodic memory, even if that decline serves a purpose. So that begs the following questions. How soon does episodic memory decline, and how dramatic is the impairment? These are the questions that the initial studies of memory and aging were trying to answer, and the answer they suggested seemed like bad news indeed. Yes episodic memory declined. Its decline began as early as 50 or 60 years of age and, relative to the memory of younger participants, the decline was pretty dramatic. If baby boomers were worried about their memory decline before the late 1980s, they were even more worried as the results of these new studies came in.

But here is where the first twist occurs. About a decade ago a researcher named Lynn Hasher was a little worried about the previous studies on memory and aging. In addition to being interested in aging effects, Hasher was also a researcher on what's called the "time-of-day" effects, and she was worried that the previous studies might have mixed these two. Before explaining that worry in detail, let's first talk about time-of-day effects, then we'll come back to the memory issue.

Our bodies all show evidence of something called circadian rhythms. These are natural rhythms in our bodies that orchestrate the flow of hormones and other neurochemicals which, in turn, directly affect both physical and cognitive cycles. So, for example, if I may venture into the generally less talked about aspects of life, we all tend to have bowel movements at roughly the same time or times every day. That would be a physical cycle. Similarly, on the cognitive side of things, we all tend to be more alert at certain times of day. For example, we tend all to be the most tired at 3 am, but we also feel drowsy at 3 pm. These cycles also underlie our sleep patterns.

Normally we don't really notice these cycles until they are disturbed. Of course the classic disturbance is travel across time zones, which leads to what we call "jet lag." What is jet lag? Well, quite simply, it's when the cycles of your body do not match the time of day anymore. You want to sleep, but its daylight. And you cannot use the washroom at your normal time either. You have become what we elegantly refer to as "irregular." I kind of like that term. It strikes me as funny for some reason. But really, it directly reflects the notion that your body has certain temporal regularities, and these regularities are being disturbed by the travel.

Here's the really interesting part. Our circadian rhythms shift as we age. Think for a moment of a typical teenager, especially if you know one. When would they like to go to bed? If it were up to them, what time would they choose to go to bed? Really late, right? Like, maybe midnight or even later? And when would they like to wake up? Late again, probably 10 or 11 am, maybe even noon. Now think of some older person, maybe you? I can't tell how old you are from here, but if not you, then maybe your parents or your grandparents. When do they like to go to bed? Much earlier, right? Maybe 8 or 9 pm? And when do they like to wake up? Well, again, earlier, right? Maybe 6 am, maybe 7 am, likely no later than 8. Why is there such a difference?

The answer is actually quite simple. For whatever reason, as we age our natural circadian rhythms shift earlier. We are alert earlier in the day, and we get drowsy sooner in the day. As a result, older and younger people are essentially living within different time zones even though they're living in the same context.

You've likely heard about this disconnect with respect to public schooling. Let's think about this for a moment. Who runs the schools? Older people do. So when do they set the hours for learning? They set them at times that make sense for them. They start the students early in the day, when the older people are feeling alert, and they let them leave in mid- to late-afternoon. Of course, the problem is that students are still really tired early in the day. They don't even begin to really be alert until almost lunch time. Then school ends just as they are starting to feel cognitively strong.

Because of this some people have suggested we should shift the school day, the school hours, to match the young people's rhythms. After all, school is about their learning, right? It's about them. So maybe school should start at about 11 am or noon, and maybe it should end at 7 or 8 pm. How many older teachers do you think would be comfortable with that schedule? How many parents? Well, not many it seems because this kind of change in schooling has definitely not caught on. Yes, we want our youth to learn, but we want them to do so on our schedule.

So what does all this have to do with memory? Well, as Hasher found out, studies of memory work almost the opposite as school days. That is, who actually collects the data in psychology experiments? Well, usually it's the relatively young, say 19 to 22 year olds. So if they are charged with running an experiment, they decide when to invite participants into the lab.

When do they do that? Well, Hasher asked exactly that question to a number of the labs who were conducting research on aging effects on memory. The logs were checked, and it was revealed that most of the studies were conducted during a period that ranged from approximately early afternoon to mid evening. This really shouldn't be surprising. This is when the young researchers felt alert.

Given this, let's think about the research again. They are testing the memory of young participants rather late in the day, at a time when these young participants feel maximally alert, and they're comparing them to older participants who are also tested late in the day, a time when they are feeling really drowsy. Now we find that the older participants are performing worse than the younger participants. Why is that? Is it because they're older, or is it simply because they are tired?

This situation is what scientists like to refer to as a "confound." They want to assess the effects of age, but age is not the only difference between the groups. Another variable, in this case general alertness, also varies across those two age groups. So we end up comparing the young and alert to the old and tired, and when we do that we don't know if any differences we see are due to age, alertness, or some combination of the two.

Luckily, variables can be un-confounded; that is, you can redo the experiment in a way that can avoid the confound. And that's exactly what Hasher did next. She assessed memory performance for both young and old participants, but she did so both early in the day and late in the day. This allows a comparison of memory performance when both groups are their most alert, later in the day for young participants, and earlier in the day for older participants. It also allows one to compare old and young at both early and late times. What did she find?

Well, when you compare old to young late in the day, you see the standard finding: The older people perform far worse than the younger people. So that replicates the finding we knew about for many years. However, when you compare older people at their optimal time, which for them is early in the day, to younger people at their optimal time, which is late in the day, the difference in memory is far less. Yes old people still perform worse than the young, but the difference is far less than those initial studies suggested. So a little bit of good news there.

The decline of memory with aging is not nearly as dramatic as the initial studies suggested. The other interesting thing that came out of this study is the following: If you actually compare older and younger participants in the morning, the older participants actually do better than the young. So the time-of-day effect is actually stronger than the aging effect. The moral here is if you are a little older and let's say you ever want to challenge your grandkids to some sort of game that has a mental cognitive component, do it first thing in the morning. Get them out of bed at 6 am. You'll kick their butts. I almost guarantee it.

All right, at any rate, this is better news. Episodic memory does not decline as much as we thought, but it still does decline. But is it actually wrong, or perhaps maybe we should say shortsighted, to think about it this way? Consider the following study also conducted by Hasher and her colleagues.

The experiment began with a study phase in which a pair of words was presented on each trial; one just to the left and another just to the right. Participants, some of whom were young and some of whom were older, were asked to study the left words for a later memory test but to ignore the words on the right. Once the study list was over, the memory test began. It was a standard recognition test. A sort of standard; there was a trick. Psychologists sometimes have these tricks.

Memory was tested for both the left and the right items despite the instructions that were given to the subjects. So participants were told that they only had to worry about the left items, but they were lied to. The question was though, in both cases, "Was this word presented earlier?" And sometimes the words came from the left, and sometimes they came from the right. But either way, the person was to say "yes" if they thought the word was presented earlier.

If you look at the memory performance for the words on the left, the words that participants were told to attend to, then you see that the younger participants in fact remember these words much better than the older participants. So that's the expected memory advantage. And you see it here too. However, if you look at the performance for the words on the right, the words that participants were told to ignore, the older participants actually remember these items better than the young participants do.

What this implies is that, really, the better memory for younger people is a result of them being better able to focus in on the important information. They remembered what they were supposed to, and they ignored, and didn't remember so well, what they were told was unimportant. In contrast, the older people seemed to attend to the list in a more general way, less focused, more likely to process both the things they were told were important and the things that were not supposed to be important. So older people were not as good at focusing in on the information they were told was relevant.

Here's something that makes this finding interesting. If you do the same study, but instead of using younger and older people, and you instead so-called "normal people," whatever they are, and people who are known to be creative, so people who do well on tests of creativity. Creative people attend to the world more generally. They are less focused. They remember, just like the older people, the things that they were told were irrelevant. So they show a pattern very much like the older participants do. And one suggestion to come from this is that maybe old people interact with the world in a way that creative people interact with the world. Is this coincidence?

Hasher argues it's not. She argues that it's merely something called cognitive transition. When we are young our lives are filled with a million details that we need to keep track of. This report is due on Friday. I have to e-mail that client. The kids have ballet later tonight. I must stop at the store for milk. There's a meeting at 2, and on and on the list goes. You all know that list quite well.

To remember all those details we have to really focus our attention regularly. Well, we do until we retire. But as we approach retirement, these little details of life fade away. Fewer things need to be done at specific times. Our schedule becomes much more free and much less imposed by our environment. As a result we may literally change the way we interact with the world, and we may spend less time thinking about details. In a sense, we become less "left brained," as they like to say, not always talking to ourselves to remind ourselves of these little details. Instead we spend more time looking at and thinking about the bigger picture. The details become much less relevant and, as a result, our brain changes to match this new way of interacting.

Accurate episodic memory, of course, is all about the details. Our last lecture really made that point clear. If we want to remember the details of some event well, we really need to focus on it. So if we spend less time focusing on details, less time encoding details, then our episodic memory will appear to degrade. We will forget people's names after just meeting them, because we didn't really pay much attention to them in the first place. We will tell the same stories to the same people, because we weren't really paying that much attention to who it was we were telling the stories to in the first place. If we don't focus on the details, we won't remember the details.

But, and this is a big but, this is only part of the story, that is, the part that talks about what gets worse as we age. The other side is this: We are spending more time on the big picture. We are, often in a very real sense, becoming more creative. In fact, it's not at all unusual for older people to take up hobbies as they age. Perhaps these are things they've always wanted to do but just didn't have the time. Some might take up photography, or they learn to use computers, or they paint, or knit, or a myriad of other activities that allow them to exercise their new creative inclinations. This is the positive side of the cognitive transition, a side that is often overlooked.

I'm thinking, for example, of a situation involving a young boy. As a young boy goes through puberty he may lose the sweetness of their young voice, but they may gain in height to the point where he becomes a better basketball player than they did before. Transitions include both losses and gains, and aging may be no different. I personally find this really satisfying, sensible, and just generally a really nice way to think about the effects of aging. Some things get better; some things not so much. Aging is not really about deterioration; it's about transition. And as the way we interact with the world changes, it should come as no surprise that our mental processes change along with that. Well, maybe you're now saying to yourself, that's a really nice way to spin all this aging stuff Joordens, but if we could avoid the memory decline part, that would make this whole transition even better. Is there anything we could be doing to keep our memories sharp?

I'm sure many of you have been told to do crossword puzzles or Sudoku, or that sort of thing, to keep your brains working hard and, therefore, to keep your cognitive processes in good shape. I think this is sort of correct. There's definitely nothing harmful in it. But it's not quite right. These are enjoyable things, and if you do them a lot, you will get better at them. You will be exercising your semantic memory at the same time. But, of course, semantic memory doesn't decline with age.

If you're really hoping that your general world memory skills would stay sharp, especially your episodic memory, then I recommend something a little more complex, something a little more general, especially something that might allow you to develop or use that creative instinct that we've just been talking about. So perhaps you might take up something like dancing, or painting, or photography, or writing, any other hobby that includes the need to learn new things, and to repeatedly bring to mind what you have learned. That's the episodic memory at work.

Let me stress that. The best thing to do is to learn things that you will later need to recall. And I can't help but point out that that's exactly what you are doing right now, by the way. To expose yourself to new information, new lectures, then think about them, and hopefully to retell some of what you've been learning to other people, well when you do all that, you are exercising your episodic and semantic memories in a really fantastic way.

Learning means using your memory, remembering what was taught last class, then putting new learning on top of that, all the while putting the learning you have done to use through practice. This approach works with the transition, and the learning and the exercise is less specific to a given task.

I would especially recommend learning something like dance, something that involves muscle skills and physical exercise. So when you combine that with a constant need to remember the steps you learned, for example, and use them to perform the dance, you're really maximizing the experience. So procedural memory is exercising and getting a workout, episodic memory is working, working memory is working, and heck, you're getting exercise, which is always good. And if you perhaps take the time go even further, you could learn the history behind dancing, which would be enhancing your semantic memory as well. So really, it's a fantastic, all-round cross-training for the mind, if you will. And it's social too. Dancing your way into old age? Isn't that a great image?

So let's sum up. The subject of memory and aging is a far more lively subject than was once believed. First of all, some of our memory systems continue to function quite effectively into normal old age. What appeared to be problems with procedural memory were actually problems with motor function, and we now know (not from studies of memory, but from physiology) that even motor function can be maintained by exercise into old age, far more than was realized even a few generations ago.

Second, while originally it looked like there were some dramatic effects of aging on some memory systems, especially episodic memory, a lot of those original, dramatic effects turned out to be due to time-of-day effects. When you factor those out, yes, you still see a decrement, but it's not nearly as big as we once thought it was.

And third, should we even really think about that as a decrement in memory, or is it more reflective of a general change in our cognitive approach to the world, one that, yes, may have some negatives but may also have some positives: Cognitive transition, not cognitive decline.

The conclusion seems to be that if we find ways of embracing the positives and working on the negatives simultaneously, then we can have the best of all worlds. Oh, and if you do sometimes repeat the same story, or if someone does that to you, that's really not so bad either.

The Monster at the End of the Book
Lecture 24

Now that you understand much more about the many-headed beast that is human memory, you can dismiss the simple question "Can I improve my memory?" and replace it with the more sophisticated "Can I remember what I want, and forget what I want?" In suitably complex fashion, the answer is "sometimes"; more important may be the question of whether or not you really want to change your memory skills at all.

By now, you're aware that the simple way you may have thought of memory before taking this course was wrong. Memory takes many different forms, some of which you might never have even recognized as memory. You also know that the different memory systems interact in complex ways that defy most people's preconceptions. Therefore, you also know that the simple question "Can I improve my memory?" and the simple answer "yes" don't even start to cover the issue.

What's more, we can't ask the question until we define what we mean by "improve." If all you want is to remember more, then there are several options. You can exercise your memory the same way you exercise a muscle—by using it. The best mental exercises involve memory cross-training—that is, tasks that work as many declarative and nondeclarative memory systems at once as possible. Memory consolidation benefits from getting good sleep. Eating the right foods—foods rich in omega-3 fatty acids, thiamine, and vitamin B_{12}—are good for brain health in general and memory in particular. But our initial goal begs the question: Do you really want to increase how much you remember?

Before you answer, consider the case of Jill Price, a woman with a specific type of obsessive-compulsive disorder that causes her to obsessively encode her episodic memories. She has near-perfect recall for everything that she has ever experienced, including the painful incidents most of us would rather forget, which haunt her life and relationships as if they happened yesterday.

How about the famous "mnemonist" known only as S., who had a condition called **synesthesia** that, in laymen's terms, cross-wired his senses. Every word S. heard also registered as a visual image, usually a color. In other words, his brain automatically performed the sort of dual coding we have to train ourselves to use. Sounds like a good thing, except like Jill Price, he had trouble forgetting painful or trivial things he'd rather dismiss. His unique perspective on reality also made him something of a social misfit and even made it hard for him to hold down a job. For most of us, the price of this kind of memory would be too great.

Can we break the strong links the amygdala and hippocampus forged in the heat of crisis?

The lesson is clear: We don't want to have a stronger memory; we want to have a selectively stronger memory. You've already learned a bit about how and why to take up active encoding, but how do you decide what to encode? It may seem obvious that you'd want to encode the details of your wedding day strongly—unless the marriage doesn't work out. What we wanted to remember in the past isn't always what we want or need to remember in the future.

So can we forget things we've made an effort to encode, or can we forget painful or paralyzing flashbulb memories of the sort that cause **post-traumatic stress disorder (PTSD)**? Can we break the strong links the amygdala and hippocampus forged in the heat of crisis?

For some strong, painful memories, you can avoid the cues that trigger them—avoid the people, places, songs, and so forth that bring them to mind. Unfortunately, that's not viable for people with PTSD, who can have unavoidable triggers like loud noises or bright lights. Researchers are therefore looking for a way to block the emotional response to these memories, even if they can't remove the memories themselves. Drugs called **beta-blockers** show a lot of potential in this area.

Still, there may be times when we want to remember an event we did not deeply encode originally. Often, this means you have made a choice (consciously or subconsciously) about what to pay attention to in a situation, only to be disappointed that you have lost a "more important" detail. Our brains are performing a delicate balancing act all the time. Is this an act we want to interfere with? Maybe you don't have to "improve" your memory at all.

Throughout this course, we have challenged the notion of a single thing called memory and talked about memory as a collection of systems that exist within a single body. So let's end this course by challenging that notion as well: Memories are passed from person to person, implicitly by example, explicitly with the help of language. Memories also are transmitted across time and space thanks to the printed word and, increasingly, digital media. We can even point to something like communal memories, existing in diverse formats from museums to urban legends. Memories like these allow us a glimpse of what it means to be immortal. To be remembered is to be alive, even if that new life is in the mind and body of another. Thus memory not only guides us through life; it sustains us even after death. ∎

Important Terms

beta-blocker: A drug that blocks certain neurological signals to the heart, preventing it from speeding up under conditions of stress.

post-traumatic stress disorder (PTSD): A disorder characterized by extreme anxiety and fear in response to remembering a traumatic event.

synesthesia: A condition in which a sensory stimulus (say, a sound) is perceived by more than one sense (say, as both a sound and a color).

Suggested Reading

McGaugh, *Memory and Emotion.*

Nelson and Gilbert, *Harvard Medical School Guide to Achieving Optimal Memory.*

Woll, *Everyday Thinking.*

1. Now that you understand the many different ways that memory systems contribute to human behavior, what answer will you give the next time someone asks if it is possible to improve memory? What if the person wants a quick answer, something you can express in a minute or two?

2. At encoding, we identify details we want preserved in memory; the more details we encode deeply, the more our memory of the event will match the actual event. But deep encoding takes time and effort, so we only worry about so many details. For comparison, let's say you have a good friend who is willing to shop for you. Suppose in one case you give your shopper very few details about what you would like ("I'd like a medium shirt."), but in another case, you give a lot of details ("I'd like a blue shirt with some white striping and an Asian-style collar that is fitted and made of a material that can be easily washed."). In either case, the shopper ultimately comes back with a shirt for you. How closely will the shirt match with what you hoped for? Compare this process with the way memory works.

Exercise

You just invested a lot of time listening to this course on memory, and I hope you have learned a lot. But now what can you do to maximize the chance that you will remember all you have learned?

One sort of mnemonic that is sometimes used in educational contexts like this is called a concept map. First, you think of all the concepts you have learned in a course and write them down. You might include such concepts as episodic memory, semantic memory, procedural memory, implicit memory, sensory memory, familiarity, frontal lobes, hippocampus, amnesia, Alzheimer's disease, reconstruction, déjà vu, animals, and so forth. Next, take these concepts and link them in ways that represent connections, perhaps also labeling the links in ways that make the connections explicit. These connections, or associations, allow one to see the concepts at a higher level, seeing interconnections and lacks of connections.

If you really want to remember a course, the conclusion is a perfect time to create a concept map. We've even provided a blank space on the page for you to use.

Use this page to draw your own concept map.

The Monster at the End of the Book
Lecture 24—Transcript

Wow. The last lecture. Let me share with you one more memory. It's a memory from my youth. It's a memory about my first book or at least the first book I can remember. It was a Sesame Street book, and it featured my favorite character: Grover. The book was called *The Monster at the End of the Book*, and all through this book Grover was warning me—I was the reader, he was my narrator—and he kept telling me there was going to be a monster at the end of the book. He was very worried. He was terrified of the monster, and throughout the pages he would be worrying and fretting, and he was trying hard to prepare me for what was about to come. But then when the two of us got to the end, there was an amazing revelation: Grover himself was the monster at the end of the book. All our worries were for naught. I still remember how happy and relieved Grover was.

Well, to some extent, it seems to me that throughout this lecture series I've been trying to tell you that the simple way you may have thought of memory was wrong, and that memory was, in reality, a bit of a monster. OK, maybe I used the word "party," but that's just because I didn't want to scare you. I also highlighted, though, that memory could take many different forms, some of which you might never have even recognized as part of that monster. I also suggested that these forms of memory interacted in complex ways that defied many of your preconceptions.

And, of course, I did discuss one type of memory—habits—as being a lot like Frankenstein's monster, perhaps a nice, misunderstood monster but, in that case, we were looking at nondeclarative memories, specifically those that were so durable that we can lose conscious control of them.

But now here we are, at the end of the book, at least in the figurative sense, and now you have a clear vision of what the monster actually is. I think you'll all agree that, just like Grover himself, the monster of memory is more interesting than it is scary.

And what's really gratifying from my perspective is this. There are relatively few people who have actually taken the time to understand the monster of memory as you now do. When I give short talks, by contrast, and people ask me relatively simple sounding questions about memory, I often feel confined to reply with relatively simple answers, answers that are more true than not, but answers that aren't as rich as they really could be.

But that's not the case now. I honestly feel like you and I, we've shared virtually everything I know about memory. So I feel that we now share a common knowledge base, a knowledge base that will allow us to think about the true complexity of memory and really kind of come to those rich answers.

So what I'd like to do is this in the final lecture of the course: I'd like to take what we learned from the various experiments and theories that I've been describing, and think about what these findings tell us about memory in the context of one single question. What question? Well, it may even be the question that influenced you to be interested in this lecture series in the first place. It is perhaps the main question that is most commonly asked about memory. Ready? Here goes: Can I improve my memory? Well, you know the answer. The simple answer is yes. And you know the longer answer, too. You know that the question about improving memory is potentially multiple, depending on which memory systems we're talking about.

But we also know that when people ask this question, the part of the monster that they mean is the episodic part, so let's restrict our answer to just episodic memory. Can I improve episodic memory? Well, sure. We've been drilling into our heads with repetition that the answer is yes. If I use organization, association, and dual coding, I can improve my episodic memory. And that answer is right at some level. But even that is too simple of an answer. That is not the monster-at-the-end-of-the-book answer.

So now, here is the way I always wanted to answer that question, but never felt I could without confusing people. The first step to a full answer is to be clearer about the word "improve." Typically when people say they want to improve their memory, what they think they want is to remember more. But do they really? If so, then there are indeed various things that we can do, simple things like the following.

First, exercise your memory. And again, we do need to be clear about which memory. So many people fail to make this distinction and then suggest some simple activities like, for example, crossword puzzles. Crossword puzzles do indeed exercise your memory, your semantic memory. Remember this: Even the patient HM loved to do crossword puzzles, and he was unable to create any new episodic memories at all. So if it's episodic memory you're really interested in improving, the typical crossword puzzle sort of exercise just won't do.

Instead, as discussed in the last lecture, I would suggest that the best way to exercise your episodic memory is with some sort of memory cross-training exercise that includes as many different memory systems, or as many parts of the monster, if you will, as possible. At that point I really didn't emphasize the nondeclarative contribution, but it is clearly there as well. For example, when you hear speech or music as part of some episodic memory, it is not the case that the speech is suddenly non-grammatical or that the music no longer follows the scales we know. So really the best way to keep the episodic part of the monster fit it to keep all parts of the monster fit, including the nondeclarative systems. I suggested that learning dance as an activity that does just that. Given that episodic memory is the system we are most worried about, an important consideration should be whether you will stick with your activity long enough to reap the benefits from retrieving things that you are learning. This is a memory-based reason to find some activity you would really enjoy. Maybe that's dance. Maybe it's not. So just learn something that you might actually wish to use. Using your learning will require retrieval of episodic memories, and that will keep it fit and strong.

Second, of course, memory also benefits from some pretty simple lifestyle things, like sleeping and eating the right foods, and these also include habits you might want to cultivate a little bit more fully. Foods rich in Omega-3 acids, thiamine, and B_{12} are especially good for brain health in general, and for memory in particular. If you don't want to do all the research, here's a mnemonic. Go to your produce section and pick up fruits and vegetables that have rich dark colors. Deep rich colors support deep rich memories. How's that?

But now let's give the real monster-at-the-end-of-the-book answer. That answer begins by restating the answer as a question. Do you really want to increase how much you remember? Well, not so fast. Let me introduce you to Jill Price. Jill is an obsessive-compulsive, but a very interesting and unique one. Most people who suffer from obsessive-compulsive disorder are obsessive-compulsive with respect to some behavior. Maybe they must wash their hands every few minutes for fear of germs, or maybe they continually check to ensure the iron is off or the door is locked.

Jill, however, is what might be called a cognitive obsessive-compulsive. Just as others might wash their hands over and over, Jill relives every experience in her life over and over. In her words, she hordes episodic memories. Since she was just a child, Jill's mental life has consisted almost entirely of reliving events that occurred in her life, and she does so compulsively.

You and I? We use our working memory for all sorts of things: We daydream, we worry, we fantasize, we plan, we revisit old memories, those sorts of things. I'm not saying that Jill doesn't do these things as well. She likely does but probably to a much less extent than most of us. Instead it seems that most of the simulations she performs in her working memory involve reliving the events of her day over and over. She doesn't do this intentionally, by the way, she just can't help herself. She is compelled to do this. She is a rote memory machine locked into some automatic setting. What's the result?

Jill has an absolutely incredible episodic memory. For example, a reporter tried to stump Jill by asking her if she recognized a tiny snippet of a theme song from a show that only aired for a single season when Jill was a child. Jill was not only able to remember the show, but she also recalled other details related to the experience of watching the show. I think she was about 4 or 5 at the time, and that's the age where most of us are just exiting the clouds of childhood amnesia.

So if we take the initial question at face value, then this is what we all want, right? Well, be careful what you wish for. You see, there were times in Jill's life when her mother said some things to her that were a little hurtful, things about Jill's weight. No big deal, right? All of our mothers probably said hurtful things to us at one time or another, perhaps even deservedly at times.

We might have said hurtful things to them, and sometimes a war of words just escalates.

But Jill replayed those words over and over, and they were ingrained in her mind. Forgive and forget? Well, when you can't forget, then the sentiment of forgiveness becomes rather fanciful. What Jill is to rote memory, others are to deep encoding.

There was a famous case of a so-called mnemonist only referred to as S. And S. was documented extensively by a Russian doctor named Luria. S. had a condition called synesthesia, which means that neurons in the different parts of the brain, especially the sensory parts of the brain, seem to be cross-wired in a strange way that made him, for example, see words in colors, or that automatically generated images when he heard certain stimuli. As a result, the sorts of techniques that I suggested you consciously perform in my lecture on mnemonics were things that S.'s brain just did automatically.

It shouldn't surprise you that S. had an amazing memory. However he was also sometimes annoyed by how much trouble he had forgetting things, and he was never able to hold down a good job, even when he tried being a journalist, the sort of profession one would think would be easy for one with a good memory. Luria himself described S. as a "somewhat anchorless person" who was unable to hold down any steady job. Apparently the price of this fantastic memory was some sort of a problem being a social misfit. While having a great memory could be helpful at times, being socially accepted may actually provide much greater success and happiness.

What Jill and S. show us is that our original question is that our original question is really too simple. We really do not want to have a stronger memory. We want to have a selectively stronger memory. That is, we want to remember some things really well, while still being able to forget other things, the things that are either less important or are potentially negative in some non-useful way.

Now that the question is posed in this way, I can say that we partly answered it a couple of lectures ago. That is, I devoted an entire lecture to a consideration of the factors that govern which details of some experience are encoded in a way that ensures that certain information is later remembered. I also discussed the notion of how to downplay negative experiences in a way that reduced the likelihood of them being subsequently remembered. I encouraged you to take control of encoding as much as you can to ensure this happens, and I gave you some suggestions on how to do that.

All that is great if you have a good sense of what you want to remember at the time of encoding, but often the priorities of encoding are not sustained over time. For example, I have a bit of a joke that I tell my freshman students on the first day of class. The idea is to encourage them to protect their privacy, in general, and in terms of their university student number specifically but, of course, I want to do so in a way that has some personal relevance. Here's the joke:

"Be careful who you share your personal information with, because today's boyfriend or girlfriend may be tomorrow's stalker." Perhaps a pretty graphic image but, hey, images are memorable right?

Perhaps because I teach memory, over the years, I have repeatedly had some student come to my office looking for a very specific kind of advice. They say things like the following. "Dr. Joordens, I have exams coming up, and I know how important they are. However, I just broke up with my boyfriend or girlfriend and now I find I can't think about anything else. So studying feels impossible. What can I do to ensure I don't fail my exams?"

For those of us who know the monster of memory, let me translate that for you: "I filled my working memory with thoughts of this person, and I formed all sorts of associations between them and virtually every other stimulus in my life, but then suddenly it was over, and now everything I see or hear reminds me of what is lost." The translation of that: "These associations I have formed now keep filling up my working memory with distracting images of the twit that dumped me when it should be filled with the things I need to study."

This really highlights a sub-question of the initial question. So if the initial question is how can I improve my memory? That is, how can I forget things that I had encoded with the thoughts that I would want to remember them, only to subsequently find out that I don't. This is like the problem of those people who get tattoos, thinking it's a great idea at the time then suddenly they don't want the tattoos any more. Whoops. What do you do?

Really, this is a question about how can I forget things that I have encoded deeply? Now this is a question we haven't yet tackled in this lecture series, and it is one that has implications that go well beyond the effect of break-ups on exam performance. So let's look at a much more serious version of this question. A lot of people are going through what is called post traumatic stress disorder. For example, let's think about someone who went and found themselves in the front lines of a war situation. Well, when you are in that situation, deep encoding of all sorts of issues is very important. For example, it makes a lot of sense to spend a lot of time getting to know those people you are on the front lines with. You need to know who you can rely on, and what you can rely on them for. It also makes sense to form strong bonds with your comrades to ensure they are there for you when you need them.

If you find yourself in the heat of battle, well now all of those aspects of the emotional-binding hypothesis are probably in play in a big way. You are paying attention to everything that is happening around you, encoding and binding all sorts of details relevant to that situation of high personal threat. And you may even experience one or more of your brothers or sisters in arms being killed. This is a very personally relevant flashbulb memory, perhaps the deepest sort of encoding one can experience. And thanks to the emotional binding produced by the amygdala and hippocampus, it is linked to a variety of things like the sounds of gunfire or explosions, perhaps to sudden bright lights, whatever stimulus was present at the time of your friend's death.

In this case, you didn't encode all that intentionally, as my swooning undergraduate might have, but you definitely encoded it deeply, very deeply. And once you are back home and away from the battle, that memory may replay anytime any similar stimulus triggers it.

Again, we are not always in control of what we encode deeply, and even when we are, we may encode deeply only to later find that the resulting memory is something we would rather not continue to experience. So here, how we "improve" our memory is actually by forgetting. If there is some persistent unwanted memory, perhaps persistent because I encoded it deeply, what I can do to forget it?

Well, once a memory is deeply encoded and strongly bound to cues, the first thing you can try to do is avoid the cues that trigger it. So for my heartbroken student I might have suggested that they avoid the locations, people, songs, and anything else that they might have associated with their lost love. For the soldier, though, that advice seems insufficient. Sure, avoid loud noises, bright lights, and war movies.

But there is some recent research that sounds like something out of a science fiction movie. Wait, it actually is out of a science fiction movie, a somewhat hokey, romantic, science fiction movie called *The Eternal Sunshine of the Spotless Mind*. In that movie a couple breaks up, and the girlfriend goes to a doctor to have her memories of her ex-boyfriend removed from her brain. This is ridiculous, right? You can't just remove unwanted emotional memories, can you?

Well, it turns out that very recent studies suggest that maybe we can. One Dutch study from 2009 worked as follows. Participants were first shown pictures of spiders, and they were given brief electric shocks at the same time. (Perhaps I should mention, by the way, that in most parts of the world, North America included, it is no longer considered ethical to give participants electric shocks in the context of psychology experiments. Holland's a little more liberal.)

At any rate, in that study they found that participants who had formed a fearful memory of spiders could have that fearful memory dissolved if they were given so-called beta-blockers. Beta-blockers are drugs that prevent a fear response. The fear switch can literally be locked down, and the beta blockers do just that. So participants on beta-blockers forget to become fearful. They are actually incapable of becoming fearful, even in fearful situations.

The suggestion is that we while we may not be able to prevent certain memories from coming to mind, we may be able to "de-emotionalize" them by presenting the normal cues that would prompt them while preventing emotional response using, for example, beta blockers. So perhaps it's impossible to forget painful memories that were deeply encoded, but you may be able to lose the pain of them.

Let's see. We've taken the original question, "Can I improve my memory?" We've changed it to the much more reasonable, "Can I remember what I want, and forget what I want?" And we provided strategies we can use to do so, at both the time of encoding, and even after encoding, when we subsequently want to forget an event that was even initially deeply encoded.

What we've left out so far are the cases when we might want to remember an event that was not deeply encoded originally. Here, maybe I can at least provide a better understanding of the problem, and maybe even question whether it really is such a problem at all.

Autistic children are often known to have really incredible memories. In the book *The Curious Incident of the Dog in the Night Time*, by Mark Haddon, we are given a glimpse into the mind of one such autistic child. The book is fiction, but Mark did spend many years working with autistic children so, artistic license aside, it seems his account is accurate, at least for some children.

According to the protagonist in that book, what many people just saw as a field of cows, he sees a highly organized and vivid representation of the world, kind of like the following: 52 cows over all, 12 cows over there, 3 that are more black than white, 5 that are more white than black, 4 that are kind of balanced, certain ones are facing left, others are facing forward, one is lying down, then another cluster of 7 over there. Well, you get the idea. He has exceptional perception of, and subsequent memory for, the details of what he is seeing.

However, at the same time, he has a horrible time interacting socially with humans. Why? Well, how do you tell the difference between someone who is angry and someone who is happy? For most of us, that's trivial. But if you think about it, it turns out that anger and happiness are actually quite similar at the level of specific details, and no one detail really tells you the difference. Both reflect energized, animated people, speaking loud, gesticulating widely.

The answer is not in the details. It's in the way those details come together to form some whole. That's where the social relevance of the signal is. This is the sort of thing the fusiform gyrus does. It helps us interpret these kinds of holistic representations. And often this is the level at which social cues are communicated.

So to really remember details like names well, you need to focus on those details, the trees as it were. But social interactions are shared at the level of holistic representations the, forest. So whenever we find ourselves in some social interaction, we are presented with both the trees and the forest.

Remember, humans are largely single minded. We cannot load both the forest and the trees into our working memory. We must choose a level to attend to. If you really want to remember details like names, the simple answer is to focus on the trees. Interact with the world in a way that more closely resembles the way autistic children do. You will remember the details better that way.

But again, is this really what you want? If you focus on the trees, you will miss aspects of the forest. Your social interactions will likely become less fluent, and that could lead to consequences that are even more embarrassing or awkward than forgetting someone's name. So it is a balancing act, and perhaps it is one where errors of some sort are bound to happen. It's a question of finding a balance that minimizes errors; eliminating errors may be just impossible.

So maybe, just maybe, the balance that you currently use is the right balance, or anyway is very close to the right balance for you. Maybe your brain has used its implicit memory, that is, its knowledge of the structure of the world, to find the optimal balance for you. Sure, you might want to tweak this with intentional strategies every now and then, especially when you come across some information that has some very clear future relevance. But overall, maybe you really do not want to make any major changes to how your memory works. Maybe the big improvement would be realizing that you do not have to worry about how to "improve your memory" at all.

OK. That's the answer I've always wanted to give to the simple question, "Can I improve my memory?" Given everything we've covered, you now know enough to decide for yourself how much thought and effort you would like to exert and devote to improving your memory. This also means that we are really nearing the end of the book, or the end of the lecture series anyway.

Perhaps I have time for just one more point. What I'd like to free the monster from its cage. Yeah, dramatic I know, but here is what I mean. So far I have been talking about memory, including all the various systems that make up the colloquial single noun of memory, as though it lived in the brain, imprisoned within the skull. But already we know from a couple lectures ago that the monster of memory is bigger than our brains, working intricately together with our sympathetic and parasympathetic nervous systems throughout our body. Moreover, memory cannot be caged within the confines of an individual body.

Memories are, of course, passed from person to person. Memories also are transmitted across time and across space, thanks to the printed word, and increasingly, thanks to digital media. It may not even be a stretch to think of memories as existing at another level entirely, a level sometimes described as communal memories.

Perhaps the most concrete form of such communal memories, and I mean that literally in some senses, are the libraries and museums we build. We build museums of natural history to share our knowledge of the earth and museums of the Holocaust to ensure that we remember the capacity within us all of us to commit horrible acts. In fact, we have museums for almost every endeavor humans have engaged in. Recently, when I was driving on a highway near Ottawa, I saw a sign for a canoe museum, a museum devoted to the history and art of canoe making. Our knowledge and experiences certainly are not confined to our biology.

When I told you about working memory, I said that each time we repeat some item we are trying to remember to ourselves, it is like we are breathing life into that item, keeping it alive for a little longer. Well I think this is true of memory in general. Every time we remember some event or person it is like we are breathing life into that event or person.

In Dante's *Inferno*, Dante travels through the various levels of hell and meets a number of tormented souls as he does. Upon learning that Dante was actually flesh and blood, and therefore that he might actually return to the land of the living, the strongest desire of many of the souls in hell was to be remembered by those who were still alive. They would plead with Dante to have others remember them. Hell or no, I think we all have a desire to live on in the memories of those who know and love us. To be remembered is to still be alive, even if that new life is in the mind and body of another. Thus memory does not only guide us through life, but memory even sustains us after death.

On that note then, I'd like to dedicate this lecture series to the loving memory I have of my Dad, a father who taught me as much through his deeds as through his words, and through all the memories I have of him. I thank you all for watching. I hope you learned a lot. And who knows? Maybe we'll get to do this again sometime. Goodbye for now.

Glossary

agnosia: The failure to comprehend the meaning or function of things otherwise correctly and accurately perceived.

Alzheimer's disease: A degenerative neurological disorder characterized by memory loss caused by loss of cortical neurons, amyloid plaque formation, and neurofibrillary tangles.

amygdala: An almond-shaped region of the brain involved in the processing of emotions, particularly fear.

amyloid plaque: Abnormal clumps of beta amyloid protein found in the brains of patients with Alzheimer's disease.

anterograde amnesia: The inability to form new memories after a neurological event.

basal ganglia: A group of brain regions associated with motor control, both voluntary and involuntary.

beta-blocker: A drug that blocks certain neurological signals to the heart, preventing it from speeding up under conditions of stress.

Broca's area: The brain region involved in speech production.

Capgras delusions: A failure of memory that allows a person to recognize objects or people they have encountered before, but recognition is accompanied by a strong sensation that those objects or people are unfamiliar.

capture error: A situation in which we are consciously trying to not perform a strong procedural memory (i.e., a habit) but are unable to stop.

catharsis: In psychoanalytic theory, the release of blocked psychic energy, typically by way of free-association and sustained talk.

childhood amnesia: The human inability to encode episodic memories before about the age of 3.

circadian rhythms: The daily ebb and flow cycles of hormones and neurotransmitters.

classical conditioning: The encoding of procedural memory via the implicit memory system.

cognitive prosthetics: Technologies that help replace lost cognitive functions.

constructivist learning: The principle that it is easier to learn structure through direct experience of the structure rather than by explanation.

cortex: The outer mantle of the cerebrum.

declarative memory: Memory systems used deliberately to produce a clear, conscious answer to some query; these systems include episodic and semantic memory.

déjà vu: A disquietingly strong sense that a new event has already been experienced; from the French term meaning "already seen."

dorsolateral prefrontal cortex: The area of the frontal lobe where current theory indicates that working memory resides.

dual coding: The process of relating a new piece of information we wish to remember with both an image and a word to increase the ways we can retrieve the information later.

echoic memory: The ability to hold or recall a sound in one's mind; the auditory form of sensory memory.

emotional binding hypothesis: The notion that memories with powerful emotional content are more strongly encoded than those without.

episodic memory: Memories of specific, individual events, as opposed to general knowledge.

flashbulb memory: A brief and highly detailed memory usually associated with a traumatic experience; often found in patients with post-traumatic stress disorder.

forgetting curve: A mathematical function that predicts the time required to memorize, forget, and re-encode a set of data through rote memorization.

frontal lobe: The lobe at the front of the cortex involved in decision making, impulse control, and long-term planning.

functional magnetic resonance imaging (fMRI): An imaging process that uses magnets to create detailed images of which areas of the brain are active during certain tasks by showing the blood flow to each region.

habit: A form of procedural memory that is so well formed the actor is no longer in control of whether or not he or she performs it.

habituation: An acquired tolerance for a stimulus in an environment.

hippocampus: A region of the midbrain that allows the transfer of working memory into permanent storage and may coordinate the simultaneous activation of various memory systems.

iconic memory: The ability to hold or recall an image in one's mind; the visual form of sensory memory.

implicit memory: Memories encoded by repeated experience within some context but without a deliberate attempt at encoding; contrast with **rote memorization**.

jamais vu: A disquietingly strong sense that a familiar event has never been experienced before; from the French term meaning "never seen."

long-term potentiation: Enhanced connectivity between brain regions as a result of new experiences. *See* **neural plasticity**.

mere exposure effect: The surprisingly strong memory effect of brief exposure to a stimulus, even when no effort was made to remember the stimulus.

method of loci: A memory-encoding technique that relates an unfamiliar set of data to a familiar set of connected data, the most common example being places along a route; by recalling the familiar information, we can quickly bring to mind the new information.

modeling: Learning by imitation; specifically, an infant's mimicry of others' facial expressions.

neural network: A system of on/off switches interconnected in such a way as to imitate the structure of the brain or a region of the brain.

neural plasticity: The idea that the brain undergoes physical changes, specifically enhanced connections between brain regions, as a result of learning. *See* **long-term potentiation**.

neurofibrillary tangles: Clumps of tau protein that are found in the brains of patients with Alzheimer's disease.

nodes: The switches in a neural network that stand in for the brain's neurons.

nondeclarative memory: Memory systems used with little or no conscious mediation, such asd procedural and implicit memory.

parahippocampus: A brain region involved in sensations of familiarity.

parallel distributed processing: A form of neural network processing where the overall pattern of ons and offs is more important than the on/off state of any one node.

parasympathetic mode: The state of the nervous system during periods of calm, associated with "rest and digest" functions.

parietal lobe: The lobe at the top of the cortex that contains areas for processing sensory and spatial information.

perceptual fluency: Familiarity; the resonance between present and past experience.

phonological loop: The ability of the working memory system to recall and repeat a sound; one's inner voice.

post-traumatic stress disorder (PTSD): A disorder characterized by extreme anxiety and fear in response to remembering a traumatic event.

primacy effect: Better encoding and recall of the beginning of a list or series of events.

priming: A process of being prepared for a stimulus by some previous experience.

proactive interference: A previous experience that prevents successful encoding or recall of a similar piece of information.

procedural memory: The body's mastery of a physical routine; often called muscle memory.

prosopagnosia: The inability to recognize faces, despite being able to recognize other objects without difficulty, caused by damage to the fusiform gyrus.

prospective memory: Giving oneself instructions to remember or do something in the future.

rapid eye movement (REM) sleep: The sleep state during which dreaming occurs.

rapid serial visual presentation: A technique used in memory experiments wherein a set of words is flashed before a subject so quickly that the subject feels he or she hasn't seen most of them.

recency effect: Better recall of the most recently encoded information.

recovered memory: The retrieval of a memory, usually a traumatic one, thought unrecoverable, usually with the aid of hypnosis or psychoanalytic techniques.

REM atonia: The temporary state of paralysis that occurs during REM sleep that prevents us from acting out our dreams.

retrieval failure: Forgetting; that is, when we cannot recall a piece of information, usually because it was encoded without good retrieval cues.

retroactive interference: An experience that weakens the encoding or recall of a previously memorized piece of information.

retrograde amnesia: The loss of memories from before a triggering neurological event.

rote memorization: Memorization through repetition.

saccades: Swift glances moving from object to object in a scene that our iconic memories use to piece together a whole.

script theory: The idea that social theory is learned via implicit memory.

semantic memory: General knowledge about the world learned through repeated exposure to the information, as opposed to memories of specific events.

semantic overlap: In a recognition test, a word that evokes a sense of familiarity because it has a meaning similar to or belongs in a category with a word presented earlier (e.g., red and crimson; rose and tulip).

sensory memory: A temporarily retained impression of a sensory stimulus.

slow-wave sleep: The deepest stage of sleep, in which memory consolidation occurs.

state-dependent memory: A memory whose recall is improved by re-creating the emotional context in which it was learned.

striatum: A brain region associated with procedural memory.

sympathetic mode: The state of the nervous system during crisis situations, associated with the "fight or flight" response.

synaptic pruning: The removal of weak brain cell connections to make way for new ones that occurs at least twice in normal, healthy humans: once in adolescence and once in old age.

synesthesia: A condition in which a sensory stimulus (say, a sound) is perceived by more than one sense (say, as both a sound and a color).

tactile memory (a.k.a. **haptic memory**): The lingering impression of something we have touched or been touched by; a form of sensory memory.

temporary graded amnesia: The temporary loss of memory of events leading up to the triggering neurological event; the victim's older memories return before the more recent ones, and events immediately before the event may never return (e.g., a concussion patient may never remember being hit on the head).

visual-spatial sketchpad: The ability of the working memory system to re-create and explore a place or object in iconic memory.

weapon focus effect: The tendency of a witness to or victim of a crime to be able to recall details of a weapon (i.e., the immediate perceived threat) more clearly than he or she can recall the perpetrator.

Wernicke's area: The brain region involved in language recognition.

working memory: Sometimes called short-term memory, a memory system used for both temporary storage and as a mental workspace where information from other systems is processed.

Note: For those wondering where to begin, there are 4 books below that would provide a great starting point. Each has a different style and focus. Baddeley's *Essentials of Human Memory* provides a great overview of all memory systems; Graf and Masson's *Implicit Memory* focuses more specifically on one of the most overlooked aspects of memory; Foer's *Moonwalking with Einstein* is aimed at a general audience and focuses on mnemonic techniques; and Matthews and McQuain's *Bard on the Brain* provides a witty and informative look at brain imaging and memory. Together, they offer a fresh sampling from the complex and fascinating world of memory.

Baddeley, Alan D. *Essentials of Human Memory*. Hove, UK: Psychology Press, 1999. A good general overview of memory with an especially strong discussion of working memory, the form of memory that was and remains the focus of much of Baddeley's work.

————. *Working Memory, Thought, and Action*. Oxford: Oxford University Press, 2007. A book on working memory from the researcher who is most strongly associated with it. This highlights in detail the research of Baddeley and all it tells us about working memory.

Baddeley, Alan, Michael W. Eysenck, and Michael C. Anderson. *Memory*. Hove, UK: Psychology Press, 2009. A general book on memory systems that includes a good overview of the distinction between episodic and semantic memory in the context of memory systems more generally.

Baddeley Alan D., Michael D. Kopelman, and Barbara A. Wilson. *The Handbook of Memory Disorders*. 2nd ed. New York: Wiley, 2002. Written primarily for a scientific audience, this book outlines various memory disorders and describes the sorts of brain damage linked to each.

Bauer, Patricia J. *Varieties of Early Experience: Implications for the Development of Declarative Memory in Infancy*. London: Academic

Press, 2010. An interesting book highlighting the potential effects of early childhood experiences on the development of declarative memory systems.

Benjamin, Arthur. *Secrets of Mental Math*. DVD. Chantilly, VA: The Great Courses, 2011. Mostly a course about mental arithmetic, but Lecture 9, "Memorizing Numbers," gives a thorough introduction to the so-called major system for remembering numbers by converting them into more memorable strings of words.

Best, Deborah L., and Margaret Jean Intons-Peterson. *Memory Distortions and Their Prevention*. Hove, UK: Psychology Press, 1998. This book describes the process of memory reconstruction and the manner in which it is open to distortions. It further provides some advice on how to be aware of, and potentially minimize, such distortions.

Bjorklund, David F. *False-Memory Creation in Children and Adults: Theory, Research, and Implications*. Mahwah, NJ: Lawrence Erlbaum Associates, 2000. This book considers false memory in a great detail, providing a description of links to the recovered memory issue, descriptions of lab-based research, and implications for courtroom testimony from both children and adults.

Brainerd, C. J., and V. F. Reyna. *The Science of False Memory*. New York: Oxford University Press, 2005. This book brings together and organizes research related to the creation of false memories and the variables relevant to that process.

Braisby, Nick, and Angus Gellatly. *Cognitive Psychology*. Oxford: Oxford University Press, 2005. An overview of cognitive psychology that includes a discussion of sensory memory in the context of other memory systems.

Cermack, Laird S. *Human Memory and Amnesia*. Hillsdale, NJ: Lawrence Erlbaum Associates, 1981. This book provides a strong and clear description of amnesia, describing many interesting patient cases as well as research projects that take a more group-based approach. If you want to understand the amnesias better, this would be a good place to start.

Cole, Elliot, and Ron Baecker. *Cognitive Prosthetics for Brain Injury: Lessons Learned over Two Decades*. San Rafael, CA: Morgan & Claypool Publishers, in press. A nice review of the development, research, and application of various forms of cognitive prosthetics. This book highlights the promise of such prosthetics while also highlighting the importance of thorough research for the development of effective technologies.

Covey, Stephen R. *The 7 Habits of Highly Effective People: Powerful Lessons in Personal Change*. New York: Free Press, 1990. A popular book that highlights how one can intentionally form habits that might lead to success. Thus, it shows the potential applied value of intentionally creating specific habits rather than simply allowing the habits to form on their own.

Craik, Fergus I. M., and Timothy A. Salthouse. *The Handbook of Aging and Cognition*. 3rd ed. New York: Psychology Press, 2007. This book provides a fantastic and thorough, though already slightly dated, description of research related to the effects of aging on cognitive functioning in general. The authors are both very highly respected researchers in the fields of memory and aging.

Davies, Graham M., and Tim Dalgleish. *Recovered Memories: Seeking the Middle Ground*. Chichester, UK: Wiley, 2001. This book provides another consideration of the recovered memory issue and provides a case for not dismissing the possibility of recovered memories completely.

Dere, Ekrem, Alexander Easton, Lynn Nadel, and Joe P Huston. *Handbook of Episodic Memory*. Amsterdam: Elsevier Science, 2008. A shorter book focusing on episodic memory that hits the highlights without going as deeply into background research.

Dill, Karen E. *How Fantasy Becomes Reality: Seeing through Media Influence*. Oxford: Oxford University Press, 2009. This book considers the influence, intended or otherwise, of the media on human thought and behavior. It includes a discussion of memorial influences such as those discussed in the lectures, but it does so within an even broader analysis of media influence.

Ebbinghaus, Hermann. *Memory: A Contribution to Experimental Psychology*. Translated by Henry A. Ruger and Clara E. Bussenius. New York: Columbia University Press, 1913. Ebbinghaus' original book detailing his experiments on memory and how they show that even something as abstract as memory can be studied in a highly scientific manner.

Eichenbaum, Howard. *The Cognitive Neuroscience of Memory: An Introduction*. New York: Oxford University Press, 2002. This is a shorter book that gives a very good overall picture of links between the brain and memory.

Eichenbaum, Howard, and Neal J. Cohen. *From Conditioning to Conscious Recollection: Memory Systems of the Brain*. New York: Oxford University Press, 2004. Conditioning results in nondeclarative memories, and while this book does not focus specifically on how these memories interact with declarative memory systems, it does provide a good overview of the players in those interactions.

Emilien, Gérard, Cécile Durlach, Elena Antoniadis, Martial Van Der Linden, and Jean-Marie Maloteaux. *Memory: Neuropsychological, Imaging, and Psychopharmacological Perspectives*. New York: Psychology Press, 2004. This book discusses neuropsychological approaches to understanding links between the brain and memory, but it does so in a way that integrates it with imaging techniques and techniques that focus on the neurotransmitters used by the brain. Thus, it provides an interesting, more integrated perspective on brain-memory relations.

Fennis, Bob M., and Wolfgang Stroebe. *The Psychology of Advertising*. Hove, UK: Psychology Press, 2010. Good advertising both catches the mind and leaves a memorable trace, conscious or otherwise. This book considers the manner in which advertisers apply psychological research toward the goal of increasing sales.

Foer, Jonathan. *Moonwalking with Einstein*. New York: Penguin Press, 2011. A book written for a popular audience that considers the techniques of memory enhancement as motivated through interactions with people who compete in the annual World Memory Championships.

Forgas, Joseph P., Kipling D. Williams, and Simon M. Laham. *Social Motivation: Conscious and Unconscious Processes*. Cambridge: Cambridge University Press, 2009. An interesting book that considers the interplay between conscious and unconscious (declarative and nondeclarative) systems in social contexts.

Foster, Jonathan K. *Memory: A Very Short Introduction*. Oxford: Oxford University Press 2008. As advertised, a brief overview of memory that includes a good discussion of sensory memory systems.

Gilhooly, Kenneth J., and Robert H. Logie. *Working Memory and Thinking*. Hove, UK: Psychology Press, 1998. Another good book on working memory, one that highlights the link between working memory and conscious thought.

Graf, Peter, and Michael E. J. Masson. *Implicit Memory: New Directions in Cognition, Development and Neuropsychology*. Hove, UK: Psychology Press, 1993. An excellent book that provides both an overview of classic work on implicit memory and a clear description of more recent research trends.

Gruetzner, Howard. *Alzheimer's: A Caregiver's Guide and Sourcebook*. 3rd ed. New York: Wiley, 2001. A resource for caregivers that both describes the general course of the disease and offers best practices for care related to various stages.

Gurney, Kevin. *An Introduction to Neural Networks*. London: CRC Press, 1997. This book provides a nice introductory-level description of neural networks and the data they have attempted to model. For any who would like to try creating some basic models themselves, this book would be the best place to start.

Haberlandt, Karl. *Human Memory: Exploration and Application*. Upper Saddle River, NJ: Pearson Education, 1998. While not focused as strongly as other books on mnemonic techniques per se, this book provides a broader overview of memory research that has relevance to daily life. As such, it considers the relevance of research related to memory systems beyond just episodic memory.

Haykin, Simon. *Neural Networks and Learning Machines*. 3rd ed. New York: Prentice Hall, 2008. While this book might be a little more challenging for the complete novice, its strong organization allows it to remain accessible. For one who wants to gain a deeper understanding of neural networks, this is a great book.

Herbert, Wray. *On Second Thought: Outsmarting Your Mind's Hardwired Habits*. New York: Crown, 2010. This book discusses some of our mostly deeply rooted mental habits and explains how they affect almost every decision we make in some manner or another. Sometimes these effects are helpful, but in some highlighted cases they produce tragic results. By knowing these habits of mind, perhaps they can be more readily controlled, or so goes the premise of this book.

Herrmann, Douglas J., and Roger Chaffin. *Memory in Historical Perspective: The Literature before Ebbinghaus*. New York: Springer-Verlag, 1988. This book highlights some of the ideas about memory that predated Hermann Ebbinghaus's research, which also explains the intellectual context within which Ebbinghaus worked.

Hiby, Lydia, and Bonnie Weintraub. *Conversations with Animals: Cherished Messages and Memories as Told by an Animal Communicator*. Troutdale, OR: NewSage Press, 1998. While less scientific than some of the other selections here, this book provides a more liberal approach to learning about animal cognition, an approach based on a learned ability to read the signals that animals send. The resulting claims are thus more speculative but very interesting and thought provoking.

Higbee, Kenneth. *Your Memory: How It Works and How to Improve It*. New York: Prentice Hall, 1988. This book provides a brief overview of memory systems and then focuses more specifically on mnemonic techniques.

Howard, Robert W. *Learning and Memory: Major Ideas, Principles, Issues and Applications*. Westport, CT: Praeger, 1995. Another good overview with a heavier emphasis on knowledge acquisition and real-world applications.

Kausler, Donald H. *Learning and Memory in Normal Aging*. San Diego: Academic Press, 1994. The book provides a more general description of the effects of aging on learning and memory, but it does not consider the more recent work of Lynn Hasher that I highlighted in lecture.

Kendrick, Donald F., Mark E. Rilling, and M. Ray Denny. *Theories of Animal Memory*. Hove, UK: Psychology Press, 1986. This book highlights current views on the extent and types of memory in animal species, emphasizing current theories as well as the data that support them.

Konar, Amit. *Artificial Intelligence and Soft Computing: Behavioral and Cognitive Modeling of the Human Brain*. Boca Raton, FL: CRC Press, 1999. A good description of various approaches to cognitive modeling. This book provides some historical perspective and considers neural network approaches within this larger framework.

Koonce, Jeffrey. *The Déjà Vu Experience*. Camp Sherman, OR: Deep River Books, in press. This book defines the déjà vu experience, discusses how to study it, then presents both materialistic and parapsychological accounts of it.

Langone, John. *Growing Older: What Young People Should Know about Aging*. Boston: Little Brown & Co, 1991. This book considers both cognitive changes and lifestyle changes that are common as people age. As suggested, it is meant to provide young people with some perspective about what they will value and what sort of life they should expect when they are older.

Lewandowsky, Stephan, John C. Dunn, and Kim Kirsner. *Implicit Memory: Theoretical Issues*. Hove, UK: Psychology Press, 1989. As implied by the title, while also describing some empirical findings related to implicit memory, this book delves deep into several of the leading theories and their implications for memory and cognition in general.

Loftus, Geoffrey R., and Elizabeth F. Loftus. *Human Memory: The Processing of Information*. Hillsdale, NJ: Lawrence Erlbaum Associates, 1976. Although somewhat dated, this book provides another great overview from 2 of the major players in the world of memory research. This book includes some very nice examples of experiments that have direct relation to the influences of memory in real-world contexts, especially the legal context.

Lorayne, Harry, and Jerry Lucas. *The Memory Book: The Classic Guide to Improving Your Memory at Work, at School, and at Play.* New York: Ballantine, 1974. Another book on mnemonic techniques, one that situates these techniques more specifically in the suggested contexts: work, school and play.

Luck, Steven J., and Andrew Hollingworth. *Visual Memory.* Oxford: Oxford University Press, 2008. This book focuses on memory for visual stimuli, and while it is not limited to sensory memory systems, it does describe iconic memory and the research supporting it in some detail.

Markowitsch, Hans J., and Harald Welzer. *The Development of Autobiographical Memory.* Hove, UK: Psychology Press, 2009. This book focuses more specifically on the development of episodic or autobiographical memories and includes a good discussion on the development of a sense of self.

Marsick, Victoria J., and Karen E. Watkins. *Informal and Incidental Learning in the Workplace.* London: Routledge, 1990. While other books listed about implicit memory focus primarily on lab-based findings and their implications, this book shows how common and important implicit memory is by analyzing the effects it has in the typical workplace.

Mason, Douglas J., Michael Lee Kohn, and Karen A. Clark. *The Memory Workbook: Breakthrough Techniques to Exercise Your Brain and Improve Your Memory.* Oakland, CA: New Harbinger Publications, 2001. This book provides a range of both general and specific habits and techniques one can use to keep memory systems working well.

Mason, Douglas J., and Spencer Xavier Smith. *The Memory Doctor: Fun, Simple Techniques to Improve Memory and Boost Your Brain Power.* Oakland, CA: New Harbinger Publications, 2005. While this is a general book on improving memory and cognition, it emphasizes the importance of encoding and techniques that can make it more powerful.

Matthews, Paul M., and Jeffrey McQuain. *The Bard on the Brain: Understanding the Mind through the Art of Shakespeare and the Science of Brain Imaging*. New York: Dana Press, 2003. A whimsical, and extremely interesting, description of brain imaging and brain science in general.

McGaugh, James L. *Memory and Emotion: The Making of Lasting Memories (Maps of the Mind)*. New York: Columbia University Press, 2006. This book highlights the manner in which attention and emotion naturally allow us to remember certain events better than others, and it does so in the context of a general appreciation of memory systems and all we know about them. The focus is on emotion, but many of the themes discussed in this lecture series are also discussed in this book.

Medina, John. *Brain Rules: 12 Principles for Surviving and Thriving at Work, Home and School*. Seattle, WA: Pear Press, 2008. This easy-to-read book contains a number tips for healthy cognitive functioning, including a chapter on sleep.

Memon, Amina, Aldert Vrij, and Ray Bull. *Psychology and Law: Truthfulness, Accuracy and Credibility*. 2nd ed. Chichester, UK: Wiley, 2003. This book is often used as a text for courses on psychology and the law. It considers the myriad ways that psychological research is relevant to the legal setting, including a large discussion on memory. It provides both statistics from the legal system as well as clear and organized descriptions of psychological research relevant to various issues.

Nelson, Aaron, and Susan Gilbert. *Harvard Medical School Guide to Achieving Optimal Memory*. New York: McGraw Hill, 2005. In addition to providing a general description of many of the same issues addressed in this course, this book also provides many recommendations on health issues and tips and exercises for keeping your memory abilities at their optimal level.

Nelson, Charles A. *Memory and Affect in Development*. Hove, UK: Psychology Press, 1993. A general overview of the developmental stages related to memory and emotion.

Parker, Amanda, Timothy J. Bussey, and Edward L. Wilding. *The Cognitive Neuroscience of Memory: Encoding and Retrieval.* New York: Psychology Press, 1996. This book considers the interaction between encoding and subsequent memory retrieval from 3 different research perspectives; functional magnetic resonance imaging, lesion studies, and computational modeling. Thus, it considers encoding in the context of brain systems.

Payne, David G., and Frederick G. Conrad. *Intersections in Basic and Applied Memory Research.* Mahwah, NJ: Lawrence Erlbaum Associates, 1997. The focus on applied work in this book highlights the importance of strong encoding for successful memory.

Plihal, Werner. *Differential Effects of Early and Late Nocturnal Sleep on the Consolidation of Declarative and Nondeclarative Memory.* Frankfurt: Peter Lang Publishing, 1997. This book details the relationship between different stages of sleep and the consolidation of declarative versus nondeclarative memories.

Reder, Lynne M. *Implicit Memory and Metacognition.* Hove, UK: Psychology Press, 1996. This book focuses on the relation, and sometimes lack thereof, between implicit memory and deep conscious thought.

Sandler, Joseph, Peter Fonagy, and Alan D. Baddeley. *Recovered Memories of Abuse: True or False?* Madison, CT: International Universities Press, 1997. This book focuses more specifically on the potential validity of recovered memories, but does so in the context of the false memory debate.

Schacter, Daniel L. *Searching for Memory: The Brain, the Mind, and the Past.* New York: Basic Books, 1996. A strong and detailed book describing the link between brain anatomy and memory processes. This book is written by one of the leaders in the field of implicit memory research.

———. *The Seven Sins of Memory: How the Mind Forgets and Remembers.* New York: Mariner Books, 2002. This book, written by one of the leaders of memory research, describes the various ways in which memory can fail us and the current state of theory underlying each form of memory error.

Spear, Norman E., and Ralph R. Miller. *Information Processing in Animals: Memory Mechanisms*. Hillsdale, NJ: Lawrence Erlbaum Associates, 1982. This book considers the issue of animal cognition more generally, including discussion of cognitive processes other than, and including, those related to memory.

Tulving, Endel. *Elements of Episodic Memory*. New York: Oxford University Press, 1985. This is a book from the master. Tulving was instrumental in defining and championing the difference between semantic and episodic memory. This book focuses on episodic memory and the research related to it.

Tulving, Endel, and Fergus I. M. Craik. *The Oxford Handbook of Memory*. New York: Oxford University Press, 2000. This book provides a somewhat encyclopedic description of memory systems in general that includes strong sections on procedural memory.

Uttl, Bob, Nobuo Ohta, and Amy Siegenthaler. *Memory and Emotion: Interdisciplinary Perspectives*. Malden, MA: Wiley-Blackwell, 2006. As implied by the title, this book includes considerations of the link between emotion and memory from a wide range of scientific perspectives. It provides a great example of how different researchers may approach the same general issue in quite different specific ways.

Vanderwolf, C. H. *The Evolving Brain: The Mind and the Neural Control of Behavior*. New York: Springer, 2010. This book focuses primarily on the link between the brain and the systems it uses to voluntarily control behavior.

Vandierendonck, Andre, and Arnaud Szmalec. *Spatial Working Memory*. New York: Psychology Press, 2011. In contrast to other books in this bibliography about working memory, this one really focuses on the visuo-spatial scratchpad, what others sometimes term spatial working memory.

Wayman, Laura. *A Loving Approach to Dementia Care: Making Meaningful Connections with the Person Who Has Alzheimer's Disease or Other Dementia or Memory Loss*. Baltimore, MD: The Johns Hopkins University Press, 2011. Advice from someone who has provided care for Alzheimer's patients and for patients of memory loss generally, and who has also worked with other caregivers. This book represents accumulated wisdom about how best to deal with the challenges that arise in a manner that attempts to preserve the loving connections between caregiver and patient.

Weingartner, Herbert, and Elizabeth S. Parker. *Memory Consolidation: Psychobiology of Cognition*. Hove, UK: Psychology Press, 1984. This book outlines some of the neurochemical interactions that may underlie the consolidation of memories over time.

Woll, Stanley. *Everyday Thinking: Memory, Reasoning, and Judgment in the Real World*. Hove, UK: Psychology Press, 2001. This book starts from the real world, highlighting various situations and how they map onto research on memory, reasoning, and decision making. As such, it provides a larger cognitive perspective on how basic processes, including but not exclusively those related to memory, play out when considered outside of laboratory contexts.

Internet Resources:

The Brain from Top to Bottom. http://thebrain.mcgill.ca. This site focuses on the link between your brain and various cognitive abilities, memory included. It also allows you to vary the level of explanation from beginner to advanced.

"Memory Improvement Techniques." *Mindtools*. http://www.mindtools. com/memory.html. This site focuses on strategies for memory improvement. It includes a detailed description of a number of mnemonic techniques.

"Psych Basics: Memory" *Psychology Today Online*. http://www. psychologytoday.com/basics/memory. A nice collection of articles originally published in *Psychology Today* that are relevant to memory issues. It includes advice on how to maximize your memory along with general information about memory presented for a lay audience.

On Memory: A Caregiver's Guide to Alzheimer's Disease. http://www. onmemory.ca/en/home. This site provides a very rich caregivers guide to

Alzheimer's disease and is especially useful for those who might be worried that a loved one is in the early stages. It includes a discussion of signs to look for, when one should consult a doctor, and the sort of information the doctor will want to know. However, it also includes many videos, stories, and advice relevant not only to caring for patients, but also for care for the caregiver.

The Memory Exhibition: Memory Games and More. http://www.exploratorium.edu/memory. This site is now more than 10 years old, but it contains many really nice demonstrations and animations related to memory.

"Memory." *Medline Plus.* http://www.nlm.nih.gov/medlineplus/memory.html. This medical resource focuses on problems with memory, ranging from Alzheimer's disease to common forms of forgetting. It offers information, tips, and advice, as well as information about the medical processes related to various disorders.

"Learning and Memory." *Big Dog & Little Dog's Performance Juxtaposition.* http://www.nwlink.com/~donclark/hrd/learning/memory.html. A concise and very general overview of scientific results and theories related to memory.

"Effective Memory Strategies." *The University of Western Ontario Student Development Centre.* http://www.sdc.uwo.ca/learning/memory.html. A short document describing strategies one can use to enhance their memory.

"Signs and Symptoms." *On Memory: A Caregiver's Guide to Alzheimer's Disease* http://www.memorytest.ca/english/index/default.asp?s=1. A short checklist people can use to assess whether they or a loved one are experiencing memory problems to a level that deserves medical attention.

"Using Memory Effectively." *Study Guides and Strategies.* http://www.studygs.net/memory. Another site providing tips on memory improvement, but this site does so within the context of studying for an exam.